Understanding Sleep and Dreaming

William H. Moorcroft

Understanding Sleep and Dreaming

Second Edition

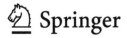 Springer

William H. Moorcroft
Emeritus Professor
Sleep and Dreaming Laboratory,
    Psychology Department
Luther College
Decorah, IA
USA

and

Founder and Chief Consultant
Northern Colorado Sleep Consultants, LLC
Fort Collins, CO
USA

ISBN 978-1-4614-6466-2   ISBN 978-1-4614-6467-9   (eBook)
DOI 10.1007/978-1-4614-6467-9
Springer Boston Heidelberg New York Dordrecht London

Library of Congress Control Number: 2013931749

Printed on acid-free paper

Springer is part of Springer Science+Business Media (www.springer.com)

Foreword

The Art of Sleeping Well

Like everything else in life, sleeping has become more complicated.

Living used to be simple. People awoke from their sleep to face the day; they worked, learned, ate, had fun, worried, rested, shared ideas or gossip, entertained themselves, procreated and raised families, hunted, planted and harvested, got ill, and got hurt or killed. Life was difficult but living was less complicated. Now, particularly in industrialized nations people can select among many types of lifestyles, careers, amusements, habits, goods, food, drink, clothes, and dwellings. There is so much work to do each day that much of it is left to be done the following day. People can choose how to live and how to end that life, but seeming never having enough time to do anything, much less anything worth doing, in between.

Sleeping used to be simple as well. People fell asleep wherever and whenever their weary bodies took them. They slept on cave floors softened by grass, leaves or animal fur; on hammocks located high on treetops; or in wooden huts or teepees. In their slumber, the unknown dangers of the darkened external world are replaced by unknowable, sometimes equally dark and frightening, visions in their dreams. In the morning, they rose with the sun.

Now, things are more complicated. The layperson is increasingly more knowledgeable, and equally increasingly more misinformed, about sleep. Individuals interested in learning more can easily access a multitude of resources, but without knowing how to distinguish credible science from emerging science or pseudoscience. Like everything else in love and life, the art of sleeping has been commoditized and transformed into a marketable item that can be purchased or practiced to satisfy an individual's wants or needs, whether he wants or needs them or not.

It is time to return the acts of sleeping and waking into their proper settings—as part of the daily rhythm of biological life, much like an ebb and flow, rise and fall, or waning and waxing of physiologic processes that are essential to maintain the balance necessary for health and living. It is time to allow falling asleep to be "natural" again. It is time to be familiar with scientific studies that help distinguish what is fact or fiction about sleep, to provide a personalized approach to managing persons with sleep-related complaints, and to have meaningful discussions with the public regarding dysfunctional beliefs, irrational expectations, and unrealistic concerns about sleep, sleep disorders and sleep loss. It is time for the science of sleep and the art of clinical sleep medicine to be well known. This textbook, *Understanding Sleep and Dreaming*, 2nd edition, is a good way to start.

Recipient of the American Association of Sleep Medicine Excellence in Education Award 2012, Author/Editor of Sleep: A Comprehensive Handbook (2006) and several sleep medicine textbooks.

Teofilo Lee-Chiong
Professor of Medicine
School of Medicine
National Jewish Health
University of Colorado Denver
Denver, CO, USA

Preface

As I am writing this, the 60th anniversary of a pivotal moment in the field of sleep is approaching. For it was in 1953 that Aserinsky and Kleitman discovered REMS in a lab at the University of Chicago. They were surprised to notice that eye movements occurred periodically even when their subject was, by all indicators, completely asleep. Four years later, Bill Dement—then a student of Kleitman—discovered the connection between these eye movements during sleep and dreaming (Dement and Kleitman 1957). These startling observations set in motion a whole new era of interest in the laboratory study of sleep, dreaming, and subsequently sleep disorders. From these pioneering investigations came an explosion of discoveries and surprises, frequently leading to revision and even outright rejection of established notions about sleep, sleeping, dreams, and dreaming.

This explosion of new information continues today. The number of articles in scientific journals about sleep, dreaming, and sleep disorders in the past few decades easily outnumbers all those that preceded them. New journals devoted to sleep and dreams have been born and are thriving. A number of very fine technical books have been published. This book is intended to distill all of this information into a textbook or course supplement suitable for use by students in higher education, but also useful for anyone wanting to know about sleep and dreaming.

I have written this book from several perspectives. One perspective is from the vantage point of a researcher in each of the three areas of sleep, dreaming, and sleep disorders. I have included the results of some of my research in order to show how knowledge about these many facets of sleep has been discovered.

The second perspective is out of my experiences with sleep disorders in sleep disorder centers and more recently my experience doing clinical treatment of sleep problems using behavioral methods. I have included many actual experiences with sleep disorder patients so that students can better understand the problems that sleep disorders present to their suffers.

Finally, I have written this book from the perspective of my experience as a college professor who has frequently taught courses on sleep, dreaming, and sleep disorders for more than 30 years.

This book is written for college students with no prior knowledge of sleep and related phenomena. At the same time, it is also informative for those students who already have some knowledge in these areas. Most people have a natural fascination about sleep and dreams. From this starting place I build to an even greater fascination for, as well as increased understanding of, all aspects of sleep and dreams. I have avoided using technical jargon as much as possible unless the terms are critical to understanding the material. At the same time I have tried to avoid overgeneralization and oversimplification. In addition, I have endeavored to involve readers as much as possible by talking about aspects of their own sleep and dreaming; as well as taking them to a sleep laboratory during an all-night recording session; and having them feel like they are present while sleep disorder cases are being reviewed in a sleep disorders clinic.

The organization of the book is designed as a journey. Together readers will travel with me first to a modern sleep laboratory to see the cardinal way that sleep and dreaming is studied. From there I will guide you on a climb through the mountains of information that has accumulated about sleep and dreaming. We will travel on an efficient route through these mountains, pointing out the important and scenic highlights along the way. We start the journey with the twin peaks of what is known about sleep and of what causes us to sleep. Next, we visit the dreams and dreaming mountain. Then we from a vantage point looking back at these mountains of information we have explored, we can contemplate what might be the functions of sleep and dreaming. We conclude our journey by traveling over to the mountain of sleep disorders.

More specifically, after our visit to a sleep lab in Chapter 1, Part I of this book starts with a chapter on the basics of sleep (Chapter 2) that describes the specific criteria for sleep and its substages as measured in the lab, what a typical night of sleep is like, and how it changes with age. It includes information on sleep in animals. This is followed by Chapter 3 that discusses the need to sleep and sleep as a rhythmic process. Chapter 4 looks at variations from these basics including the effects of sleep loss.

Part II focuses on the brain in sleep and the body in sleep. Chapter 5 presents an overview of the structure, basic chemistry, and functioning of the brain, with an emphasis on those aspects most important for sleeping and dreaming. Chapter 6 discusses how sleep affects the body and how the body affects sleep.

Part III turns to dreams and dreaming. Chapter 7 looks at what is known about the nature and content of dreams. Chapter 8 then focuses our attention on the process of dreaming. In Chapter 9, the key aspects of the major theories about dreaming are summarized and also includes a section summarizing methods of dream interpretation.

Part IV uses what we have learned so far to explore the probable functions of sleep and dreaming. Chapter 10 includes functions of sleep and non-REM sleep. Chapter 11 continues with functions of REM sleep and dreaming.

Finally, Part V brings us to problems people can encounter with their sleep. In Chapter 13 the major types of disorders treated at sleep disorder centers are presented, usually introduced by illustrative case examples that bring the problems to life for the reader. Before that in Chapter 12, we look at other difficulties people may have with sleeping and dreaming.

In the end, I hope that readers will gain increasing fascination with and knowledge about sleep and dreaming from reading this book. I know I have, while writing it.

Fort Collins, CO, October 22, 2012   William H. Moorcroft

P. S. I like to hear from instructors and students who have used this book in a course. For that matter, I also like to hear from any others who may have read it or parts of it. I will try to keep updating the book as new information comes to my awareness and will try to pass it along to those who may be interested. Try contacting me at Bill@sleeplessincolorado.com. Meanwhile, I wish you the best of sleep and pleasant dreams.

References

Aserinsky, E., & Kleitman, N. (1953). Regularly occurring periods of eye mobility and concomitant phenomena during sleep. *Science, 18*, 273–274.

Dement, W., & Kleitman, N. (1957). The relation of eye movements during sleep to dream activity. *Journal of Experimental Psychology, 53*, 89–97.

Acknowledgments

There are many people and institutions to which I owe a big debt of gratitude. Over the years many have helped me know and understand sleep and dreams in many ways. For opening their labs for visits: Alex Borbély, MD and associates Irene Tobler, Ph.D. and Peter Acherman, Ph.D. in Switzerland; Jim Horne, Ph.D. in England; Eva Svanborg, MD, Ph.D. in Sweden; Helmuth Rauscher, MD in Austria; Tom Roth, Ph.D. and associates in my home town, Detroit; Ida Karmanova, D.Sc. in Russia; Harvey Moldolsky, MD in Toronto; Mark Mahowald, MD and associates, especially Andrea Patterson, in Minneapolis; Peter Hauri, Ph.D. at the Mayo Clinic in Minnesota; Mark Solms, Ph.D. in London; and Mark Petrun, MD, his manager of the lab, Cindy Crosby, and polysomnographic technicians Chiquita Robinson and Diane Black. Also the Sigmund Freud Foundation and Sigmund Freud Museum in Vienna, Austria. For so readily and helpfully corresponding with me by mail or email: Mary Carskadon, Ph.D., Kathy Lee, Ph.D., RN, Mike Bonnett, Ph.D., Monika Woolsey, MS, RD, Bob Stickgold, Ph.D., Eve Van Cauter, Ph.D., Bob Sack, MD, Ernie Hartmann, MD, Lee Kavanau, Ph.D., and Robert Ogilvie, Ph.D. For visiting and speaking where I taught at Luther College in Decorah, Iowa: Bill Dement, MD, Ph.D., Gayle Delaney, Ph.D., and Peter Hauri, Ph.D. For sharing rooms while at sleep meetings: Dr. I. N. Pigarev, Barry Krakow, MD, and Larry Scrima, Ph.D. For extended conversations at meetings: Bill Domhoff, Ph.D., Kelley Bulkeley, Ph.D., John Shepard, MD, Alan Siegel, Ph.D., Jerry Rosen, MD, Carlyle Smith, Ph.D., Henry Lahmeyer, MD, Carol Landis, Ph.D., Bob McCarley, MD, Merrill Mitler, Ph.D., Misha Radulovacki, MD, Tim Roehrs, Ph.D., and Barry Sterman, MD. For corresponding with me with suggestions for updates and improvements to the first edition of this book: John Harrington, MD, Jim Horne, Ph.D., Teofilo Lee-Chiong, MD, Mark Mahowald, MD, Jodi Mindell, Ph.D., Tore Nielsen, Ph.D., Bill Orr, Ph.D., Amy Wolfson, Ph.D., Dan Lee, MD, and Linda White, MD. For hosting me on sabbatical: Roz Cartwright, Ph.D. at Rush Medical College in Chicago and Phil Westbrook, MD at The Mayo Clinic in Minnesota. And finally, I also thank the many students over the years who have worked with me on research and asked insightful questions in class.

Special thanks to Kathy Buzza of the Luther College Library for assistance in providing research articles through Interlibrary Loan. She was always very helpful and prompt in fulfilling my many requests. Thanks also to the Poudre River Public Library District in Fort Collins, Colorado and the library at National Jewish Health in Denver, Colorado.

My thanks also go to the editor at Springer Science+Business Media, Sharon Panulla and her assistant Sylvana Ruggirello for their assistance and guidance and readiness to quickly respond with answers to my questions.

If there are others that I have forgotten to acknowledge, my apologies and my thanks.

And finally, thank you to my loving wife and friend, Christina, who for over 40 years has supported and encouraged me in my endeavors. She has also been a wonderful academic colleague and traveling companion in so many ways. And I am forever indebted to her for so carefully editing my writing in this edition and giving advice on its content.

Contents

Chapter 1
A Visit to a Sleep and Dreams Lab

Contents

If you were asked to determine whether someone is asleep, what would you look for? You probably would check the person's eyes to see if they were closed, note if the person is relaxed and still, be sure they are not very responsive to stimuli, look to see if they were breathing regularly, and so on. But you like just about everyone, have at one time or another done all of these things to fool other people into believing you were asleep. Then, too, someone in a coma shows all of these signs, appearing to be asleep. It is apparent that you cannot tell very accurately if a person is asleep simply by observation. Alternatively, you could wake the person up and ask if they were asleep, but you then depend on that person's ability to willingly and accurately tell you, and of course the person is then no longer asleep. It is rather like the joke my father used to tell: "Says one Englishman to another, 'Were you in the boat when the boat tipped over?' 'No, you blithering idiot, I was in the water!'".

There are two important implications of this inability to observe whether or not another person is asleep. First, until the middle of the twentieth century, there was little scientific study of sleep. Thus, much of what is known about sleep is relatively new knowledge, and some of it is surprising since it is contrary to popular beliefs. Second, most studies of sleep have taken place in a sleep lab where the sleeper is attached to sensitive instruments, allowing objective determination of sleep without disturbing it. However, the recent development of miniaturized portable equipment has allowed increasingly more sleep research to be conducted outside the lab. Sleep labs have only been in existence since 1953 when Aserinsky

---

Adapted from Moorcroft (1993), with permission of the publisher.

W. H. Moorcroft, *Understanding Sleep and Dreaming*,
DOI: 10.1007/978-1-4614-6467-9_1,
© Springer Science+Business Media New York 2013

and Kleitman first reported that sleeping people have two different kinds of sleep. Today, there are many sleep labs all over the world engaged in exploring the mysteries of sleep every night. Let us first take a visit to a sleep lab before we discuss what is known about basic sleep processes.

1.1 A Visit to a Sleep Lab: Sleep Stages

We arrive at the sleep lab a little before 9 p.m. and walk down a pleasant, carpeted hallway that has several doors on either side. We are met by a man in his mid-30s in a white lab coat. He is on the tall side and slender, with a neatly trimmed dark mustache. He walks up to us and says, "Hi. I'm Sam, the sleep lab technician. I'm happy to show you how sleep is studied in this kind of lab."

We follow Sam through one of the doors into what, at first, looks like a motel room with a big, comfortable looking bed with an attractive quilt on it and several pillows, an overstuffed recliner, a small, plain desk with a desk chair, a flat screen TV on the wall, a ceiling fan, and a door to an adjoining bathroom. Curiously, most of the floor is carpeted, but the area between the door and the bed, about 4 feet wide, is synthetic wood flooring. Then, we also notice some unusual things in the room: an IV stand with a lot of multi-colored wires with golden disklike enlargements on one end hanging from it and a box about the size of a paperback novel into which the wires all lead. There is also a couple of what look like woven belts hanging from the stand. We also see a small, closed-circuit TV camera mounted on the wall that is pointed at the bed. There is an infrared light next to the camera, also pointed at the bed. On the night stand next to the bed, there is a microphone and a speaker. Finally, there is the cart. The top is about 2 and a half feet square and is about 3 feet off the ground. There are a series of 4 drawers on one side above which is a bar for pushing the cart that spans the width of the top.

On the top of the cart are several tubes, a plastic sheet the size of a piece of copy paper with a large number of thin white gauze squares about an inch and a quarter by 2 and a half inches stuck on it, a few long metal hair clips, some cotton-tipped applicators, a small tape measure, scissors, and a pencil with a broad wax filling instead of lead.

The "subject" for tonight's study is a young, adult female, a paid volunteer who has changed into her pajamas is sitting on the bed. "This is Joan," Sam says. "She will be our sleeper tonight. Joan has been here before, so she knows what we are about to do. As I get her ready, I will describe what I am doing and why I am doing it."

"First we have to apply several wires to Joan's head. They are called electrodes, but think of them more as antennae that pick up the electrical activity of the nearby brain cells." As he is talking, he has us inspect one of the wires. Up close, the disk end looks about the size and shape of half a pea and is hollow. "This disc is a gold plated electrode."

Meanwhile, he has started to make precise measurements of Joan's scalp with the miniature tape measure and marks it with the special, soft, red wax pencil. "The electrodes have to be placed on specific locations on the side of the head called C3 on the left side and C4 on the right side, and others at the back of the head called O1 and O2 and at the front of the top of each side of the head at F3 and F4. The same measurement technique is used worldwide to apply electrodes. That way results from any lab can be directly compared." He carefully marks a spot on each side of the head about one-third of the way down from the center of the top of the head toward each ear. He picks up the comb and several hair clips and parts the hair over the marked area on the right side. Then, he picks up a cotton-tipped stick and one of the tubes.

"Our bodies are covered with a layer of dead skin plus oil." Turning back to Joan, he proceeds to moisten the cotton tip with a cleansing gel from one of the tubes and then gently rubs the exposed marked area. "This process removes the dead skin and oils to enable better electrical reception by the electrode." With a smile, he turns to Joan and says, "The green color in your hair will grow out in about 9 months."

Laughing, Joan replies, "You can't fool me. I've been through this before."

Turning to us, Sam explains, "Actually, all of this stuff is very harmless and easily washes out." He then picks up the toothpaste-like tube. "This substance is electrode gel. It also helps to hold the electrode to the head and to make better electrical contact." As he is talking, he puts a glob of the gel near one of the places he has marked and then mashes an electrode into its center. Excess gel is all around the edges of the electrode. Then, he removes one of the fabric rectangles from the plastic sheet and carefully places it on top of the electrode. "This fabric is very sticky on one side and will help hold the electrode in place all night now. If I were to give a gentle but firm tug on the attached wire, Joan's head would tilt toward me."

"He thinks I'm a puppet on a string," she complains.

"Not to worry. I will easily remove it in the morning with soap and water."

"What does the electrode do?" you ask.

While repeating the application procedure on the other marked spots on Joan's head, he tells us, "this allows us to record her brain waves on what is technically called the electroencephalogram or EEG. As you will see, there are brain waves specific to sleep."

Having finished applying the four scalp electrodes, Sam turns his attention to the skin 1 cm below the outer corner of the left eye and proceeds as he did with the scalp areas. Next, he adds a piece of hypoallergenic surgical tape over the electrode and the wire leading from it extending well into the surrounding skin. The wire is directed across the temples toward the back of the head. Giving a little jerk on the wire he says, "That one will also stay in place all night."

As he similarly applies another adhesive electrode 1 cm above the outer corner of the right eye, he explains, "These electrodes will enable us to measure her eye movements. The eyes are like little batteries with the positive end in front. When the eyes move, the positive front moves closer or farther from the nearby electrode, thus changing the electrical influence on the electrode. In this way, we get what you might call 'eye movement waves', actually the electrooculogram or EOG. Like brain waves, eye movements help us to determine when Joan is asleep and what kind of sleep she is in."

He then similarly attaches three additional electrodes: one 1 cm above the middle of Joan's chin, and one 2 cm on each side of that one and 2 cm lower. He explains, "These electrodes let us record neck muscle tension. Electrical changes occur when muscles contract. The more contracted or tense a muscle, the more electrical activity. This procedure enables us to assess how relaxed the muscles of the neck are. You see, as long as we are awake, our neck muscles maintain tension in order to hold our head up, even when we are resting our heads on a pillow. This neck muscle tension or electromyogram (EMG) gives us another indicator of the presence of sleep and the stage of sleep." Turning to me, he asks, "How can you tell when students fall asleep during your lectures, Dr. Moorcroft?"

I reply, "Well, of course they never do." After a few seconds of silence accompanied by stares of disbelief, I continue. "OK, so once in a while a student may doze off. How do I know? Well, let me see. Ah, they don't answer my questions or take notes and their heads are dropped."

"That's it! Their heads drop because during sleep the neck muscles relax. Also, as we shall see, in one kind of sleep the muscles are almost totally relaxed."

"You mean there is more than one kind of sleep?"

"Yes. We all cycle in and out of different kinds of sleep each night!"

"Is she ready now?"

"Not quite." Sam replies, as he reaches for three more electrodes. "These pieces of equipment are called ground and reference electrodes." As he prepares and attaches one to the middle of Joan's forehead, he continues, "This one prevents other electrical 'noise' from interfering with our recordings. Have you ever had a portable radio get louder and clearer as you reach out to adjust the knobs?"

"Yes."

"That happens because you are acting as an antenna for the radio. You see, your body is constantly receiving all sorts of electrical signals—from radio, TV, and all sorts of electrical appliances and motors. Many of these signals are stronger than brain waves and the rest of what we measure. By applying this electrode, we can get rid of this electrical garbage."

He then proceeds to put the final two electrodes on the bony knob behind the bottom of each ear.

"What do those electrodes do?" you ask.

"They are called reference electrodes. Anything we record needs input from two electrodes. Activity on one is actually compared to activity on the other. Sometimes both electrodes are from active areas such as two parts of the brain, and the resulting record is the difference in activity between the two. A lot of other times, it is better if the comparison electrode has no electrical input of its own so that the record shows all of the activity from the active electrode. There is not much electrical activity from this spot, so they work well for comparisons. One of these reference electrodes that I'm applying now is used as a comparison to the eye and scalp electrodes and sometimes to one chin electrode."

"Wait a minute. What about the other scalp electrodes and reference electrode?"

"They are back-ups. We usually don't use all of the electrodes at one time. If something goes wrong with the recording from an electrode, we can easily switch to the back-up for it without disturbing Joan. Otherwise, we might have to wake her up to attach another electrode."

"Can I go to sleep now?" asks Joan, barely stifling a yawn.

"Soon. Just a few more things to do." He tapes some of the loose wires to her face, directing them all to the back of her head, shaping them into a ponytail with a piece of two foot long cloth that is velcroed together around the wires. Sam proudly mentions that he made this "electrode wire sock."[1]

"All set."

"Great. (Yawn) I'm tired."

After Joan uses the toilet, she lies down in bed. Into a receptacle in the wall, Sam plugs a cable from the box into which the color-coded electrode wires are attached. The wires are long enough to allow Joan to move around easily in bed.

"Are you comfortable?" he asks.

"Very much," she replies.

Sam leads us out of the room and closes the door.

"How can she sleep with all those wires on her?"

"Most people have little trouble, especially after the first night. Think how hard it is to stay awake all night, especially in a quiet room and in a comfortable bed."

We walk across the hall to another room labeled control room. As Sam opens the door, we see a room about the size of the bedroom except lined with several computers, speakers, microphones, manuals, and papers. There are trails of various colored horizontal lines on the computer screens, some of which are straight and others showing various constantly changing waveforms. The wires from each bedroom feed into one of these computers. This one here is showing the recordings, called a polysomnogram, from Joan. I previously made careful adjustments and calibrations for the five channels we will be using. The top two lines are the brain waves—one from above one ear (C3) and the other from the back of the head (O1), the third line is from her left eye the fourth line from her right. The bottom line is the muscular activity from the chin electrodes. There is also a little image of the sleeper in a corner of the screen.

Sam flips a switch on an intercom next to the computer. "Joan, can you hear me?"

"Just barely." He adjusts the volume.

"How about now?"

---

[1] Diane Black, a polysomnography technician at the Sleep Disorders Center of the Rockies in Fort Collins, Colorado, is actually the person who came up with the idea of "sock" to contain the electrode wires.

"Fine. Real fine."

"OK. Remember to stay awake while I make adjustments to the machine."

"OK, but don't take too long or I might be gone."

As Sam types on the keyboard, the lines on the computer get larger or smaller. He can also adjust how fast they move across the screen with the mouse but usually he sets it so that 30 s of record appear at a time. He can also move the display to an earlier portion of the record if he needs to check on something. Meanwhile, the data are being continuously recorded for later review. The keyboard can also be used to type observations and comments onto the screen.

The *eye movement* lines look like mirror images of hills and mountains.

The *brainwaves* on the screen are small, rapidly but irregularly oscillating lines, like a very nervous person might make if trying to draw a straight line. This low, fast, random pattern of brain waves is called beta waves, and they indicate wakefulness.

The *muscle tension* recording does not look like a line at all, but rather a thick band made up of many vertical lines of random heights, somewhat like a magnified side view of a shag carpet.

Suddenly, all the lines become very wide, irregular, thick tracings. This pattern stops after a second or two as abruptly as it started, and the lines return to what they looked like previously.

"What was that?" you blurt out.

"She moved. She probably was trying to get more comfortable. We'll occasionally see that all through the night. It actually is useful, because it tells us how restless the sleep is."

Sam continues to look at the record while making some adjustments using the keyboard. Finally satisfied, he turns to us and says, "Now, we will see if everything is working as it should." Pulling on the intercom switch he says into the microphone, "Joan, I'd like you to do a few things for me now."

"OK."

"First, look up." Pause. "Look down." Pause. "Look up." Pause. "Look down." Pause. "Look right." Pause. "Look left." Pause. "Look right." Pause. "Look left." Each time he gives a command, he types a notation of it on the screen. The eye movement lines seemingly respond to his commands, moving toward each other, almost touching when Joan moves her eyes up or to the right and away from each other when the eyes move down or to the left.

"Now blink five times." Again the top two lines respond but this time producing what looks like a row of five dunce hats. Again, Sam notes his instruction to Joan on the screen.

"Now grit your teeth." This time, the thickness of the muscle line triples. "That's fine." Now addressing us he says, "The muscles of the neck contract when a person grits their teeth and the polysomnography shows it. Next, we'll check the EEG and at the same time get a sample of another kind of brain wave."

"Joan, close your eyes and blank your mind, but don't fall asleep."

"(Yawn) I'll try," came the sleepy voice in return. As Sam makes a notation on the screen, the EEG lines begin to change from their low, fast, random pattern of *beta waves* to higher, slightly slower, but very rhythmic and regular patterns, looking somewhat like a folded ribbon candy viewed from the side. ⋁⋀⋁⋀⋁⋀

"These patterns are *alpha waves*. They occur when a person's mind is awake but relaxed and not particularly concentrating on anything." When he flips the intercom switch and tells Joan to open her eyes, the alpha waves change back to the beta waves.

"Alpha waves also occur when a person is drifting into sleep. What you saw before the alpha waves, and are seeing now, are the beta waves of an awake, alert mind."

"Well, Joan, it's time. Call me if you want to get up or need anything, OK?"

"OK."

"Goodnight." He types a notation into the computer as he switches off Joan's sleep room lights with a remote switch near the intercom.

We all watch the screen closely. Not much happens at first, other than an occasional body movement. In several minutes, the EMG becomes less thick to about half its original size, more alpha waves appear, and fewer eye movements can be noted. Then, the eye channels trace out lines that look like mirror images of rolling hills, and the EEG becomes much more jagged, but the waves are not as rapid as beta nor as rhythmic as alpha. "These waves are the signs of the start of sleep—so called slow rolling eye movements and the replacement of alpha waves with slower, less regular *theta waves* in the EEG. ⋀⋁⋀⋁ It's a light sleep called *N1* short for NREM 1; it was formerly called stage 1. She will probably spend very little sleep time in this stage. It's more of a transition between stages."

Soon Joan's eyes stop moving, and the EEG line gradually oscillates less rapidly than before, but it is still rather jagged. Then, it more rapidly and regularly oscillates for about a second, producing a wave that looks like compact alpha. "That's a *sleep spindle*, ⋀⋀⋀⋀ a sure sign of *N2* sleep formerly called stage 2 sleep." Soon there is a sudden, large, upward movement, then down past midline, then back to its previous activity level, resulting in a pattern resembling an upside-down pointed ice cream cone next to a smaller but right side up cone. ∧⋁ "That's a *K-complex*, another characteristic of N2."

This pattern continues for another 10 min—occasional spindles and K-complexes on a background of irregular but slower and slower activity. Then, the EEG begins to show occasional large sonorous movements ⋀⋁⋀⋀ and fewer spindles and K-complexes. When about 20 % of the record is of this pattern, Sam explains, "These are *slow waves*, also called *delta waves*. They indicate the presence of *N3* sleep previously called slow wave sleep. In many ways, this sleep is the deepest sleep." Soon much of the record contains delta waves and continues this way with little change for about half an hour.

Suddenly, all of the lines become large and blurred indicating a body movement. We confirm this recording when we look up at the TV that is monitoring Joan and see that she is rolling over. When things settle down, the record again resembles N2 with moderate, jagged background and spindles and Ks.

Exactly 93 min after sleep onset, the EMG becomes almost a thin, straight line. Suddenly, the eye movement channels burst into activity, showing large, jagged, mirror-image mountains for a few seconds, and then falling silent. "That recording is a burst of rapid eye movements. Joan is now in another kind of sleep called *REMS* for rapid eye movement sleep. Look closely at the EEG. Notice no spindles or Ks are present ᠕ᠰᠠᠰ and many of the brain waves look like the teeth of a saw blade and thus are called *saw tooth waves*." Just then there is another burst of eye movement lasting longer than the first. "As you can see, sleep is not a single entity, but is made up of several different states."

The REMS period does not last long. After a few minutes, another body movement occurs and N2 returns for 10–15 mins followed by more N3 sleep.

And so it goes throughout the night. Joan cycles between the stages, except there is less and less time spent in N3, in fact, almost none at all in the second half of the night, and more and more time in REMS. Most time, however, is spent in N2—about half of the night. Around every hour and a half, she starts a REMS period.

It is interesting to observe what is happening to us as we stay up all night to watch Joan sleep. It is especially hard for us to keep awake when nothing exciting is happening, like long periods of N2. We have to stand up and keep moving or keep talking. Otherwise, a brief sleep overtakes us. Several times we catch each other drifting off. It seems to get cold in the room between 3 and 5 a.m. We check the thermostat and find that the temperature remained unchanged. We later realized that this time was also the time when it was hardest to stay awake.

At 6:15 a.m., through blurry eyes, we can see that the pattern on the computer screen is changing. Several body movements occur, and the EMG gets thicker again. The EEG becomes low and fast and random, and Joan's eyes start moving, but not as rapidly as during REMS and more continuously. "She's awake now," Sam informs us. "Good morning," he intercoms to Joan and turns on the light.

"Ugh—oh, mornin'" (Yawn).

"I'll come in and unplug you now."

"Yeah. OK."

We follow him in. "How do you feel? Sleep well?"

"Hey, I slept like a log. How about you?"

"Oh, be quiet," he blurts out with a smile.

Now unplugged, all of the electrodes and the tape are removed from Joan's head, and the glue is wiped away with a moist cloth. We say good-bye to one another before Joan heads for the shower, and Sam returns to the control room to do some post-sleep checks on the polysomnograph. "See you again tomorrow night," he says as he disappears into the control room. We start to float out of the sleep lab in our sleepless, dazed state, toward our own beds in search of our own quota of that sweet commodity that we have been scientifically observing all night.

1.2 A Second Night in the Sleep Lab: Dream Collection

"I hope you slept well during the day today," I say, "after being up all night."

"Well, I slept but not as well as usual," you reply. "I was kind of restless and woke up a lot, but I'm OK."

"Sounds typical for daytime sleep. Tonight Sam will awaken Joan at various times during the night to collect dream reports."

"I can't wait. I hope she has some wild ones."

"You may be surprised," I comment, "at just how dull they are!"

"Hi, Sam. Here we are for another night."

"Oh, hi. I just about have Joan ready, so it won't be long now." At that moment, she came walking out of the preparation room carrying the ponytail of wires leading from the electrodes on her head and face.

"Not a bad way to earn 150 bucks—sleeping," she says to us.

"It's not all sleep tonight," Sam reminds her. "I will be waking you at various times throughout the night and asking you to report whatever is going through your mind at the time. You may be dreaming or thinking or may have nothing at all going on at that time. That's all right. I just want to know what is going on in your mind when I wake you. All reports are equally valuable."

"Oh well, it's still an easy $150. See ya in the morning."

By now she is in bed with the electrodes in place and connected from the box to the receptacle in the wall. Soon Sam has turned the machine on, made adjustments, and assured himself that everything is working fine and that Joan is asleep.

"It is thought that dreams," Sam says, can be explored much better in the sleep lab, because we can catch their recall when they are fresh. Tonight, we will wake her three times—first during N3, then during N2, and finally during REMS. Watch for differences in what she reports in each stage. The questions I ask are a bit formal, but they have to be the same every time to be sure we don't miss something.

Soon we see the signs on the moving chart that she is asleep and moving down through the stages. Then, at 12:07, 10 min into the first N3 period, Sam turns on a tape recorder and begins. "Joan… Joan… JOAN!"

"Ugh…, oh-ah…"

"Joan?"

"Yea." Yawn.

"What was taking place just at the moment you were called?"

"Nothin'. Nothin' was happenin'."

"At that moment would you say that you were awake, drowsy, in light sleep, or in a deep sleep?"

"Deep. It was good sleep."

"Was there any visual imagery? If yes, describe it."

"Well, yeah, kinda. A woods, some trees, you know."

"Were there any distortions in the way familiar people or objects were represented?"

"No, not really. It was kinda vague."

"Were you an active participant in what you experienced or just passively observing it?"

"I just saw it."

"Were there any other persons in this experience?"

"No, none; just trees."

"During this experience were you aware that you were here in the laboratory?"

"No."

"During this experience were you aware that you were observing the contents of your own mind, or did you feel that you were observing or participating in events out in the real world?"

"Sort of real world, but fuzzy."

"How vivid an experience was this: very vivid, moderately vivid, or quite vague?"

"Kinda vague."

"How realistic was this experience: very realistic, a mixture of real and unreal, or very unrealistic?"

"A mixture, I'd say."

"How emotional was this experience: very emotional, only mildly emotional, or very unemotional?"

"Not at all emotional. No emotion."

"How pleasant was this experience: very pleasant, neutral, or unpleasant?"

"Neutral."

"Were you dreaming or thinking?"

"I don't know. Kinda thinking, I guess. But not thinking hard or rationally."

"OK, you can go back to sleep now."

After Sam turns off the tape recorder you state, "That wasn't really much of a dream, was it?"

"No," he replies. "That's typical, though, of what you get in N3 sleep—something like a fuzzy photograph. Many times you get nothing."

At 3:10 a.m., 10 min into N2, Sam says, "It's time again," as he turns on the tape recorder.

"Joan."

"Ah, yeah," followed by a strain in her voice indicating that she is stretching.

"What was taking place just at the moment you were called?"

"I (yawn) could not find the classroom where I had to take the final exam. It was like I kept trying one door after another but never finding the room."

"Was there anything else?"

"No, that's pretty much it. It was not real clear."

"What about the visual imagery? Can you describe it?"

"Not very well. I just knew I was opening non-descript doors, looking for the classroom."

"At that moment would you say that you were awake, drowsy, in light sleep, or in deep sleep?"

"I was asleep alright, but it did not seem like it was deep sleep."

"Were there any distortions in the way familiar people or objects were represented?"

"It was not real clear. I just kinda knew what everything was."

"During this experience, were you aware that you were here in the laboratory?"

"No. I thought I was really there, yet it did not seem entirely real."

"During this experience, were you aware that you were observing the contents of your own mind, or did you feel that you were observing or participating in events out in the real world?"

"Neither. It was kinda dreamy. Oh, sorry about the pun."

"That's OK. I understand. How vivid was this experience: very vivid, moderately vivid, or quite vague?"

"It was moderately vivid to a bit vague."

"How realistic was this experience: very realistic, a mixture of real and unreal, or very unrealistic?"

"I did not think about it while I was experiencing it, but reflecting on it now, it seems almost unrealistic. Incomplete."

"How emotional was this experience: very emotional, only mildly emotional, or not emotional?"

"Surprisingly, not very emotional. I was concerned about missing the exam, but I did not feel emotional about it."

"How pleasant was this experience: very pleasant, neutral, or unpleasant?"

"It was OK. Kinda neutral, I guess."

"Were you dreaming or thinking?"

"More dreaming than thinking."

"You can go back to sleep now."

Sam turns the tape off as he says to us, "That was pretty typical of N2. Not much going on but often repeated over and over again. Also, the experience was not real clear. Sometimes, though, we get a real story. That kind of experience is more likely toward the end of the night."

"What happens in REMS?" you ask.

"Just wait."

5:23 a.m., 10 min into REMS.

"Joan,..., Joan."

"Ugh... yea!"

"What was taking place just at the moment you were called?"

"Well, I was in a shed—you know a tin type shed—with many people, some of whom I knew. I was standing on one side of the building around some cars with a couple of middle-aged men and a couple of girls around 20 years of age. Something had happened to one of the cars, an older model, and the girl was upset. At that point my attention was distracted to the other half of the shed where a guy about 20 years of age was showing films of—I guess it was the girl's vacation or something—while others of the same age watched. Right then, the scene shifted to some body of water like a lake or something. I was driving a speedboat, while the male who was showing the film was swimming in a scuba suit. It's crazy, but he was going the same speed as the boat. Then you woke me up."

"At that moment, would you say that you were awake, drowsy, in light sleep, or in deep sleep?"

"Oh, I was asleep alright; it was sound. I guess I would have to say somewhat deep."

"Were there any distortions in the way familiar people or objects were represented?"

"People? No. But, the cars were all funny pastel colors and kinda wavy, shimmering. That's all I can remember."

"During this experience, were you aware that you were here in the laboratory?"

"Oh no. It seemed real, like I was there."

"During this experience, were you aware that you were observing the contents of your own mind, or did you feel that you were observing or participating in events out in the real world?"

"It seemed real at the time, but now that I think about it, things were kind of flat or quiet. You know, not very emotional or something. Like spacey."

"How vivid an experience was this: very vivid, moderately vivid, or quite vague?"

"It was vivid, quite clear."

"How realistic was this experience: very realistic, a mixture of real and unreal, or very unrealistic?"

"It seemed realistic while it was happening, but now not all of it seems like it was real. A mixture I guess."

"How emotional was this experience: very emotional, only mildly emotional, or not emotional?"

"There was some emotion. Kinda like something was not right."

"How pleasant was this experience: pleasant, neutral, or unpleasant?"

"It was OK. Toward unpleasant, I guess."

"Were you dreaming or thinking?"

"Dreaming. No doubt about it, I was dreaming."

"Goodnight. You can go back to sleep again."

"Night"

Turning to us, Sam says, "That experience was a fairly typical dream—like a TV program with action and a sequence of events, but scenes can jump forward, backward, or parallel. I did not have to ask all of the standard questions either, since she had already indicated what the answers would be."

We decide to leave early, since there are to be no more dream reports collected and we are tired from the night before.

"Thanks Sam and say good-bye to Joan for me," you say on your way out of the door.

"I will" he replies. "Good-bye."

Turning to me as we walk down the hall, you ask, "Where was all the sex and violence in the dreams?"

"That's just it. There usually isn't any. Most dreams are pretty dull when you get right down to it."

"Do we always dream during REMS?" you ask.

"People will give a dream report like this one over 80 % of the time when awakened during REMS, even if they state before-hand that they never dream."

"Well, thanks again," you call out as you turn to head to your car. "I really appreciate your arranging for me to visit the sleep lab."

"Glad to do it," I respond, "and, by the way,..."

"Yes?"

"Pleasant dreams!"

References

Aserinsky, E., & Kleitman, N. (1953). Regularly occurring periods of eye mobility and concomitant phenomena during sleep. *Science, 18*, 273–274.

Moorcroft, W. H. (1993). *Sleep, dreaming, and sleep disorders: An introduction* (2nd ed.). Lanham, Md: University Press of America.

Part I

Sleep and Sleeping

Anthropologists tell us that sleep and dreams have been central foci of many ancient cultures. In some cultures, sleep was seen as a time for the soul to occupy another world. Perhaps more common in the history of the Western world was the notion that sleep is a slowing down of the body and brain, even to the point of approaching death. Akin to this idea have been the notions that the brain is forced into sleep by blood filling its vessels (Ancient Greeks), food decomposing in the stomach giving off vapors that ascended to the brain (other Ancient Greeks), the effect of "animal humors" (Middle Ages), blood putting pressure on the brain (Eighteenth century), and lack of sensory stimulation (Nineteenth century). Around the beginning of the Twentieth century, a popular notion was that sleep resulted from the buildup of one or another "hypnotoxins" (there were many that were proposed) that supposedly poisoned the brain into sleep when a critical amount had accumulated. During sleep, the hypnotoxin was thought to be eliminated gradually, and eventually wakefulness returned. The interactive website at http://healthysleep.med.harvard.edu/interactive/timeline allows you to select historical time periods that show how patterns of sleep and the understanding of sleep has changed over time.

A common thread in almost all of these notions is that sleep is viewed as the result of lowered activity of the brain. Waking up is simply the result of the brain being allowed to become fully active again or stimulated into such activity. Only in the middle of the Twentieth century was there a dramatic shift in thinking; sleep was shown to be the result of active processes within the brain itself. This shift occurred 25 years after the first use of the EEG by the German Psychiatrist Hans Berger to establish the presence of sleep without having to awaken the sleeper. By 1960, the stages of sleep had been discovered and named, and with some reluctance, the fact that sleep was an active process was accepted. This acceptance changed the scientific attitude toward sleep and sleeping. Scientists then began asking questions they never thought to ask before such as: What exactly is the nature of sleep? Does it change with age? How much do we need to sleep? How does sleep vary between individuals? This section begins the review of answers we currently have for these questions. Chapter 1 takes you on visit to a sleep and dream lab as an introduction to how sleep and dreaming can be scientifically studied. Chapter 2 more precisely explains how sleep is measured and what it is like. Chapter 3 explores two major influences on sleep—homeostatic and rhythmic. Chapter 4 looks at some of the common variations of sleep.

Chapter 2
What is Sleep and How it is Scientifically Measured

Contents

If we want to scientifically study sleep, we need to know when a person is asleep and when awake. How do we know if a person is asleep? We might be able with great certainty to determine that the person is awake using criteria such as eyes open, interactive with their surroundings, physically active, and appears alert. So, the presence of the opposite signs—little movement, steady breathing, eyes closed, not interacting with surroundings, and typical sleep posture—might indicate that the person is asleep. But, a person displaying all of these could be awake; we cannot be sure. Another way is to ask whether they were asleep after they were awakened. Two problems arise here. First, we cannot be certain that the answer is reliable, and second, the person is no longer in the state of sleep that we wish to study. It was not until the middle of the twentieth century that scientists devised more objective ways of determining whether a person was in a state of sleep using technological advances enabling the recording of brain waves and other bodily functions. To their surprise, they also discovered that there are several types of sleep called stages.

Specific references to statements in this chapter that can be found in multiple, widely available sources are not included in the text. A selection of these sources is listed below and can also be consulted for verification or more detail. (Kryger et al. 2011; Lee-Chiong, Somnology 2011; Amlaner and Fuller, Basics of Sleep 2009).

W. H. Moorcroft, *Understanding Sleep and Dreaming*,
DOI: 10.1007/978-1-4614-6467-9_2,
© Springer Science+Business Media New York 2013

2.1 Polysomnography[1]

It was not long before these methods, called *polysomnography*, became refined and universally accepted. Today, the determination of states of sleep and wakefulness is reliable and valid. Polysomnography involves the recording of three things— brain waves, eye movements, and neck muscle tension. Polysomnography works because many organs of the body generate small amounts of electrical energy as they perform their functions. Sensors placed near these organs can pick up some of this energy and transmit it via wires to powerful amplifiers whose output is permanently recorded as ink lines on paper or, more recently, as lines on a computer screen and stored in computer memory. (Sensors being applied are shown in a segment of http://www.youtube.com/watch?v=9nmVzXxdUeU&NR= 1&feature=endscreen from time 12:44 to 13:18). Brain waves or EEG, short for electroencephalogram, are visualizations of the waveform and intensity in microvolts of electrical activities of large groups of brain cells. For sleep recording, standard procedure calls for the EEG sensor to be placed on the scalp about 8 cm above the right or left ear. EEGs are the most important of all things recorded for the determination of stages of sleep. The shape of the EEG waves, their frequency, and their intensity or amplitude are the key components.

Eye movement recordings or *EOG*, short for electrooculogram, are possible because the front of the eye is electrically positive. As the eyeballs move, the distance of their positive poles change relative to sensors placed near the outer corner of each eye. Typically, the movements of each eye are recorded on a separate line on the polysomnogram. It is important to note the presence or absence of any eye movements as well as their shape and frequency when they are present.

For neck muscle tension or EMG, short for electromyogram, pairs of sensors are placed in the region of the chin or jaw. When nearby muscles contract, they generate some electrical activity whose strength is in proportion to the degree of the contraction or tension. The sensors can detect this electrical activity. The thickness of the EMG line is what is accessed; the thicker the tracing the greater the muscle tension.

At a minimum, a polysomnogram contains two rows of EOG, one of EMG, and one of EEG (see Fig. 2.1). It is becoming more common to also include two additional rows of EEG—one from the posterior brain region (the right or left occipital cortex) and another from the anterior brain region (the frontal cortex). These additional placements can better indicate the brain waves characteristic of different types, called stages, of sleep. Additional recordings from brain and other body organs may also be made, and although not essential to determine sleep, may be useful for determination of what else is going on during sleep (see Chap. 13).

Polysomnographic stages are designated as follows:

---

[1] The primary source for the material in this section is Carden 2009.

Fig. 2.1 A typical polysomnogram page of 30-s duration showing wake. Note the sharp eye movements that resemble mirror images of each other, the high thickness of the EMG tracing, and the not very intense but fast-frequency beta waves in the EEG

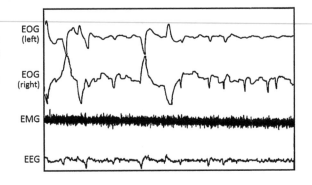

- alert wakefulness
- drowsy wakefulness
- stages *N1*, *N2*, and *N3* (pronounced N1 sleep, N2 sleep, and N3 sleep)
- N1, N2, and N3 are collectively referred to as non-REM sleep (*NREMS* pronounced "NREM sleep").
- plus rapid eye movement sleep (abbreviated *REMS* but pronounced "REM sleep").

Prior to 2007, N1 was known as stage 1, and N2 as stage 2. N3 is a combination of what was formerly known as stage 3 plus the more intense stage 4. N3 is also known as slow-wave sleep (abbreviated SWS, pronounced "slow-wave sleep") because of the presence of slower-frequency delta waves.

2.1.1 The Stages of Sleep

Figure 2.2 shows the criteria for the stages of sleep. The components most critical for determining each stage are in bold. Beta waves are irregular, low intensity, and fast frequency (>13 Hz) that typically occur in an awake, active brain. Alpha waves are regular, moderate intensity, and intermediate frequency (8–13 Hz) that typically occur in an awake but relaxed or drowsy brain. Theta waves are moderate to low intensity and intermediate frequency (4–7 Hz). Delta waves have high amplitude and low frequency (<4 Hz). A K-complex lasts at least ½ s and is a large, slow peak followed by a smaller valley. A spindle is an obvious, moderately intense, and moderately fast (12–14 Hz) rhythmic oscillation for ½–1½ s. Sawtooth waves have relatively low intensity and mixed frequency that often have a notched appearance. Left eye movement recordings look like approximate mirror images of the right eye movement recordings. Waking eye movements tend to be relatively constant and have mainly sharp peaks and valleys with some smaller peaks and rounded peaks mixed in. So called "slow rolling eye movements" are associated with sleep onset; they are mostly large with rounded peaks. The eye movements of REMS usually have sharp peaks and come in bursts of a few

Fig. 2.2 EEG, EOG, and
EMG characteristics of
waking and each stage of
sleep. The most important
aspects for determination of
each stage are shown darker
than the less important
aspects

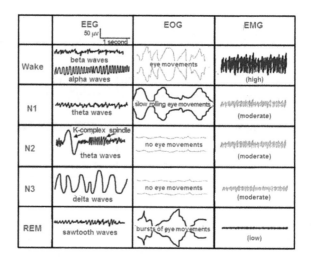

Fig. 2.3 A typical 30-s
polysomnogram page
showing N1. Note the slow
eye movements, moderate
thickness of the EMG, and
theta waves in the EEG

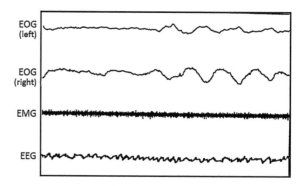

seconds each with intervening quiet periods of a few to 10 s. The thickness of the
EMG line is the key indicator of the amount of muscle tension.

Figures 2.1 and 2.3, 2.4, 2.5, and 2.6 show typical 30-s polysomnogram pages
for each stage.

Although not important for the distinguishing of the stages of sleep and waking,
during the 1990s, the importance of 20–50 Hz gamma waves became apparent.
These waves are present during waking and REMS. They are thought to be
important in synthesizing[2] various aspects of sensory-motor inputs (e.g., size of an
object with its color and shape) and/or cognitive processes.

Accurately determining the times of first falling asleep and final awakening is
also of great importance. The time between these transitions is called the sleep
period. Awakening is easier to determine; it is the sudden shift from a sleep stage

---

[2] Our brain uses sensory and other information to put together our awareness of our external
world in a process called synthesis.

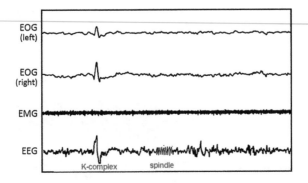

Fig. 2.4 A typical 30-s polysomnogram page showing N2. Note the absence of eye movements (the upward spikes early in the record are not eye movements since the one on the first line is not a mirror image of that on the second line), moderate EMG intensity, and theta waves in the EMG with occasional K-complexes and spindles

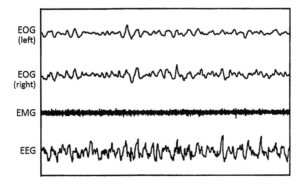

Fig. 2.5 A typical 30-s polysomnogram page showing N3. Note the moderately intense EMG, the intense but slow EEG activity, and the absence of eye movements. The peaks and valleys that appear in the EOG records during N3 are not from eye movements since they are not mirror images. Rather, they are produced by the strong slow-wave electrical activity of the brain near the eyeballs

Fig. 2.6 A typical 30-s polysomnogram page showing REMS. Note the bursts of eye movements, the low EMG (but with occasional brief muscle twitches), and the fast-frequency, low-intensity "sawtooth" pattern of the EEG

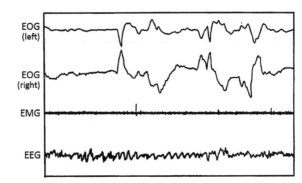

Fig. 2.7 A typical 30-s polysomnogram page showing movement artifact. Note the very thick EMG and obliterated EEG and partially obliterated EOG

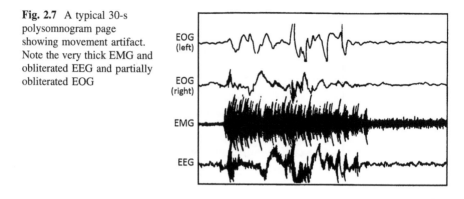

to active wake, usually accompanied by many seconds of movement artifact composed of intense, very high frequency registrations in the EEG, EOG, and EMG recordings (see Fig. 2.7). Sleep onset is more difficult to determine, because we do not suddenly fall asleep. Instead, the transition from wake to sleep is a complex succession of changes beginning with relaxed drowsiness, going through N1, and ending in the first couple of minutes of N2. While this succession may occur very rapidly, it is usually more gradual and a person may briefly dip in and out of sleep several times before maintaining it. Different sets of criteria are used to pinpoint the time of sleep onset, but most involve the replacement of drowsy waking EEG (alpha waves) with sustained theta waves plus the indicators of N1 or N2. In practice, the time of sleep onset can usually be determined within a range of several seconds.

As can be seen in Figs. 2.2 and 2.6, REMS is a very unique state. The EEG very closely resembles that of wakefulness, yet it is clear from behavioral criteria (see Sect. 2.2) and subsequent subjective reports from the person that they are asleep. At one time, REMS was called paradoxical sleep because in some ways, the person showed characteristics of both sleep and wake. Furthermore, during REMS, the muscles controlling body movements are paralyzed into a very relaxed state as shown by the very low EMG level. During REMS, the EOG shows bursts of rapid eye movements with seconds of quiescence between bursts. This phenomenon can be observed even without the aid of a polysomnograph by looking at the bulge of the eyeballs moving under the eyelids in a sleeping person early in the morning. Just be sure the person knows that they will be observed, as they may awaken only to be startled with a face a few inches away! Actually, this exercise is easier to do with a baby.

It is useful to distinguish between the components of REMS that are tonic and those that are phasic. The tonic components are those that are constant, such as the EEG and the muscle paralysis. The phasic components are the relatively short-lived clusters of events, such as the rapid eye movements and a number of changes in the body discussed in Sect. 2.1.1 and Chap. 6.

NREMS is what most people think sleep is and ought to be. The brain waves, especially in N3, are those of a brain that is idling. At the same time, the body is relaxed but capable of movement.

Let us put all this together now by following a typical young adult, Rita, as she sleeps through the night. Shortly after she turns out the lights and closes her eyes with the intention of going to sleep, her EOG is flat and her EEG begins to show fewer beta waves and more alpha waves, while her EMG thickness gets smaller as her muscles are relaxing. A few minutes later, she begins to show signs of N1—slow eye movements appear on her EOG, while her EEG alpha waves are replaced by theta waves mixed with other low-voltage fast waves. However, the alpha waves reemerge a few times before disappearing completely. At this point, if we were to ask, she would quickly say that she was not quite asleep but less conscious, maybe experiencing something like floating. On other occasions, she might say she had had a simple, short dream.

A short time later, usually less than 10 min, we see the first sign of N2—a K-complex or perhaps spindle in her EEG. If we now were to ask whether she was asleep yet, it would take longer to get a response, and she would seem a bit groggy at that, but her reply would be affirmative. The slow eye movements shortly after that disappear. After another 20 or so minutes go by, we begin to see large, slow delta waves that quickly begin to dominate the EEG. We now know she is in N3. Awakening her now would be more difficult and result in obvious grogginess. A good half hour later, the delta waves diminish and signs of N2 reemerge for about another 10 min.

It is now about 80 min since the onset of Rita's sleep and we notice that the EMG has become almost a thin, flat line. Shortly thereafter, there are sawtooth waves in the EEG, and suddenly the EOG dances with a burst of rapid eye movements signaling the appearance of REMS. We could have awakened her at this point more easily than when she was in N3 but less easily then N1. If asked, after being awakened from REMS, she probably would have said she was dreaming.

After only a couple of minutes of REMS, the lines on the polysomnography computer get very intense and scrambled. Rita has moved. Around 30 s later, she settles down again but is no longer in REMS. A brief interval of N1 is followed by solid N2 followed by a bit more N3 before again entering REMS.

This sequence continues throughout the night with the interval between REMS periods gradually increasing to closer to 100 min, the indicators of REMS on the polysomnogram getting more obvious, and the duration of each successive REMS period increasing until the last one is a half hour or more. As changes are taking place, the amount of N3 quickly diminishes such that it is hardly visible in the latter half of the night. From this point on, her NREMS is N2 with some periods of N1 and brief arousals, counted as awakenings only if lasting more than 30 s, mixed in. She has moved, often at the point of stage change, about 50 times during the 8 h sleep period.

2.1.2 Other Sleep Brainwave Patterns

There are other brainwave patterns that occur during sleep that are not a part of discerning the stages of sleep. They are associated with poor sleep or outright sleep disorders. Two of them are fast-wave intrusions during N3 and the cyclic alternating pattern (CAP).

Many years ago, some people were observed to have fast waves riding on their slow waves during N3. That is, the slow waves on the EEG were not relatively smooth lines but more like a spring that was stretched on the slow waves. At first, this was called an alpha-delta pattern because the fast waves are in the alpha-wave frequency range. However, research I and colleagues did at the Rush Medical College Sleep Disorders Center and later confirmed in other laboratories, suggested that they are not true alpha waves (Weber et al. 1983). They are more like sleep spindles because of their frequency characteristics and the fact that they originate from the anterior of the brain rather than the posterior. Although what this indicates is not clear-cut, the presence of this EEG pattern is often associated with light and unrefreshing sleep. More recently, fast waves have been sometimes noted in other stages of NREMS, so now the term alpha EEG sleep rather than alpha-delta sleep is used. Alpha EEG sleep is associated with pain and fatigue syndromes such as rheumatoid arthritis and some sleep disorders.

The term cyclic alternating pattern (CAP) designates the occurrence of bursts of a repetitive, transient, dramatic 2–60 s change in the EEG during NREMS (Parrino et al. 2012). The presence of CAP indicates unstable sleep that compromises the restorative aspect of sleep. CAP has sometimes been noted to occur in patients with pain but also occurs in others without pain.

2.2 Definition of Sleep

In spite of all of this description of scientific measurement and the stages of sleep, we have not yet defined sleep. Polysomnograms are a convenient way to measure sleep accurately but say little about what sleep is. For centuries, most people seemed to accept the intuitive notion of sleep: it is a passive phenomenon with the body, including the brain, slowed down or even stopped. Science has shown that this belief is wrong. For example, the discovery that there are different stages of sleep that alternate in a lawful way showed that an active process produces sleep. Today the accepted definition is that *sleep is simply a reversible behavioral state of low attention to the environment typically accompanied by a relaxed posture and minimal movement.*

Other than intense, discomforting, or especially meaningful stimuli can cause a sudden awakening, the sleeping person is much less aware of their surroundings and makes little response to it. This finding has been verified in experiments like the following. Sleepy subjects in a quiet environment were asked to continue doing

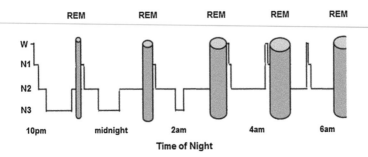

Fig. 2.8 Idealized sequence of sleep stages through the sleep period in an average young adult. Note that the first REM sleep period comes after about 80 min and then NREM and REM sleep alternate about every 100 min thereafter. Also note that SWS occurs mainly early in the night and REMS gets longer as sleep progresses

a simple behavioral task, such as alternating tapping or attending to words, visual patterns, or sound patterns. They began to falter greatly at the time the polysomnogram showed clear N1 patterns. For example, Ogilvie (e.g., Ogilvie et al. 1989) had people press a button each time they heard a sound. When awake, they performed at or near 100 % accuracy but only at about 5 % when in N2 and at 0 % in N3 and REMS. Importantly, as soon as they showed signs of N1, they averaged about 60 % (ranging from 0 to 75 %). In contrast to these behavioral observations, people are not always aware that they have just fallen asleep even when the polysomnogram shows they have.

Not only are there several states of sleep rather than a unitary state, as our intuitive experience would have us believe, the states also alternate in a pattern. NREMS is replaced with REMS about every 90–110 min. The first REMS period of the night lasts only a few minutes. This time gradually increases with each successive REMS period such that the last one is 30 or so minutes in duration. Additionally, there are changes in NREMS as the night progresses. Early in the night, there is considerable N3 (in the neighborhood of 60 min) but as the sleep period progresses, it rapidly diminishes in time and intensity in an exponential fashion such that there is little to be seen in the second half of the night. N1 sleep occupies only about 5 % of the sleep period and, other than at sleep onset, mostly follows the two to three 1 min awakenings scattered during the sleep period. Overall N2 sleep occupies around 50 % of the sleep period, but there is less of it early in the sleep period and more as N3 diminishes. N3 is typically around 20 %, but less as we get older. About 25 % of sleep is REMS. Figure 2.8 and Table 2.1 summarize these and other facts.

Three other important terms are *sleep period*, *sleep efficiency*, and *sleep latency*. The sleep period is the time from when a person first falls asleep through last awakening. Sleep efficiency is the proportion of sleep period spent asleep rather than awake. Sleep latency is the time it takes to get to sleep.

Table 2.1 Average sleep characteristics in the typical young adult

Stage	Percent	Range
W	1	0–3
N1	5	1–10
N2	50	40–60
N3	20	10–35
REM	25	15–35
Stage shifts		35 (about)
Efficiency		0.96
Sleep latency		10 min
Time in bed		7 h and 20 min
Total sleep time		7 h
Number of awakenings		2
Latency to REM		100
NREM–REM cycle		90 min
Number of REM periods		4–5

One other factor needs to be mentioned. We sometimes talk about deep sleep. In one sense, this term usually means our sleep was relatively uninterrupted, and we awakened feeling refreshed. Yet, in another sense, it is not very meaningful. It is a holdover from the notion of deep sleep being furthest away from wakefulness. In fact, neither REMS nor NREMS are quantitatively deeper sleep. Rather, they are qualitatively different kinds of sleep. Instead of thinking of sleep as being toward the lower end of a ramp leading from waking, we should think of it as being like different rooms in a house. Just as a kitchen differs from a family room and both differ from a bedroom, so too does wake differ from NREMS, and both differ from REMS. Yet, we can accurately talk about the depth or quality of sleep in general. For one thing, it is harder to awaken someone when they are in N3 than in other stages of sleep. Also, depth of sleep is measured by such things as greater intensity of delta waves, less stage one, and fewer arousals. Research has shown that sleep punctuated by arousals lasting 3–15 s that occur more frequently than every 20 min fragment sleep enough to reduce its quality resulting in sleepiness the next waking period. Arousals are indicated by bursts of faster-frequency EEG or alpha waves sometimes accompanied by increases in EMG. Typically, these arousals do not result in awakening but leave the perception that sleep was not deep.

2.3 Sleep Changes with Age

What we have been describing pertains to the sleep in the "average young adult" who is approximately between 20 and 50 years of age. Most average young adults, as carefully done studies have shown, need between 7.5 and 8.5 h of sleep each night. However, as will be pointed out in Chap. 3, not all young adults are average in this regard. This amount of sleep and the way it is patterned as just reviewed forms the basis from which comparisons can be made to different ages and to unusual sleep. It is convenient to contrast sleep in average young adults with that of newborns and infants, children, teenagers, and the elderly. (The interactive website http://healthysleep.med.harvard.edu/interactive/sleep_lab enables you to see the sleep characteristics of sleep in an average young adult. It also compares this to sleep in a newborn and an elderly person as well as some sleep problems).

2.3.1 Sleep in Newborns and Infants

Sleep in newborns and infants is markedly different from that of the average young adult. Newborn sleep does not fit the polysomnographic criteria used at other ages, because the newborn brain is too immature to produce the kinds of brain waves we have just reviewed. They are so different that the stages have their own names. *Quiet sleep (QS)* is characterized by EEG similar to that of N3 in adults, no eye movements, high EMG, plus the absence of body movements. *Active sleep (AS)* is characterized by low-voltage, irregular brain waves, eye movements, low EMG, plus the observation of body and facial movements and occasional vocalizations. The term *indeterminate sleep (IS)* is used when there is a mixture of indications of both quiet and active sleep. Newborns sleep 16–18 h of every nychthemeron[3] of which 50 % is AS. AS constitutes as much as 75 % of the sleep of late term fetuses and premature newborns. QS and AS alternate in a 50 min cycle that gradually lengthens to about 100 min by school age, and for the first several months of age, infants frequently go directly into AS. In a relatively short period of time during infancy, AS comes to resemble REMS more and more (it can be called REMS at 12 weeks of age), and QS morphs into NREMS by 6 months. This process is similar to the maturation of the coos and babbling of infants into adult language; the coos and babbling are not adult speech but are the important, immature precursors of it. Furthermore, the amount of REMS per nychthemeron drops to adult level by about 2 years of age. N3 as a percent of total sleep is as high as it ever will be in early childhood then gradually declines by around 50 % by preadolescence. REMS is also very high during childhood and shows a decline with maturation.

Another difference at this age is the distribution of sleep and wake across the nychthemeron. Rather than the characteristic adult pattern of a long period of sleep, typically at night, alternating with a long period of wake every nychthemeron plus maybe an afternoon nap, newborns alternate between sleep and wake many times during a nychthemeron. After a few weeks of age, longer periods of sleep and wake are seen with greater and greater amounts of sleep seen during the night. During the first 4 months, infant sleep rapidly merges into fewer periods

---

[3] A nychthemeron (nick-**them**-er-on) is a full period of a night and a day or 24 h. In everyday use, "day" can mean 24 h or the portion of every 24 h that is light. In science, we need to be more precise, so we eliminate ambiguity when we use nychthemeron to refer to a 24 h cycle and reserve the term "day" to refer to the light portion of this cycle.

(Henderson et al. 2010). Eventually—typically between 2 to 3 months of age, but the sooner the better in the view of the parents—most infants are "sleeping through the night" (Henderson et al. 2010) supplemented by a couple of daytime naps. By 5 months of age, over half of infants are sleeping during the same period as their parents (Henderson et al. 2010). The total sleep time drops to 14–15 h per nychthemeron by 16 weeks of age and gradually continues to drop to 10–12 h between ages 3–5. Also about this time, daytime napping ceases. However, these are averages and individuals may need more or less sleep than this. Short sleepers remain this way until adolescence, as do long sleepers. There are similar individual differences in circadian sleep phase preferences with some individuals being evening types ("night owls"), others morning types ("morning larks"), and others neither type (see Sect. 4.4 for discussion of circadian sleep phase preference). Napping diminishes until there is typically one per nychthemeron and then none by age 3–5.

Toddlers and preschool-aged children have a NREM–REM sleep cycle averaging 60 min. When they first fall asleep, they quickly (within 10 min) go into deep N3 sleep from which it is difficult to awaken them. They often stay in this stage for about an hour at which point the child's brain waves shift into a mixture of sleep and arousal. Children may change positions and show other movements such as stroking their face, vocalizing, blinking. They may even awaken briefly. Although there may be initial signs of REMS at this time, frequently the first REMS period is "skipped." Usually within a minute or two, they are back in NREMS, mainly N3. The initial REMS period lasts about 10–20 min with the duration of subsequent REMS periods increasing to around 35 min in the middle of the sleep period, gradually decreasing to 20–25 min. There may be some increase in NREMS toward the end of the sleep period.

During the rest of childhood, the changes in sleep continue but more slowly. By grade school, the NREM–REM sleep cycle is at adult levels, and by age 10, the sleep stage proportions begin to assume adult levels, but the total sleep time remains higher at about 10 h. It appears that the sleep of older children is the most intense of any other age. It is easy for children of this age to fall asleep, and they have fewer awakenings. Also, it is very difficult to awaken a preteen child from NREMS.

2.3.2 Sleep in Teens

The sleep of teenagers also differs from that of the average young adult. Although the need for sleep per nychthemeron remains higher than that of the adult, averaging 9.25 h (but some do well with 8.5 h), teens in the Western world typically get much less than this amount, especially males. Let us look at the source and implications of these statements more closely.

For several years beginning in 1976, Bill Dement (physician and one of the long time, most active, and most influential sleep researchers, now retired from the Stanford University sleep research labs) and Mary Carskadon (PhD, former student and then colleague of Dement at Stanford and now Director of Sleep and Chronobiology Research at E.P. Bradley Hospital and Professor of Psychiatry and Human Behavior at the Brown University School of Medicine) did a series of experiments with teens at what they called summer "sleep camp" (e.g., Carskadon et al. 1980). The campers were monitored with the polysomnograph while required to spend 10 h in bed every night. They were then tested for alertness and behavioral functioning in various ways during the day. It was found that, separately from the amount of sleep obtained, daytime sleepiness gradually increased from the onset to the middle of puberty then stayed level through the rest of the teen years. When given the opportunity, teens consistently slept more than the average young adult. In subsequent studies at this camp, the amount of time in bed was shortened by varying degrees. When sleep was restricted to less than the amount needed, increased signs of fatigue and drops in behavioral abilities resulted during the day, especially in the morning (see Sects. 3.1.2–3.1.4 and 12.1.2 for more on the effects of sleep deprivation).

Subsequent research showed that the amount of sleep teens were getting in their home situations was found to be considerably less than the amount the campers demonstrated was actually needed. One survey showed that about a quarter of high school students in the United States regularly sleep less than 6.5 h on school nights, while only 15 of every 100 sleep 8.5 h or more. To make up for lost sleep, teenagers tend to sleep for an additional couple of hours on weekend mornings (Wolfson and Carskadon 1998). Similar patterns in teen sleep have been noted worldwide (Gradisar et al. 2011).

So, we know that Western teens need much more sleep than they think they need and actually get. The drop in obtained sleep begins in the early teenage years. On the average, there are 2½ h less sleep than needed on school nights and over one hour less on non-school nights. Another drop of an additional ½ h occurs in college freshmen. It is not known for certain what happens to the sleep of like-aged teens who do not go on to college, but it is thought that they too under sleep to some degree. The net results of teenagers sleeping less than really needed are signs of sleep deprivation including daytime sleepiness resulting in automobile accidents, decline in grades, moodiness, and impulsivity (see Sect. 4.5 and Box 12.2). Further complicating matters is the irregularity of sleep schedules in those teens who often go to bed later on weekends and holidays, then "sleep in" the next morning. Napping returns for many adolescent and college students as schedules permit. For example, in one study about 1/3 of older adolescents averaged 4 naps per week, usually around 4 pm (Gradisar et al. 2008). To round matters out, during the rest of the college years, there is a gradual drift toward the average young adult patterns (Moorcroft, unpublished data).

These changes in the sleep of adolescents appear to be the result of several factors. Adolescents seem to be less sensitive to sleep loss and more tolerant to sleep pressure. Additionally, there is a shift of the circadian influence on sleep to later clock hours.

2.3.3 Sleep in the Elderly

Sleep in the elderly is best characterized as fraying (Webb 1975), like the way the ends of a rope can unravel with time. In a similar way, the tightly defined sleep of the average young adult may come apart with age. For some older adults, sleep frays a lot, and for others, the changes are minimal. As a consequence, there are great individual differences in the sleep of the elderly. These changes actually begin during mid- to late middle age but become more intense and noticeable in the elderly.

The amount of sleep needed may not decline with age. Both self-reports and polysomnographic studies agree that older people tend to sleep less at night (averaging 6–7 h) than when younger. However, if naps are included in the count, then it appears that there is much less difference per nychthemeron. Also, an objective test for daytime sleepiness, the MSLT (see Sect. 3.1.1.2), and other data suggest that the elderly are sleepier during the day than when they were younger. This finding can be interpreted to mean they are not getting enough sleep at night. A contrasting interpretation is that the elderly need just as much sleep as they did when younger but more evenly distributed throughout the nychthemeron. Supporting this latter conclusion are studies with elderly animals that also show a more even distribution of sleep per nychthemeron. On the other hand, the negative consequences of the loss of sleep (see Sects. 3.1.2–3.1.4) are less in elderly people than they are in younger people, suggesting less of a need for sleep. Certainly, the elderly's sleep/wake pattern changes, and the intensity of both sleep and wakefulness lessens, but the meaning of these facts is not obvious.

Sleep onset is often reported to be more difficult and it is fragmented by more and sometimes longer awakenings. The sleep of the elderly tends to be more easily interrupted by noises and other stimuli. In sum, sleep efficiency gradually declines by about 3 % per decade starting at about age 30, going from 0.96 to the low 0.80 s.

The amount of N3 sleep gradually diminishes up to 60 years of age and then remains relatively constant at only 5–10 % (or even less in males). However, some authorities say that N3 sleep does not drop that much; delta waves still occur but many do not have enough amplitude to be counted. But even if the amplitude criterion for delta waves is lowered, the amount of N3 is still a bit lower than that of the average young adult.

There is some decrease in the total amount of REMS, but the decrease in the number of rapid eye movements during REMS is even greater. Additionally, there is more REMS earlier in the night and the duration of the REMS periods may not change much as the night progresses. Accompanying these changes is a proportional increase in N1 sleep. As a result of all these changes, the elderly frequently report that their sleep is less satisfying and less restorative than when they were younger.

Other changes are common in addition to these changes. The timing of the sleep–wake cycle, which is called the circadian rhythm (see Sect. 3.2) shifts; older adults become sleepy earlier in the evening and awaken earlier in the morning. Additionally, sleep often is more fragmented because of the emergence of sleep disorders (see Part V) and illnesses common in the elderly, plus medications often used by this population can contribute to complaints of insomnia.

Box 2.1 Sleep in Other Cultures and Eras

Most of what we know about sleep is from the study of sleep in the Western industrialized world where people typically sleep at somewhat regular times, in night clothes, alone or in pairs in a bed with a comfortable mattress, and in isolated, quiet, climate-controlled indoor bedrooms. We tend to accept this as the only acceptable way to sleep. In contrast, for much of human existence, things were much different (Horne 2006; Bed 2012; Worsley 2012). People have slept in what they had been wearing for many days and between animal skins on a pile of straw, mats, wooden platforms, o the ground with a pillow made of rolled up animal skin with the fur on the inside. Eventually, carpets or rugs that lay on the floor were used to sleep on.

An improvement was to raise the sleeping surface of the floor or to place it on a bench against the wall or in a shallow chest. Even today in the non-Western world, sleep occurs on horsehair or cotton mattresses that are not placed on springs. In Persia almost 4,000 years ago, waterbeds made by filling several goat skins were in use. What we now know of as a bed with linen sheets evolved over time in some parts of the world. By the seventeenth century in the United States and Europe, a bed was most likely rope or leather stretched out on a simple wood frame with a bag containing straw or wool on top. A step up was a mattress made of sailcloth with grommets along the edges that were fastened to pegs in the frame. During the nineteenth century, mattresses that were tufted or buttoned and placed on coiled bedsprings made their appearance. It was not until the mid-twentieth century that latex mattresses began to be used.

For most of history, sleep occurred in shared spaces with constant noise and great variations in heat and cold and humidity. This is true even today in many places. These communal sleeping spaces could be malodorous and sweaty, yet they were often better and more secure than sleeping out-of-doors. Before recent times, it was typical for members of a family to even share a bed. Even colleagues from work might share the bedroom. In fact, it was not unusual for strangers to do the same in an inn. It was not until recently that people felt the need to sleep by themselves. Before this, isolated was not possible because there were not enough rooms in dwellings for this purpose. And the sleeping room might also be used for cooking, washing, and working as well as a place to eat meals and interact with others socially. One extreme example of sleeping arrangements was among the poor in Victorian England living in workhouses. They slept in a line on benches with their arms hanging over a chest high tightrope, referred to as a "hangover." And they were charged by the hour for this sleeping arrangement.

Darkness of night tended to determine bedtimes, but sleep may not have been consolidated. Western Europeans of 200–500 years ago are reported to have slept in two phases at night. "First sleep" lasting several hours was followed by a "watching period" before the "second or morning sleep." During the watching period, people often stayed in bed to contemplate, pray, converse with one another, have sex, or simply just let their wandering minds enjoy this semiconscious state. Additionally, they awakened after each REMS period. In order to explore this a bit more, Thomas A Wehr, psychiatrist at the National Institute of Mental Health in Bethesda, Maryland, had subjects spend weeks of 14-h nights during which time they had to be in bed. They soon settled into a pattern of taking a long time to fall asleep, sleeping for 2–5 h, lying quietly in bed for 1–3 h, then sleeping for 2–5 h (e.g., People in traditional societies sleep in eye-opening ways 1999).

Sleep patterns are affected by cultural beliefs, what is thought to be the function of sleep, and how important it is believed to be for things like health and social relationships (Owens 2008). For example, in some cultures, sleep is seen as something done communally with people sleeping together regardless of age. For more on fascinating cross-cultural differences of sleep in children, see Judith Owens' paper entitled Socio-Cultural Considerations and Sleep Practices in the Pediatric Population (2008).

2.4 Sleep in Animals

To this point, we have been focusing on sleep in humans. However, as far as we know, all mammals and many other animals have some form of sleep. There are no reported occurrences of sleepless animals. Sleep in over 90 species of mammals has been studied, extensively in a few species like the cat, rat, mouse, and of course human, but otherwise slightly studied in only a very small proportion of all the animals alive today. As a result, there are large gaps in our knowledge of animal sleep, and often what we can conclude is based on broad inferences from scant data. However, at least a few representatives from each of the 17 mammalian orders have been studied. There are enough data available to make some observations about sleep in animals.

There are great variations in the sleep of animals. Those animals closer to us on the evolutionary tree have sleep that more closely resembles ours, but the amount of sleep per nychthemeron varies greatly as does the proportion of sleep spent in REMS and NREMS. For example, the length of sleep per nychthemeron ranges from 1.9 h in the giraffe to 19.9 h in the little brown bat. Other examples include Asiatic elephants at 3.1 h, baboons at 9.4 h, lions at 13.5 h, and eastern chipmunks at 19.9 h. Hairy armadillos spend 16 h per nychthemeron in NREMS, but horses only 2 h, and Virginia opossums are in REMS for 7 h per nychthemeron, but sheep only ½ of an hour. The amount of sleep per nychthemeron bares no affinity to the degree of relatedness between species. Cows, sheep, deer, and other grazing animals sleep only up to 2 h per nychthemeron and even that is divided into multiple occasions. Dogs may sleep for 8 h. Cats and mice spend about 13 h asleep divided into several periods. Possums, baboons, and bats may sleep close to 20 h per nychthemeron. It appears that several factors interact to influence sleep length in mammals with some factors being more important than others for individual species. These factors are thought to be as follows:

- *The degree to which the species is predator or prey* the more likely an animal is to be preyed upon, the less it can afford to sleep. However, this factor is controversial because it is hard to measure.
- *The quality, quantity, and availability of the food supply that the species typically eats* animals that do not have an abundant supply of highly nutritious food need to spend more time awake finding and consuming food.
- *The type of sleeping habitat the species has* an animal with a safe sleeping place can safely sleep more than one that does not.
- *If the species is warm- or cold-blooded,* cold-blooded animals may use sleep as a time to avoid becoming too warm or too cold.
- *The degree to which the brain is developed at birth in the species* REMS seems to facilitate brain development (see Sect. 11.1.1.1). Thus, animals relatively immature at birth need to spend more time in this state.
- *The body size of the species* large animals are at less risk for losing or gaining too much body heat during sleep, thus can sleep for longer periods at a time.
- *Events and activities* sleep increases around the time of situations like brooding, hibernation, injury, and copulation.

The distribution of sleep in the nychthemeron varies greatly among species, too. Diurnal animals, such as humans, sleep mainly at night, while nocturnal animals do the opposite. Other animals sleep during both the day and night. Even within these patterns, there are variations. Some animals, like humans, generally have a single, consolidated period or two of sleep. Others have many small periods of sleep per nychthemeron. Then, there is the crepuscular pattern of sleep like that of the bat—asleep except at dawn and dusk.

The habits, places, and postures of animal sleep likewise vary greatly. Some animals, such as rabbits, sleep in burrows; some animals, such as gorillas, make nests to sleep in; while others, such as zebras, sleep in the open. Horses sometimes sleep standing up; some birds can apparently sleep while flying; foxes sleep curled up. Some humans have even been observed to sleep sitting at a desk in a classroom! You can probably add to the list other varieties of animal (and student) sleep habits.

All of the mammals (except possibly the sea-dwelling dolphins, porpoises, and whales) and birds so far investigated cycle between REMS and NREMS. Only a small percent of the sleep of most birds is REMS, but avian predators (e.g., eagles, hawks) have a much larger percent of sleep. For a while it appeared that the Australian spiny ant eater, echidna, did not manifest REMS. This observation was of considerable theoretical interest, because this animal is an egg-laying mammal of very ancient origin. It was thought to give a clue of how sleep developed over the ages, specifically that REMS is a newer type of sleep than NREMS. However, careful study in the 1990s by neurophysiologist Jerry Siegel (of UCLA and the VA Center in Sepulveda Medical Center in California) and colleagues using newer kinds of techniques revealed that the echidna shows signs of rudimentary REMS mixed in with its NREMS (Siegel 1997). They also found that another ancient egg-laying mammal, the platypus, has copious amounts of obvious REMS.

Smaller animals generally sleep longer than larger ones and have a shorter NREM–REM sleep cycle. Birds have much less REMS in their sleep than do mammals. Most primates have the same three NREM stages of sleep that humans have. Non-primate mammals seem to have two or just one stage of NREMS. Not all animals show all of the signs of REMS that are seen in humans. Some animals such as rabbits, dogs, and most birds do not show complete muscle paralysis. Rapid eye movements are absent in or minimal in animals such as moles, opossums, and owls that do not move their eyes when awake. Yet, in all of these animals, there is some kind of regular cycling between NREM and REMS. All mammals and birds that have REMS have more of it early in life.

Some mammals and birds show patterns of sleep not seen in humans. Some carnivores, ungulates, and insectivores spend part of their nychthemeron some-where between sleep and wake in what is called dozing (also called drowsiness, but not to be confused with human drowsiness as discussed in Chap. 3). This state is characterized by relaxed body position, partially closed eyes, slightly less responsiveness to stimuli, and a mixture of activated EEG waves and slow waves. You may have noticed cats spending a lot of time in this state, but contrary to appearances in class, college students have not been documented to exhibit this kind of drowsiness.

Mammals that live in the sea and birds that migrate over oceans have a problem. They cannot settle down to rest while sleeping. The sea mammals need to surface periodically to breathe, and the migrating birds have no place to stop. One way some of these animals have solved the problem is to sleep half of their brain at a time. Bottlenose dolphins and porpoises have been most studied by the Russian scientist L. M. Mukhametov of the Severtsov Institute of Evolution, Morphology and Ecology of Animals in Moscow. He and his colleagues have found that both sides of the brain in these animals may simultaneously show a small amount of N2-like sleep, with the animal surfacing to breathe without awakening, but such complex continuously coordinated activity is not seen during N3. Rather, EEGs show that while one half of the brain sleeps, the other half is awake. When in this state, the eye on the opposite side of the head remains open allowing the animal to monitor their surroundings. Further, the wake half enables the animal to surface periodically and then take a breath. This pattern can persist for over an hour at a time followed by awakening before the other half takes its turn to sleep. However, the total amount of sleep that each side of the brain gets is seldom equal. Addi-tionally, studies have shown that each side has its own quota of sleep each ny-chthemeron and that one half cannot sleep for the other half. Note, however, that such one-sided sleep has not been observed during REMS in these animals. Other sea mammals compensate differently; they hold their breath while sleeping for up to ½ h at a time, then awaken to surface and breathe before returning to sleep.

Many species of birds have also been found have NREMS half a brain at a time with one eye open. The riskier the environment the more they do this. Additionally, several other variants of sleep are found in birds. Vigilant sleep found in birds is an intermediate combination of NREMS and REMS. Gaze wake in birds is sleep with low-voltage fast EEG and reduced muscle tone but with open eyes manifesting slow, unique eye movements. Pigeons and other birds sometimes peep, something like a reverse blink, while sleeping. The frequency of blinks in individual pigeons is increased by predators being nearby but decreased by the presence of other pigeons or by sleep deprivation.

Even less is known about the sleep of lower animals, but of those that have been studied, the signs of sleep are even more different from those found in humans and other mammals due to their more primitive brains. In most cases, behavioral criteria are relied upon to study sleep in these animals. These criteria include: (1) periods of quiescence in a typical posture that are easily reversed by intense or sensory stimuli indicating a potential threat and (2) a compensatory increase in this state following a period of its deprivation. These indicators of sleep have been shown in at least some representatives from all orders, including lower vertebrates (e.g., reptiles, amphibians, and fish) and invertebrates (e.g., scorpions, cockroaches, and fruit flies). However, no signs of sleep have been found in other representatives of these orders.

Sleep has been clearly seen in many but not all reptiles that have been studied. Some amphibians appear to have some form of sleep, but others apparently do not. Some fish and some invertebrates have clearly been shown to have states resembling sleep. Interesting animal sleep research has been done by biological sciences Dr. Ida Karmanova, Professor and retired Director of the Laboratory of Wake-Sleep Evolution at the I.M. Sechenov Institute of Evolutionary Physiology and Biochemistry in St. Petersburg, Russia (Karmanova 1982; Karmanova and Oganesyan 1999). This research has not been widely attended to in the West. She and her associates have data that strongly suggest that reptiles have two kinds of sleep that are forerunners of NREMS and REMS in more advanced animals. Even lower vertebrates demonstrate wakefulness plus three other states of immobility or "protosleeps" according to these Russian researchers. These states are not sleep per se, but sleep as seen in higher vertebrates developed out of one of these (e.g., Karmanova and Oganesyan 1999).

Hibernation and torpor seem in some ways to be related to sleep and in other ways to differ from it. Hibernation is an extended period of quiescence, while the body temperature and metabolic rate are greatly lowered with periodic bouts every several days to every several weeks of increases in muscle tension, more than a few deep breaths, and other activity. Torpor is a similar state but not as intense and only lasting part of a day. EEG, body temperature, and arousability all line up in a continuum from quiet wake to sleep to torpor to hibernation. Torpor consists mainly of low-amplitude N3, but there are no recordable brain waves during hibernation. However, hibernation is usually achieved by going through N3 and eliminating REMS and then through torpor. During sleep, there is typically a slight drop in body temperature, a moderate one during torpor, and a great drop during hibernation. Arousal is slower from torpor than from sleep and even slower yet from hibernation. On the other hand, when animals come out of torpor or hibernation, they sleep for a long time with an increase in SWS as if they are sleep deprived. The longer the duration of the hibernation, the longer the subsequent sleep, and the greater the amount of SWS.

(Interesting research program on sleep in fruit flies can be seen at http://www.pbs.org/wgbh/nova/body/sleep.html from 0:39 to 2:05.)

2.5 Conclusion

Sleep is not as simple as it seems. Prior to the scientific study of sleep, people believed that sleep was a passive phenomenon. Our brains and bodies simply seemed to reduce their levels of functioning as we went to sleep. Indeed it seems that way, because things like noises, pains, or thoughts that keep our minds or bodies aroused can keep us from sleeping. Also, in spite of dreaming, it was believed that not much is going on mentally when we sleep. The discovery of REMS in the middle of the twentieth century changed all that. The existence of more than one kind of sleep and the regular cycling between the stages of sleep showed that there must be active mechanisms controlling sleep as well as wakefulness. Also, REMS is anything but an inactive state. The EEG shows the brain is very activated. The only reason we remain quietly in bed during REMS is because our muscles of movement are paralyzed.

Along with the change in the notion of what sleep is came a whole new scientific attitude toward it. New questions were asked that no one ever thought to ask before. More interest, especially in REMS, was generated. More scientists turned their research attention to sleep. More research money became available. More sleep research was done. With this, increase in research came even more surprise discoveries about sleep—and even more understanding of how much more there is to learn. Much of the rest of this book is filled with the knowledge and understanding, much of it surprising and some counterintuitive, gained as a result of the new attitude and understanding about sleep since the mid-twentieth century.

References

Amlaner, C. J., & Fuller, P. M. (Eds.). (2009). *Basics of sleep* (2nd ed.). Westchester, Illinois: Sleep Research Society.

Bed (2012, July 20). Retrieved August 3, 2012 from Wikipedia, the free encyclopedia: http://en.wikipedia.org/w/index.php?title=Bed&oldid=503232320.

Carden, K. A. (2009). Recording sleep: The electrodes, 10/20 recording system, and sleep system specifications. *Sleep Medicine Clinics, 4*, 333–341.

Carskadon, M., Harvey, D., Duke, P., Anders, T., Litt, J., & D, W. (1980). Pubertal changes in daytime sleepiness. *Sleep, 2*, 453–460.

Gradisar, M., Gardner, G., & Dohnt, H. (2011). Recent worldwide sleep patterns and problems during adolescence: A review and meta-analysis of age, region, and sleep. *Sleep Medicine, 12*, 110–118.

Gradisar, M., Wright, H., Robinson, J., Paine, S., & Gamble, A. L. (2008). Adolescent napping behavior: Comparisons of school week versus weekend sleep patterns. *Sleep and Biological Rhythms, 6*, 183–186.

Henderson, J., France, K. G., Owens, J. L., & Blampied, N. M. (2010). Sleeping through the night: The consolidation of self-regulated sleep across the first year of life. *Pediatrics, 126*, e1081–e1087.

Horne, J. (2006). *Sleepfaring*. New York: Oxford University Press.

Jenni, O. G., & Carskadon, M. A. (2007). Sleep behavior and sleep regulation from infancy through adolescence: Normative aspects. *Sleep Medicine Clinics*, 321–329.

Karmanova, I. G. (1982). *Evolution of sleep: Stages of the wakefulness-sleep cycle in vertebrates.* Basel: Karger.

Karmanova, I. G., & Oganesyan, G. A. (1999). *Sleep: Evolution and disorders.* Lanham, MD: University Press of America.

Kryger, M. H., Roth, T. R., & Dement, W. C. (Eds.). (2011). *Principles and practice of sleep medicine* (5th ed.). St. Louis: Elsevier.

Lee-Chiong, T. (2011). *Somnology 2*. Seattle: Amazon.

Moorcroft, W. H. (1993). *Sleep, dreaming, and sleep disorders: An introduction* (2nd ed.). Lanham, Md: University Press of America.

Nicolau, M. C., Akaarir, M., Gamundi, A., Gonzalez, J., & Rial, R. V. (2000). Why we sleep: The evolutionary pathway to the mammalian sleep. *Progress in Neurobiology, 62*, 379–406.

Ogilvie, R. D., Wilkinson, R. T., & Allison, S. (1989). The detection of sleep onset: Behavioral, physiological, and subjective convergence. *Sleep, 12*, 458–474.

Owens, J. (2008). Socio-cultural considerations and sleep practices in the pediatric population. (H. S. Driver Ed.). *Sleep Medicine Clinics, 3*, 97–107.

Parrino, L., Ferri, R., Bruni, O., & Terzano, M. (2012). Cyclic alternating pattern (CAP): The marker of sleep instability. *Sleep Medicine Reviews, 16*, 27–45.

People in traditional societies sleep in eye-opening ways. (1999, September 25). *Science news*, (pp. 205–207).

Siegel, J. M. (1997). Sleep in monotremes; implications for the evolution of REM sleep. In *Sleep and sleep disorders: From molecule to behavior* (pp. 113–128).

Webb, W. B. (1975). *Sleep: The gentle tyrant*. Englewood Cliffs, NJ: Prentice-Hall.

Weber, S., Bergan, D., Golden, H., Moorcroft, W. H., & Hansen, G. (1983). Alpha delta sleep in fibrositis patients. *Fourth International Congress of Sleep Research*. Bologna, Italy.

Wolfson, A. R., & Carskadon, M. A. (1998). Sleep schedules and daytime functioning in adolescents. *Child Development, 69*, 875–887.

Worsley, L. (2012). 'If walls could talk': A history of the home. Retrieved March 13, from http://www.npr.org/2012/03/13/148296032/if-walls-could-talk-a-history-of-the-home.

Chapter 3
The Need to Sleep

Contents

We humans are a day-night system, with sleep and waking experiences interacting continuously.

—Rosalind Cartwright (2010)

The need to sleep is compelling. You feel sleepy at regular times and even sleepier if you go without it. Bernie Webb, a psychologist who had a long and distinguished career in sleep research at the University of Florida prior to his retirement, called sleep a "gentle tyrant." As we shall see, duration of recent wakefulness and time of nychthemeron result in biological factors that interact to influence sleep/wake, but there are other less biological factors that are also important. We shall explore each of these factors separately.

Specific references to statements in this chapter that can be found in multiple, widely available sources are not included in the text. A selection of these sources is listed below and can also be consulted for verification or more detail. (Kryger et al. 2011; Lee-Chiong 2009; National Sleep Foundation web-site http://www.sleepfoundation.org/YourSleep.aasmnet.org.).

W. H. Moorcroft, *Understanding Sleep and Dreaming*,
DOI: 10.1007/978-1-4614-6467-9_3,
© Springer Science+Business Media New York 2013

Fig. 3.1 How sleep drive
affects the likelihood
of sleep

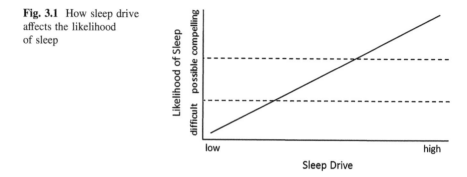

3.1 Sleep as Homeostatic

Generally speaking, the longer we are awake, the greater the intensity and/or
duration of our subsequent sleep. That is, sleep seems to compensate for wakefulness. In this way, sleep is homeostatic.[1] It is thought that sleep drive is maintained
between an upper threshold for initiating sleep and a lower threshold for terminating
sleep (see Fig. 3.1). When between these thresholds sleep may be possible but not
compelling. Above the upper threshold sleep is more compelling, and below the
lower threshold sleep is more difficult to achieve. The intensity of slow-wave (see
Sect. 2.1) activity (*SWA*) in the brain during N3 is an indicator of the level of sleep
drive. The intensity of SWA is proportional to the amount of prior wakefulness but
also depends upon the type and intensity of the waking experience.

3.1.1 Measuring Sleepiness

Generally speaking, the longer we are awake, the greater our need to sleep. During
the first several hours awake, we may not notice the urge, but as the amount of
continuous time we are awake approaches 16 h, we are much more likely to
become aware of the pressure to sleep. That is, we feel sleepy. This occurs sooner
if we are already sleep deprived. If our time awake goes well beyond 16 h, we feel
the urge to sleep getting stronger and stronger. There is some evidence that the
level of sleep drive plateaus after about 30–50 h without sleep, when we seem to
be as sleepy as we can be.

 There are three aspects of sleepiness: introspective, physiological, and manifest.
Introspective sleepiness is the self-assessment of your internal state. *Physiological
sleepiness* is your body's biological need to sleep. It can be viewed as similar to

---

[1] Homeostasis is the process of trying to compensate for deviations from a standard or norm. The
thermostat in your home engages in homeostasis when it turns on the furnace or air conditioner if
the room becomes cooler or warmer than the desired temperature set on it.

> How likely are you to doze off or fall asleep in the following situations, in contrast to feeling just tired? This refers to your usual way of life in recent times. Even if you have not done some of these things recently try to work out how they would have affected you. Use the following scale to choose the most appropriate number for each situation:
>
> $\qquad$ 0= no chance of dozing
> $\qquad$ 1= slight chance of dozing
> $\qquad$ 2= moderate chance of dozing
> $\qquad$ 3= high chance of dozing
>
> 1. Sitting and resting
> 2. Watching television
> 3. Sitting, inactive in a public place (e.g., a theater or a meeting)
> 4. As a passenger in a car for 1 h without a break
> 5. Lying down to rest in the afternoon when circumstances permit
> 6. Sitting and talking to someone
> 7. Sitting quietly after a lunch without alcohol
> 8. In a car while stopped for a few minutes in traffic

Fig. 3.2 The Epworth Sleepiness Scale

other drives such as hunger and thirst. *Manifest sleepiness* is the behavioral component as shown in performance deficits, errors, inattention, and even being overcome by sleep. There are methods of measuring each of these kinds of sleepiness, but they do not always correlate well with each other because factors like individual differences, motivation to remain awake, and being in a stimulating and distracting environment may affect each of them differently.

3.1.1.1   Introspective Sleepiness

Introspective sleepiness is measured by asking people how sleepy they think they feel in certain kinds of situations or how sleepy they feel at the moment. This is most often and best done using standardized scales rather than casually asking people how they feel. However, these scales may not always be accurate because a person may not be aware of their true sleepiness or not wish to divulge it. Here are the most commonly used introspective scales.

Epworth Sleepiness Scale The *Epworth Sleepiness Scale* (shown in Fig. 3.2) is the most widely used the standardized subjective scales to assess introspective sleepiness. It asks questions about falling asleep in situations that typically promote sleep. It has been validated on populations of people complaining of a sleep problem.

Stanford Sleepiness Scale The *Stanford Sleepiness Scale* or *SSS* (shown in Fig. 3.3) instructs a person to select one of seven items to describe the current state of alertness. While it has been shown that sleep deprivation does increase SSS scores, there are no norms available with which to compare responses.

Analog Scales Various *analog scales* have also been developed on which a person indicates how they feel by placing a mark on a line of set width, usually 10 cm, between very alert at one end and very sleepy at the other (see example in Fig. 3.4).

Choose one of the following to describe your current state:

1. Feeling active and vital, alert, wide awake

2. Functioning at a high level, but not at peak, able to concentrate

3. Awake, but relaxed; responsive but not fully alert

4. A little foggy, not at peak, let down

5. Fogginess, beginning to lose interest in remaining awake, slowed down

6. Sleepiness, prefer to be lying down, fighting sleep, woozy

7. Almost in reverie, sleep onset soon, lost struggle to remain awake

---

Fig. 3.3 The Stanford Sleepiness Scale

Place an X on the line that best describes how you feel right now.

Almost asleep _____Extremely alert

Fig. 3.4 An example of a part of an analog scale

3.1.1.2 Physiological Sleepiness

Multiple Sleep Latency Test The most commonly used assessment of physiological sleepiness is the multiple sleep latency test (MSLT). For this test, a person is given a 20-min opportunity to fall asleep in a quiet, comfortable sleep lab room every 2 h during the day. They are instructed to try to fall asleep. An average of more than 10 min to get to sleep is considered acceptable sleepiness, while less than 5 min is considered pathological indicating a significant sleep problem. The MSLT has very good validity and reliability.

Although not often used, some sleep specialists propose that measuring the theta wave activity in the brain when awake is a more direct way to assess physiological sleepiness. It is known that an increase in theta activity is associated with sleepiness; however, there is also a circadian component to levels of theta activity, and meditative states can increase theta waves showing that the MSLT is less than a pure indicator of the level of sleepiness.

3.1.1.3 Manifest Sleepiness

Maintenance of Wakefulness Test A variation of the MSLT, thought to measure manifest sleepiness, is called the maintenance of wakefulness test (MWT). It is similar to MSLT except people are instructed to remain awake while being still in a semi-reclined position in a dimly lit, quiet room. As such, it measures the ability to remain awake. High levels of sleepiness make staying awake difficult.

Psychomotor Vigilance Task Another way of measuring manifest sleepiness includes various performance measures—usually repetitive tasks such as number substitution or pressing one of several buttons in response to the nature of a light or sound pattern—that are scored for speed and accuracy. These are typically known as vigilance tests. A commonly used example is the psychomotor vigilance task (PVT) that measures button press response time to a visual display on a micro-computer. The display is presented randomly every 2–10 (or 5–12) s. To try this for yourself go to http://www.sleepdisordersflorida.com/pvt1.html.

These three ways of measuring sleepiness do not correlate well with one another because they may be measuring different aspects of sleepiness and be affected by other than the need for sleep, such as where the measurement is taken, differing test durations, and what the person taking the measurement expects it to show (Horne 2010). Furthermore, Horne cautions that these tests, especially those done in the laboratory, may show small differences in sleepiness that are of no consequence in the more stimulating real-world environment.

3.1.2 The Effects of Sleep Deprivation

Since the turn of the century, over 1,000 studies of sleep deprivation have been published. Their results have shown considerable consistency. The list of the effects of continuous sleep deprivation that have been reported is long and includes negative changes in emotions, behaviors, and mental processes as well as biological effects (see Table 3.1). (http://healthysleep.med.harvard.edu/video/sleep07_matters also shows the effects of not getting enough sleep.) Overall, the effects of sleep deprivation on mood appear to be greater than the effects on motor or cognitive performance (Pilcher and Huffcutt 1996). Additionally, sleep deprivation increases manifest and physiological sleepiness but not always introspective sleepiness showing that people may not be aware of the severity of their sleep deprivation.

Some of the effects of sleep deprivation are modulated by circadian arousal influences (see Fig. 3.8) resulting in periods when the ensuing deficits are less noticed. For example, only mildly diminished alertness may be experienced during the day, but considerably decreased alertness, slowed reactions, and errors are experienced during the night. This pattern is similar to your flashlight periodically getting dim. However, while the number and intensity of effects generally increase as the degree of sleep deprivation increases, the manifest sleepiness can be strongly influenced by the situation. For example, the psychomotor behaviors[2] most affected are long, monotonous, externally paced, newly learned tasks requiring use of memory but without providing any performance feedback. An example is driving (see Box 3.1).

---

[2] Thinking and decision making which lead to movements.

Table 3.1 The range of effects of sleep deprivation

COGNITIVE PROCESSES:

   Difficulty concentrating

   Invasive daydreaming while engaged
     in cognitive work

   errors of omission > errors of
     commission

   Disorientation

   Perceptual distortions and
     hallucinations

   Greater indecisiveness

   Slowing of mental processes such as
     reaction time

   Decrease in short-term memory

   Decrease in creativity and mental
     flexibility

   Decline in logical reasoning ability for
     complex problems

   Decreased attention

   Decreased information processing

   Interference with executive functions[a]

   Decrease in integrative ability

   Lapses of consciousness

   Confusion

   Negative impact on mood

   Difficulty multitasking

SUBJECTIVE:

   Lethargy

   Sense of partial loss of control

   Disorientation

   Irritability and negative moods

   Even paranoia in some individuals

BEHAVIORS:

   Less spontaneous

   Over responsiveness

   Microsleeps

   Decrease in vigilance

   Decreased sense of humor

   Less able to deal effectively with
     unfamiliar situations

   Involuntary sleep attacks

   Less desire to socialize

   Decreased psychomotor performance

   Clumsiness

   Slurring of speech

   Harder to "find the right word"

   Increased motor vehicle accidents

PHYSIOLOGICAL:

   Heart palpitations

   Fall in body temperature (about 0.8 °F)

   Slow eyelid closures

   Droopy eyelids

   Itchy eye

   Tremor

   Weight gain

   Greater gag and deep tendon reflexes

   Increased SNS activity

   Hormonal changes

   Increased caloric intake

   Weight gain

   Decreased resistance to infection

   Increased ghrelin

   Decreased leptin

   Increased insulin resistance (decreased
     glucose tolerance)

   Increased hunger

[a] A complex behavior involving decision making, working memory, ability to appropriately stick to task, reasonable risk taking, and so forth

Box 3.1 Effects of Sleep Deprivation on Driving

Studies that directly compared the effects of alcohol on driving to those of sleep loss on driving have consistently shown that driving, while sleepde-prived is similarly dangerous to driving under the influence. Both level of alcohol in the body and degree of the lack of sleep proportionally reduce response times, hand–eye coordination, visual tracking, and increase driving off the road in a driving simulator. It does not take much sleep deprivation to undermine performance on par with being legally drunk. Driving after 17 h without sleep is like driving with a blood alcohol level of 0.05 percent, and driving after 24 h without sleep is like driving with a blood alcohol level of 0.10, legally drunk in most states. The fatality and severe injury rate from motor vehicle crashes due to sleepiness is similar to that of crashes related to alcohol. The Center for Disease Control and Prevention in the United States concluded from a national survey that sleepy drivers cause over 1500 deaths per year and around 40,000 injuries (Hensley 2011).

Yet sleepy driving is not uncommon. Half of young adults admit to driving while drowsy once a month or more. Slightly fewer middle-aged adults do this, dropping to only about a quarter of older adults. Around 1 in 10 of all ages says this occurs one or more times a week. In another survey, it was found that 4.7 % of drivers of all ages actually fell asleep while driving, and it was more prevalent in young adults at 7.2 % (Center for Disease Control and Prevention 2011).

Many things that people do to counteract sleepiness when driving turn out to be ineffective after only a few minutes. These futile maneuvers include taking a stretch break, opening a window for cold air, turning up the radio, and tightening muscles. However, in situations where driving when sleepy is necessary, such as responding to a family emergency, pulling off the road and ingesting 200 or so mg of caffeine, equivalent to two cups of coffee, followed by 20 min of nap, time can be effective for up to several hours.

(For more on this topic, see the narrated presentation at http://www.aasmnet.org/safed.aspx. Also see http://www.sleepfoundation.org/es/video/heads-the-wheel-drowsy-driving-prevention.)

Microsleeps and Lapses There is another effect of sleep deprivation on behavior. *Microsleeps*[3] may cause brief absences of attention called *lapses*. These phenomena are equivalent to your flashlight suddenly going dark but only for several seconds. The frequency and duration of microsleeps increase with the degree of sleep deprivation, such that after about 40 continuous hours without sleep, they are unavoidable without sustained mental effort and strong external stimulation. Even then a microsleep may overwhelm a person without warning. Most sleep-deprived people also experience mild body complaints, anxiety, depression, and

---

[3] You probably have experienced a brief loss of electrical power that temporarily shuts everything off, including your computer. This occurrence is similar to microsleeps that are intrusions of a few seconds of sleep causing the absence of alertness in the midst of waking. During a microsleep, a person appears to be staring off into space or the head may droop a bit.

paranoia. Serious delusions, paranoid thoughts, and depersonalization may occur after four continuous nychthemerons without sleep, especially in persons of weak psychological stability.

On the other hand, not everything appears to be affected by less severe sleep deprivation. Objective measurements show that sheer physical exertion and exercise not requiring much mental effort, such as weight lifting, running, or swimming, do not seem to be diminished by mild sleep deprivation. However, sleep-deprived people *feel* that they are doing worse or are exercising harder than they would if they had had adequate sleep, and the exercise takes more effort as reflected in increased heart and respiration rates. Also, recovery after exercise takes longer. In contrast, sports that require more attention, thinking, and rapid changes in coordination, such as basketball, tennis, or soccer, are more likely to be negatively affected by sleep deprivation. Tasks involving logic are slowed but otherwise not affected.

Many people believe sleep deprivation does not affect their performance. In fact, until the late 1950s, scientists were not able to demonstrate any performance deficits resulting from sleep deprivation. This was because the scientists were not looking at the right kinds of tasks. Only when they used tasks whose timing was not determined by the subject that went on for longer than 10 min and was rather boring and repetitive, did the effects of sleep deprivation become noticeable. A typical experiment using the PVT showed that compared to non-deprived subjects, the sleep-deprived individuals gradually became slower and slower in their response times and even occasionally failed to respond. Furthermore, while their best responses were as fast as those of the controls, they had more slow responses and eventually outright lapses during the last minutes of the 10-min test.

Masking The effects of sleep deprivation can, however, be overcome or, more technically, *masked* by activity, bright light, noise, posture, stress, motivation, and some drugs. Masking occurs when extraneous influences override sleep propensity. For instance, in a 1985 experiment (Horne and Pettit 1985), volunteers doing a vigilance task involving monetary rewards for correct responses but fines for false alarms performed better than volunteers without such motivation for the first 36 h of sleep deprivation. However, during the next 24 h, the performance decreased in the incentive group but was still above that of the no incentive group. As sleep deprivation continued beyond this point, no difference occurred between the incentive and no incentive groups. In another study (Haslam 1983), soldiers without sleep for three days showed a performance drop of 55 % compared to their performance before the deprivation. But when they were simply told that the deprivation would end in a few hours, their performance jumped back to 85 %.

Several things can be concluded from such studies: not all performance is detrimentally affected by sleep deprivation; some kinds of performance are more affected than others; and when the deficits are present, they may be quantitative, such as a general slowing down, or qualitative, such as committing errors. Furthermore, sleep-deprived subjects can compensate for short periods of time even on tasks that are affected if they apply extra effort, especially when motivated by being given an incentive or immediate feedback. However, the ability of people to compensate by applying extra effort diminishes with greater sleep deprivation. Interestingly, external stimulation such as loud noise has been shown to impair the performance of non-sleep-deprived subjects but can result in small improvements in the performance of sleep-deprived subjects. The noise is distracting to the non-deprived subjects but arousing to the deprived ones.

Paradoxically, sleep-deprived people are both more easily distracted and more easily irritated by irrelevant stimuli, yet often fail to attend to important, relevant stimuli outside of their immediate focus. For example, according to Anderson and Horne (2006), people were tested on a 30-minute monotonous task. Sometimes there was an appealing video being shown off to the side, and sometimes the participants were also allowed only 5 h of sleep the night before. Task performance was worse after the restricted sleep. There was also an increase in head turns toward the video with the distraction present as well as some increase in lapses.

Even so, there are individual differences in both alertness and performance following sleep loss. For example, extroverts and people who are sensitive to caffeine tend to be more sensitive to sleep loss. A genetic basis for such differences has been demonstrated. Also, while people often believe they adjust to sleep loss, the truth is their performance becomes steadily worse. Older adults are less affected by sleep deprivation than younger adults. Overall, some people are greatly impaired by even moderate sleep loss; others are only impaired when sleep loss becomes severe.

The reason why there are so many mental and behavioral effects of sleep deprivation can be traced to changes in physiology. Most notable are decrements in brain functioning, changes in the functioning of the autonomic nervous system, biochemical changes, increased sensitivity to pain, and even how some genes are expressed. For example, there are global decreases in brain activation proportional to the degree of sleep loss plus even greater changes in specific areas of the brain (see Sect. 12.1.2.2).

Section 12.1.2 further explores the effects of sleep deprivation, especially how it can disrupt people's lives.

It is widely shown that recovery from sleep loss, even for as long as 10 nychthemerons, is quick—occurring within one to three nights of sleep. Thus, an amount of recovery sleep that is equal to the amount of lost sleep is far from necessary. The reason is that recovery sleep is deeper, that is containing more SWA. Furthermore, during sleep deprivation, SWA intrudes into waking hours, which may replace the amount needed during recovery sleep. It is noteworthy that N3 sleep recovers first, typically on the first recovery night, and then REMS on the subsequent night or two.

Box 3.2 Consequences of Sleep Loss in Children (Sadeh 2007)
Although not as well studied as in adults, there are correlative studies and some experimental studies that are consistent with the observations of many

parents, school teachers, and others of the negative consequences of sleep loss in children. Daytime sleepiness, agitation, hyperactivity, and diminished alertness are the most commonly demonstrated problems resulting from insufficient sleep in children. Additionally, cognitive problems, especially those involving executive control, the regulation of attention, working memory, and behavior regulation, especially regulation of attention but also other behavioral problems, are also compromised by sleep debt in children of all ages. Although there is less evidence, emotion regulation and mood regulation can also be compromised in overtired children. Even modest but accumulated loss of sleep, such as resulting from "one more book or TV show," can compromise cognitive skills.

The effects of insufficient sleep on academic achievements have been well researched. For example, one study showed that restricting sleep to 8 h for second graders and 6.5 h for those in higher grades for one week of school resulted in greater academic problems including problems with the quality of work, amount of work completed, rate of learning, recall difficulties, and sloppiness of the work.

Effects of a lack of sufficient sleep in children are often bidirectional, especially for temperament. That is, sleep debt results in agitation and hyperarousal that in turn makes getting to sleep more difficult.

The lack of enough sleep in children can result in both short-term and long-term effects. In the short term, the reinvigorating result of sleep is insufficient. In the long term, insufficient sleep can negatively affect the functioning, maturation, and biological maintenance of the brain.

On a positive note, one study showed that with more sleep, toddlers' behavior greatly improved.

3.1.3 The Effects of Chronic Sleep Restriction

Sleep Debt More common than missing an entire night of sleep is getting some sleep but not enough, night after night. Most sleep experts maintain that sleep deprivation is a chronic and serious problem in the U.S. resulting in what has been called *sleep debt*. They cite data such as that provided by the National Sleep Foundation.

Every year this foundation conducts a national poll on some aspect of sleep. The poll results published in 2011 provided a lot of information about the amount of sleep that people in the United States are not getting (National Sleep Foundation 2011). An astonishing almost two-thirds of respondents aged 13–64 years said they do not get enough sleep on week nights to meet their needs. For the adults, rather than the seven and a half hours that enables them to feel their best, they get a bit less than seven on the average weeknight. The situation is even worse for the teenagers; they report averaging one and three quarters less sleep per night than the recommended nine hours and 15 min. (Sect. 12.1 presents additional information on insufficient sleep).

But things may be even worse than the self-report surveys show. For example, in an extensive series of experiments reported on by Adler (1993), Tom Roth and colleagues at the Henry Ford Hospital in Detroit tested 300 healthy, young adult, normal sleepers. All slept about 7 h per night outside the laboratory, and none said they felt particularly sleepy during the day. However, when tested in the sleep lab, one quarter of them regularly fell asleep within only 6 min. When the others were allowed one hour less of sleep than they normally get for five nights, they too then fell asleep within 6 min. The quarter of the subjects who normally fell asleep within 6 min also did worse on performance tasks, had slower reaction times, and was more affected by alcohol. All subjects did better when they had slept for 10 h per night for 6 days, but the improvement was greater for the people who earlier had fallen asleep more quickly. These same people also got 7 more hours of sleep than the others when asked to sleep as much as they could. It appears that about a quarter of people biologically require more sleep than average and are sleep deprived when they try to get along on an average amount of sleep, although they may not be aware of this fact.

The result is near chronic sleepiness in many of the respondents with differences between generations. The older the generation going from people born just before the turn of the century to those born between 1946 and 1964, the so-called baby boomers, the lesser the percent reporting sleepiness, ranging from 9 to 22 %. The vast majority of those with chronic sleepiness say it affects their mood, responsibilities at home or with family life, and social life. Most adults also reported that their work and sexual relations were negatively affected.

Most sleep experts also cite other sources of data showing that many people need alarm clocks to awaken (see Box 4.2) and do not feel well rested upon awakening. Additionally, some experts believe that people average less sleep than they did at the turn of the twentieth century (e.g., Leproult and Van Cauter 2010). They also point to the fact that given the opportunity, people will and do sleep more, mood is elevated by more sleep, and MSLT scores improve with more sleep. Finally, these experts point out, as reviewed in this chapter, that not sleeping enough results in chronic symptoms of sleep deprivation with potentially serious consequences.

The effects of multiple nights of partial sleep deprivation accumulate. Most people can function well the next day after a couple of nights of missing an hour or two of sleep, but the effects are increasingly noticeable for most people when the amount of sleep per nychthemeron drops below 6 h night after night. Yet as time goes on, chronically sleep-deprived people become less aware of just how sleepy they are. At this point, people would say that they have "adapted" to getting less sleep (see Sect. 3.1.3 and Box 10.3 for experimental results on this; also Sect. 12.1.2.4). Yet, measurements of physiological and manifest sleepiness show that they are affected in many ways by this accumulating loss of sleep. As the sleep debt accumulates, alertness diminishes, resulting in increased risk of errors at work, injuries, motor vehicle accidents, conflicts with others, and health problems.

In some ways, the effects of partial sleep deprivation are similar to those of total sleep deprivation. Sleep onset generally becomes quicker, and sleep is more efficient, which is beneficial. Yet, there are many deficits. The most noticeable effect is a decline in mood, but there is also a noticeable decline in mental skills similar to those found with total sleep deprivation.

In other ways, partial sleep deprivation is somewhat akin to selective REMS deprivation, because it is the end of the night that is typically cut off. The exception may be if you go to bed very late on a couple of short nights, then you might have a lot of REM sleep due to its rising circadian phase late in the morning. With successive nights of partial sleep, *REM pressure* (the number of times REMS is begun during a period of sleep) accumulates resulting in a tendency for more REMS to occur early in the night. Nevertheless, the total amount of REMS is still diminished. N3 sleep is not totally spared either for there are elevations in SWA indicative of a greater pressure to achieve N3.

Figure 3.5 shows the effect on physiological sleepiness of obtaining partial sleep. People slept in the lab for two successive nights. Some were allowed to sleep for 9 h, others 7, 5, 4, or 0 h. The data shown are from MSLTs done after the second night. Physiological sleepiness increases as the length of sleep decreases. However, this trend is not linear; for example, there is little difference between the 7- and 5-h groups but a big jump in sleepiness in the 4-h group. Also, apparent is the mid-afternoon dip in sleepiness (see Sect. 3.2.2) in all but the 0-h group which bottomed out across all time trials—something called a basement effect. That is, the 0 h may have been even more tired than the test is capable of showing. Finally, the 5- and 4-h groups were sleepier in the morning than they were at almost all

Fig. 3.5 MSLTs from after second night of 9, 7, 5, 4, or 0 h of sleep per night (Reprinted from Kryger et al. 1989, with permission from Elsevier Science)

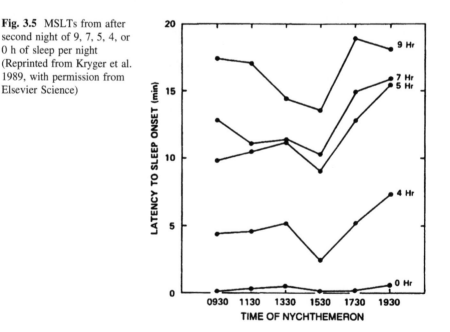

other times except during the mid-afternoon dip. This result was not seen in the 9- and 7-h groups. Similar effects were shown in a related experiment in which young adults were allowed only 5 h sleep for 7 consecutive nychthemerons (Dement and Carskadon 1981).

Sleep debt also has cognitive and physiological consequences. For most people, habitually sleeping less than seven hours per nychthemeron results in cognitive deficits that become increasingly worse over time. The greater the nightly deficit, the more rapid the rate of the cognitive decline. The deficits can accumulate to the point that they are equivalent to total sleep deprivation of 1–2 nychthemerons.

Two large experiments done in 2003 (Belenky et al. 2003; Van Dongen et al. 2003) show the cumulative effects of less than an adequate amount of sleep on cognitive performance. One study used truck drivers and the other young adults. In both studies, subjects were restricted to less than optimal sleep for several consecutive nights and compared to subjects allowed an optimal amount of sleep. Those subjects in both experiments whose nightly sleep was shortened showed decreases in standard cognitive performance measures in spite of the fact that they were not aware this was happening. The performance problems became increasingly worse as the restricted sleep progressed, through 14 consecutive nychthemerons in one of the experiments. Fourteen days of only 4 h of sleep per night caused performance deficits comparable to people who have gone without sleep for 1–2 nychthemerons. Interestingly, careful analysis of the data showed that it was not only the accumulated sleep loss that resulted in the deficits but also the accumulation of homeostatic sleep drive (see Sect. 3.1) that extended wakefulness places on the brain. The second study also showed that these deficits did not fully recover for several days even when adequate sleep was subsequently obtained. The conclusion drawn from these two studies and others like them is that for most people, less than 7 h of sleep per nychthemeron in healthy adults 21–64 years old results in an accumulation of deficits in a number of cognitive performance areas. Furthermore, this occurs without awareness and thus leads to the widely, but wrongly held assumption that chronic sleep restriction has little effect on behavior.

A very different type of experiment involved studying cumulative, partial sleep deprivation in military personnel. Least affected were tasks requiring manual effort. However, the personnel experienced considerable problems with tasks requiring mental effort—up to a 50 % increase in errors following four days of sleep deprivation. A specific example comes from the study (Pleban et al. 1990) of U.S. Army Rangers in training who averaged 3.2 h of sleep per nychthemeron for 8 weeks. After a few weeks, their instructors said it was not unusual to observe what they called "droning"—unresponsiveness and the inability to process information while performing a task. Similar behavior is more commonly called "automatic behavior" when it has been observed in night shift workers such as nurses.

Nevertheless, there are great individual differences in tolerance to restricted sleep, just as there are to continuous sleep deprivation. Some people are much more able to tolerate lack of sleep than others. This appears to be a stable trait possibly because brains of such people have more flexibility in being able to compensate by using additional areas to accomplish tasks. On the other hand, some people show greater deficits more quickly than the average.

Many people desire to learn how to sleep less. Some claim they have been successful by shortening their nights of sleep. In one classic experiment (Mullaney et al. 1977 and Freidmann et al. 1977), eight 7–8 h sleepers were asked to decrease their sleep by ½ or 1 h every few weeks. After a several weeks, they were asked to maintain their sleep at this new level before returning to whatever amount of sleep they desired. Each time the subjects made a reduction, they reported feeling sleepy but said this feeling passed after a few days. However, by the time they had reduced their sleep by 1½–2 h to about 3 NREM/REMS cycles, they voiced complaints about having trouble waking up in the morning and were unable to reduce their sleep time any further. Their sleep onset times decreased, and their sleep efficiency increased. Their N3 actually increased, while N2 and REMS decreased. Tests of performance revealed no deficits. Several weeks after the experiment ended, some of the subjects were again studied, revealing they were still getting about 1 h less sleep than before they started the experiment.

More recently 42 older people, 50–70 years old, who typically slept around 8½ h per nychthemeron had their sleep reduced by 90 min per nychthemeron for 8 weeks (Youngstedt et al. 2009). There were no observed changes in mood, lasting sleepiness, "health-related quality of life," or performance. There was some reduction in time to get to sleep and sleep efficiency. When assessed a year later, they still averaged one hour less sleep per nychthemeron than before the experiment started.

Nevertheless, careful psychometric and psychomotor testing following multiple nights of partial sleep restriction strongly counters the conclusion that people can successfully reduce the amount of sleep that they require each night.

Also, there are physiological effects of insufficient sleep. Until recently, only relatively minor effects of sleep deprivation on the body have been reported. For a long time, research showed that mild sleep deprivation has a small but measurable negative effect on the immune system (see Box 6.3). Going without sleep for over a week also results in effects such as mild vibration of the eyeballs from side to side, hand trembling, some slurring of speech, drooping eyelids, greater gagging, and increased sensitivity to pain, all of which quickly reverse with sleep. More recently, careful studies by Eve Van Cauter and colleagues of the Department of Medicine at the University of Chicago (Leproult and Van Cauter 2010) have shown more serious and potentially permanent effects of chronic sleep reduction in hormone levels (see Sect. 6.1.7 and Box 6.3). Others have confirmed that deficits occur in immune functions.

Box 3.3 An Opposing View: Most People Are Not Chronically Sleep Deprived

Psychologist and prominent sleep researcher Jim Horne of Loughborough University in England has argued against the notion of widespread chronic sleep debt (e.g., Horne 2011 and Harrison and Horne 1995). He questions the data presented above, saying it is either flawed or can be explained in other ways. For example, at the turn of the century prior to the widespread use of electric lights people reported sleeping for 9 h compared to 7½ h today. The evidence for this statement is based on one survey report from 1910 to 1911, but ignores a number of other surveys from that era that do not show such a high average amount of sleep. In addition, it is not clear that similar groups of people are being compared. Along another line, Horne points out that although people, given the opportunity to sleep more, can and will do so does not necessarily mean that they need this extra sleep. People given the opportunity to eat more food will often do so but not necessarily because they are starving. He calls such extra sleep "optional sleep" that is beyond physiological need that he calls "core" but others call "basal" sleep (see Box 10.4 for more on this theory). Horne maintains that while *core sleep* is necessary and highly beneficial, optional sleep historically only serves to keep the person asleep because of factors such as darkness, safety needs, and "socioeconomic pressures." Otherwise, the benefits of optional sleep beyond the core requirement are minimal, such as a slight improvement in MSLT and performance scores, particularly considering the costs of less wake time, longer time to sleep onset, and an increase in waking during sleep. Further, a short 20-min or so mid-day nap will give the same benefits as much longer extended nighttime sleep (see Sect. 4.9). Likewise, although he does concede that the afternoon dip (described in Sect. 3.2.2) could be attenuated with more sleep, the same effect could also be achieved by a short nap. In sum, people who are regularly getting their core sleep but less than what is commonly cited as the average amount of sleep need "are not necessarily affected by 'sleep debt' as there may be little or nothing to repay." Most people are stimulated enough to not feel sleepy in their typical daily lives, in contrast to an artificial, bland laboratory environment in which most "sleep debt" is demonstrated.

Horne (1988) also cites several experiments showing that people can learn to sleep less, including those reported in this chapter. Horne interprets these results differently, though, saying that they show people can successfully reduce sleep by eliminating their optional sleep. However, others in the sleep field have noted that it took several weeks of following rigid schedules of sleep without napping—although some subjects admitted that they did nap at times—or sleeping in on weekends. Often they had to endure bouts of discomfort from sleepiness and difficulty getting out of bed in the morning (see Box 3.3). Also, there was a lot of encouragement and attention from the experimenters for the subjects to continue. They conclude that it is doubtful that persons not involved in a formal experiment could achieve the same results, especially if they could not discipline themselves to rigidly adhere to the schedule. Other studies point to the effects of sleepiness on the body (see Table 3.1 and Box 6.3) and the increased likelihood of having a serious accident (see Box 3.1) when sleep deprived. Finally, in one experiment of this type, the subjects reported that their extra time awake was wasted doing nothing important. In the end, they actually felt they had gained little.

Given the difficulty and the risks of sleep deprivation as presented in this chapter and the limited benefits of a bit more time awake, I do not advise trying to shorten your sleep to any great extent, if at all. "But wait a minute," you might be asking at this point. "How do I know if I am getting too little or too much sleep?" We will explore the answer to this question in Box 4.1.

3.1.4 The Effects of Deprivation of Different Stages of Sleep

Research has been done on depriving people of the different stages of sleep.

3.1.4.1 REMS Deprivation

Following the discovery of REMS, there was considerable interest in determining the effects of depriving people of it. The theoretical basis for this interest was the association of REMS with dreaming and the prevailing notion, from psychoanalytic theory, that dreaming was a safety valve necessary to keep us from going crazy. Researchers saw REMS deprivation as a chance to test this theory. As sometimes happens in science, the theory was wrong, but the data generated were useful in other ways.

Interestingly, some of the earliest research was on sleep deprivation, considered dream deprivation at the time, that seemed to support the psychoanalytic theory. A commonly cited example is the experience of disc jockey Peter Tripp who went without sleep for over 8 days as a fund-raising effort (see Box 3.4). Subsequently, the research went into the sleep lab where subjects could be selectively deprived of REMS by awakening them every time the polysomnogram showed them entering this stage. This procedure is difficult because of the accelerating increase in REM pressure. For example, a typical study might show 17 awakenings from REMS were required on the first night, 42 on the fourth, and 68 on the seventh. Another indicator of increased REM pressure occurs during recovery sleep following REMS deprivation when there is a dramatic increase in REMS over baseline. However, only about 40 % of the lost REMS is recovered.

Box 3.4 Classic Sleep Deprivation Reports
Sometimes research gets poorly reported and then repeated so often that it becomes a kind of legend. The sleep deprivation "experiments" done by Peter Tripp and Randy Gardner (Coren 1998) are examples of these kinds of

studies, the first of which is used as evidence of the grave psychological problems that result from sleep deprivation and the second as evidence that is exactly the opposite.

Peter was a New York disk jockey in the late 1950s who went without sleep for 200 h as a fund-raising effort while psychologists and physicians monitored him. The reports emphasized the mental deterioration he experienced, including irrationality, hallucinations, and outright paranoia, yet ignoring the fact that he did his radio show every night so well that listeners could not tell any difference. And, following the 13 h of sleep that terminated the marathon, he awoke without any of these symptoms. Reports of Peter's experience with sleep deprivation tend to conclude that people will "go crazy" while they go without sleep.

Several things are often ignored in the descriptions of Peter Tripp's heroic sleep deprivation. First, he had a history of prior psychological problems. The stress of the sleep deprivation caused them to reemerge. Second, during the deprivation, he was taking large amounts of an amphetamine-like stimulant that is known to cause changes in personality.

Randy was a high school student in the early 1960s who decided, as a science fair project, to set the Guinness World Record for going without sleep. After he was underway, the local press did a story that caused a team of physicians and sleep researchers to get involved, observing and testing Randy. Most reports of his efforts to stay awake successfully for 264 continuous hours, that is, 11 days, offer glowing accounts of how easy and relatively uneventful it was for Randy to accomplish this task. Casual observations by a researcher who spent much of day 10 with Randy doing normal things led to the conclusion that Randy did not hallucinate, have other sensory problems, or experience any negative mood changes. Among other things, near the end of his sleep deprivation, Randy beat one of the researchers at a game of pinball. In contrast, the actual scientific reports of the experiment lead to quite different conclusions. Careful psychological and neurological testing showed that Randy was greatly affected while sleep deprived. A partial list includes trouble focusing, poor coordination, moodiness, problems concentrating, hallucinations, muscular weakness, difficulty speaking, and occasional paranoia. He recovered completely following one night of extended sleep.

The truth is somewhere between the contradictory way these two famous attempts at sleep deprivation are usually reported. There have been other sleep deprivation experiments that were more scientifically done. They show that continuous long duration sleep deprivation is not easy or comfortable and does result in temporary psychological (illusions, decreased vigilance, increased daydreaming) and neurological effects (microsleeps, slower reaction time). In contrast, the physiological consequences are minor. Yet, all the problems go away quickly, leaving no apparent permanent damage as soon as ample sleep, about ¼ of the sleep lost, is obtained.

Apparently, we need REMS but not for the psychoanalytic reasons proposed. Although some bizarre thinking and behavior happen in REMS-deprived people, these symptoms resolve quickly with the resumption of REMS. Today, it is agreed that REMS deprivation may result in any one of a number of temporary symptoms, including changes in emotions, increased liveliness, greater appetite, more interest in sex, and memory impairment. One curious finding is that REMS deprivation can temporarily lessen the degree of depression in some depressed individuals, which is consistent with the fact that many antidepressant drugs reduce REMS.

3.1.4.2 N3 Deprivation

Although there was greater initial interest and research activity directed toward the deprivation of REMS, there has also been some research done on the effects of N3 sleep deprivation. It is a bit harder to do, however, because if you awaken the subjects every time they initiate N3, the amounts of other sleep, especially REMS, are also greatly disrupted since NREMS normally is the doorway to REMS. Before reading on, what do you think is the solution to experimentally depriving subjects of N3 while minimizing REMS disruption?

Instead of awakening a sleeping person, a tone is sounded just loud enough to drive them out of N3 but not loud enough to awaken them. With this procedure, considerable REMS is still obtained, as are N1 and N2. Overall, it is more difficult to eliminate N3 than to eliminate REMS, taking about 6 times as many sleep interruptions. The result is an increase in *N3 pressure*—increasing attempts to begin it, a temporary increase in the density of delta waves, and some increase in N3 time on the first night when unimpeded sleep is again allowed to occur. Interestingly, there typically is also an increase in REMS on recovery nights 2 and 3. N3-deprived people do not report experiencing any behavioral deficits but complain about being lethargic and having muscle aches. They do tend to be more subdued and withdrawn.

3.1.4.3 Deprivation of N1 and N2

It would be informative to do studies of deprivation of N1 and N2 and determining the effects, but so far nobody has determined just how to do this without awakening the sleeper and disrupting other stages of sleep. Meanwhile, we will keep watching the research literature in the hopes that someday, someone can get the job done.

3.1.5 Recovery from Lost Sleep

Only sleep can reverse the effects of lost sleep. Caffeine, exercise, stimulation, and the like can ameliorate the effects a bit for a period of time but not reverse the loss. However, makeup sleep does not have to equal hour for hour the time lost, since recovery sleep is of greater intensity and efficiency. Recovery sleep is more intense sleep in the sense that it is harder to awaken the sleeper. Additionally, N3 intensity is shown by the percent and amplitude of the delta waves. Total recovery sleep time is somewhat longer if a person can sleep as long as desired.

Recovery from sleep deprivation is relatively quick and complete. It typically takes 1 to possibly 3 nights—shorter if the recovery nights are extended, longer if the degree of prior sleep deprivation is greater. However, as the proportion of sleep loss goes up, the proportion of it that has to be recovered goes down. The early recovery sleep preferentially emphasizes N3, so much so that REMS may be less than normal while N3 recovers. Rate of recovery of N3 has been described as "a saturating exponential curve"; that is, there is proportionally more recovery in the first few hours of N3 than the last few hours. It is only later in the night or even during the next night or two that REMS recovers. Its recovery seems to depend on increasing the amount of time in this stage more than increasing its intensity.

3.1.6 Extended Sleep

Extended sleep can contribute to recovery from sleep deprivation, but sometimes people extend their sleep even when not deprived. What are the effects of extending sleep when not sleep deprived? First, the extra sleep itself has a low efficiency and contains little, if any, N3 unless sleep is extended beyond 12 h, at which point, some N3 begins to reoccur. Instead of extra sleep making people super-alert and able to function at above normal levels, the opposite appears to be true. Too much sleep on one night has been described as making people under responsive, lethargic, and "thick headed." Additionally, such extended sleep results in emotional letdown and irritability plus deficits of performance. These effects may be an exaggeration of what is called *sleep inertia* (see Sect. 4.10).

In addition to the information in this chapter, more information on sleeping too little or too much is presented in Sect. 4.1.

3.2 Sleep as Rhythmic

Circadian Rhythm Most animals seem to have fairly regular sleeping schedules during the nychthemeron. We humans tend to be most sleepy at night and, more often than not, sleep then. This pattern is an important example of the *circadian rhythms* of the body, near 24-h cycles of behavior and physiology. Circadian rhythms influence sleep as well as our sensory processing, short-term memory, cognitive performance, alertness, and many other behaviors. Likewise, our body temperature, which is important for sleep, hormones, urine production, and other biological processes also follow a circadian schedule. Our internal biological clock(s) enable us to be in synchrony with the 24-h external world, just as the

Fig. 3.6 Important terms for describing circadian rhythms. Also, phase = position of the curve—often determined by its peaks—relative to some other curve or to time

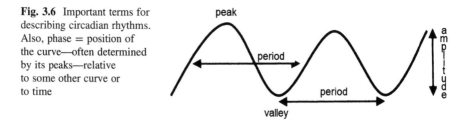

clocks on our walls and wrists enable us to synchronize our schedules with those of many individuals for collective work and social activities. In fact, our circadian rhythms enable us to have an internal biological (subjective) day and night that usually enables us to mirror and prepare for the forthcoming change between external (objective) day and night.

Before we go any further, it is important to become familiar with the terms shown in Fig. 3.6. They are useful for describing circadian rhythms.

3.2.1 Methods for Studying Circadian Rhythms

The circadian rhythms for sleep and wake are studied in a variety of ways including entrained 24-h, free-run, forced desynchrony, and constant routine experiments.

Entrained In the *entrained 24-hour protocol*, subjects live in a laboratory for a period of time. They are aware of the time of day but are on a rigid schedule of bedtime, wakeup time, meal time, and timed activities. Biological and/or behavioral measurements may be regularly taken to assess their 24-h rhythms under "normal" conditions.

For many other experiments, there needs to be a situation in which the subject can be isolated from environmental time cues. The original experiments of this type were done in caves, but, subsequently, special sleep labs with no windows, clocks, radios, phones, or any other direct links with the outside world that could give an indication, however, subtle, of the time have been used. Inside these labs, one of three types of experiments can be undertaken: free-run, forced desynchrony, or constant routine.

Free-run *Free-run* experiments were the earliest conducted. The subjects are free to sleep whenever they feel like it. They have control over the lighting, when they eat meals, and engage in leisure activities. Their sleep and wake patterns are recorded. These studies typically go on for weeks, and without any time clues, the subjects rely on their own internal circadian clocks. Free-running subjects eventually have an average circadian period of slightly *longer* than 24 h.

Forced Desynchrony In contrast, *forced desynchrony* requires subjects to be on a sleep/wake cycle that is outside the bounds of what most people are capable of achieving. For one-third of every cycle, they are required to be in bed in the dark followed by 2/3 of the cycle out of bed in light. Typical cycles that are used are short, such as 20 or 90 min, or long, such as 28 h. For example, on the 20-min cycle, the subject has to be in bed trying to sleep for 7 min. Then, they must get out of bed and be awake for 13 min before returning to bed. This might go on for anywhere from 24 to 48 h for the shorter cycles to days or weeks for the longer cycles. The amount of sleep obtained during each in-bed portion is measured. A forced desynchrony protocol causes the sleep/wake cycle to become desynchronized, that is, separated from the circadian temperature cycle, meaning that subjects will be sleeping and awake at different phases of their temperature cycle over the duration of the experiment.

Constant Routine In the *constant routine*, the subject remains in a quiet environment in a semi-recumbent position, but continuously awake with the illumination low and constant. Small meals are eaten every hour. Constant routine studies are typically done for more than 24 h but less than 48. During this protocol, changes in physiological indicators, such as melatonin and body temperature, and performance on psychometric tests, can be measured hourly to assess their circadian rhythms.

3.2.2 Results from Studying Circadian Rhythms

There are a number of major findings from these protocols about our circadian sleep rhythm. The sleep/wake cycle is dependent on the circadian clock, not vice versa. Left to its own devices, our internal sleep/wake cycle for 75–80 % of people would be close to but greater than 24 h. The best information comes from constant routine studies that show the clock averaging 24.2 h with a range from 23.9 to 24.5 h.

Entrainment Most of us live successfully in a 24-h world because our internal rhythms are regularly reset, *entrained*, primarily by stimuli from outside the body acting as *zeitgebers,* German for "time giver". Entrainment is like if you, the zeitgeber, were to daily reset your watch that runs a bit slow. The major zeitgeber for our sleep and wake cycle is the nychthemeral alternation of light and dark that occurs on the planet we inhabit. Things like exercise, social stimulation, mealtimes, room temperature, and knowledge of what time it is also help but are largely thought to play a minor role compared to that of light. Yet, the effect of the various zeitgebers may be additive. The right amount of properly timed light can either *phase advance* (move to an earlier setting) or *phase delay* (move to a later setting) our circadian rhythm for sleep to any new setting in usually two to three nychthemerons. The brighter the light, the greater the entrainment effect. However, even room light, that is, generally about 20 times dimmer than outside light on a somewhat cloudy day, can also have some entrainment influence. Our circadian rhythm for sleep can be easily entrained to shorter, up to 22 h, or longer, up to 26 h periods—even longer or shorter if approached gradually.

Pause for a moment and try to predict what would happen to your sleep in the absence of any strong zeitgebers.

PAUSE

Answer: Your sleep/wake rhythm would become "desynchronized" from the 24-h world. You would alternate something like every few weeks between wanting to sleep during the night with wanting to sleep during the day. If you were to try to sleep always at night, you would have a couple of weeks of good sleep followed by a week of fair sleep, then a couple weeks of poor sleep, then a week of fair sleep, and so on. This pattern is in fact what happens to up to ¾ of totally blind people. For the other one-fourth, either other zeitgebers are strong enough to entrain their circadian rhythm or they have a type of blindness that allows some light information to get through to the brain even though they have no awareness of light sensation.

A *phase response curve* (PRC) shows the times when we are sensitive to a zeitgeber that is able to entrain the circadian clock as well as the direction and intensity of the change. Figure 3.7 shows a PRC for light in humans. It is called phase response because how our clock responds to light depends on what part, or phase, of the 24-h cycle it is in. Exposure to light for a few hours before and after our regular time of falling asleep will delay the clock, but exposure a few hours before and after our regular arising time will advance the clock. PRCs are related to our body time, not the real time, but since most people sleep when it is dark out, it has become common to describe the phases of the PRC in terms of subjective night, subjective dawn, subjective day, and subjective dusk. Some, but not all, researchers also see a "Dead Zone" during much of the subjective day where the light has no effect.

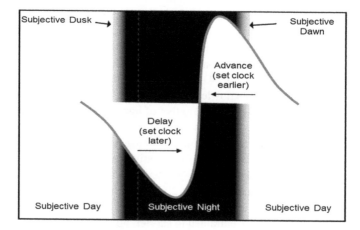

Fig. 3.7 The phase response curve, PRC, to light for resetting the phase of the circadian clock in humans. (Redrawn from Eastman and Burgess 2009)

Take a careful look at the PRC for light in Fig. 3.7. Notice that at subjective dawn, we are nudged a bit toward phase advance, and at subjective dusk, we are nudged a bit toward phase delay. Each of these effects is stronger in subjective day after subjective dawn and in subjective night before subjective dusk. In the midst of subjective night, there is a sharp "crossover point" where the effect quickly reverses. This crossover point is close to the core body temperature valley. Typically, since our circadian clock tends to run slow, that is, longer than 24 h, we need to be advanced a bit every nychthemeron to keep in phase with our external, objective world. This occurs when we open our eyes, turn on lights, and open blinds after awakening in the morning.

The circadian rhythm for sleep actually has two peaks and two valleys every cycle in most but not all people. This pattern is shown in Fig. 3.8, a composite summary of several kinds of research, especially experimental 20-min nychthemerons, MSLT studies, and some free-running conditions. It also reinforces the subjective reports of many people. Notice that about 12 h after maximal sleep propensity at night, there is a less intense increase in sleep propensity that is called the "mid-afternoon dip" because of a dip in alertness that many people have experienced in the middle of the afternoon. It is also called the "post lunch dip," which is a misnomer since it has nothing to do with consuming that meal. It is much easier to fall asleep and stay asleep during the times when sleep propensity is high but more difficult when sleep propensity is low. Notice that there is a sharp transition in just a couple of hours between our time of maximal alertness early in the evening and our time of maximal sleepiness during the night.

Your circadian rhythm, in addition to influencing when you sleep, also affects aspects of sleep according to Djik and Czeisler (1994). Generally speaking, REMS is strongly influenced, but NREMS is not. REMS latency, duration, and propensity are all at their peak in the early morning hours when circadian arousal is at its lowest. Additionally, there is a weak effect of sleep length on REMS propensity and there is a homeostatic influence on REMS propensity as shown by an increase in REM pressure if REMS is deprived. Things are much the opposite for N3, however. N3 propensity and strength are strongly affected by the amount of preceding wakefulness but only weakly, if at all, influenced by circadian phase. Additionally, the occurrence of sleep spindles is governed by weak circadian

Fig. 3.8 Typical sleepiness during a nychthemeron. (From Moorcroft 1993 with permission of the publisher)

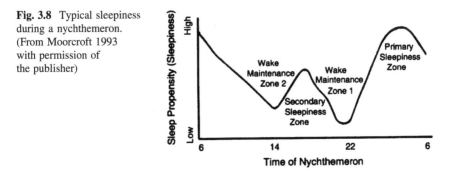

influence that is high when circadian arousal drive is lowest, and strongly inhibited by sleep drive. Since spindles function to help prevent sounds and lights from awakening us (see Sect. 5.3.5), they are an important factor that helps us to sleep in one long, consolidated period.

Circadian rhythms are not the only kind of rhythm involved with sleep and wake. The rhythmic cycling that occurs between NREMS and REMS about every 90 min is called an *ultradian*, meaning less than a day, rhythm.

3.3 Interaction of Homeostatic and Circadian Effects: The Two-process Model

By now you may be asking how the homeostatic drive to sleep and the circadian control of wakefulness both influence our sleep at the same time. One answer comes in the form of a model. Models are used in science to summarize and integrate a great deal of data in an attempt to show the way things are and how they work. The best models are based on a higher ratio of facts to assumptions. Good models are then used to formulate new research to attempt to verify some of the predictions of the model. Subsequently, models tend to be modified to encompass new data or abandoned if the new data simply do not fit.

Two-process Model Alex Borbély of Switzerland, a prominent sleep researcher, formulated what is currently the most widely accepted model of sleep called the "two-process model" of sleep/wake propensity (see Fig. 3.9). One process in this model is homeostatic which was presented earlier as sleep drive, but Borbély calls *process S*. The other process is circadian, called *process C*. You can think of the level of process S as the intensity of homeostatic sleep drive. Process S builds up while awake but declines more rapidly during N3. Naps also produce a reduction in process S, while sleep loss causes an increase in process S. In sum, the

Fig. 3.9 The "two-process model" of sleep/wake propensity

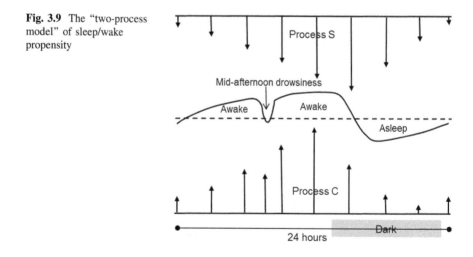

level of process S is directly related to amount of recent wakefulness and inversely proportional to amount of recent sleep.

Process C is a circadian process that is in phase to the core body temperature rhythm (see Sect. 5.3.7.1), but its exact shape and phase were derived empirically from sleep propensities at different circadian phases. Process C as represented in Borbély's model is intensity of alertness or arousal.

Think of each process in this model as a different kind of timer. Process S is like an hourglass indicating degree of sleepiness with a 30- to 50-h capacity. When awake, sand flows from one end to the other; sleep is like inverting the hourglass, so that sand flows the other way but somehow twice as fast. Process C is like a 24-h wall clock that displays the current level of circadian strength of alertness instead of what time it is. The degree of sleep propensity and sleep duration at any time result from the interaction of both timers.

The two-process model has gained considerable empirical support. It is consistent with the characteristics of recovery from sleep deprivation, how sleep duration changes in concert with the phase of the circadian rhythm, sleep during shift work, and more. For example, it is consistent with the analysis of data from a forced desynchrony experiment of Charles Czeisler, a MD/PhD sleep researcher at Harvard Medical School and Derk-Jan Dijk, a Dutch psychologist who has been a part of the research endeavors in several laboratories in Europe and the US including Borbély's lab in Zurich and Czeisler's lab at Harvard (Dijk and Czeisler 1994). They had eight young males maintain a 28-h forced desynchrony protocol with encouragement to sleep during the one-third of the cycle, or 9.33 h, that was dark. Each subject's circadian sleep/wake cycle soon became desynchronized, running at 24.18 h, from this 28 h dark/light schedule. As a result, every sleep period began almost 4 h later in their circadian cycle, while prior wakefulness length was nearly constant at almost 19 h. This allowed Dijk and Czeisler to separate the circadian influence from the homeostatic influence, so that the contribution of each to sleeping and waking could be assessed. Just as the two-process model predicted, sleep propensity was maximal when circadian alertness was at its minimum and gradually decreased as circadian alertness increased. Sleep propensity was also shown to be directly proportional to the length of the preceding period of wakefulness and diminished in proportion to the length of subsequent sleep.

If you look only at process C in the two-process model, it seems paradoxical that its arousal influence is greatest just prior to the normal sleep period and lowest prior to awakening. Likewise, if you look only at process S, it seems paradoxical that we continue to sleep near the end of the sleep period when homeostatic sleepiness is very low. But when considered together, it can be seen that the circadian and homeostatic factors oppose each other for long periods of time (see Fig. 3.9). Several hours of sleep happen when you fall asleep at the normal time, because the strength of process S is great but, as this diminishes during sleep, the process C also gets weaker. The net result is that you stay asleep until morning when process S is weak and process C begins to increase. Likewise, when you are awake, the process S builds up, but process C alertness also gets stronger, opposing process S until process C starts to weaken again about the time sleep onset typically starts. This allows one long period of sleep to be followed by one long period of wake during each circadian cycle. Without the circadian influence, total sleep amount would not change during the nychthemeron, but it would be taken in multiple naps rather than all together at night.

The effects of the two-process model on sleep may not always be obvious—both in everyday life and in the research laboratory—because of what may be considered a third and very different factor. Our immediate situation including our surroundings and what is happening in our bodies and our minds can influence the outcome of the two-process components, sometimes facilitating sleep and sometimes hindering it. A comfortable bed and bedroom, for example, while not putting us to sleep may make sleeping easier to obtain at the times that the two-process model shows a readiness to sleep. So, it is not that boring middle of the afternoon class in a warm room with dimmed lights that causes you to frequently fall asleep. Rather that situation helps the sleep-deprived student brain to fall asleep. In contrast, things like high bodily activity, bright lights, loud noise, and even body postures can mask sleepiness even when the components of the two-process model promote it.

(The interactive website http://healthysleep.med.harvard.edu/interactive/circadian shows the two-process model and how the factors interact with one another to produce normal sleep. It then allows you to select situations to see how they affect the normal pattern.)

3.4 Conclusion

Sleep is not as simple a process as it seems. The length of sleep and when it occurs depends on an interaction between two factors: (1) homeostatic sleep drive whose level at any given time is dependent on the amount of recent sleep and recent wake, and (2) the circadian clock that tends to vary the level of arousal over a 24-h period of time. The result is a long period of sleep during the night of about 8 h followed by a long period of wakefulness of about 16 h, but sometimes with a small nap in the middle.

Horne (2006) explains how sleep drive and the circadian clock interact. Wakefulness is like filling a bathtub with water with a somewhat constant flow. The rise of water in the tub represents the duration of wakefulness and an increase in sleepiness. Going to sleep is like opening the drain. At first, the water rushes out representing intense, deep N3. But as the water drains out, the flow reduces and eventually becomes just a trickle and we awaken. If we had been awake longer, such as for 24 h, the water in the tub would be higher, and at first, the rush of water would be stronger, representing deeper sleep, and it would take longer for the tub to fully drain, representing longer sleep. I would add that the influence of the circadian clock would be as if it were harder to open the drain during the day but easier at night.

I add another aspect to this metaphor. If the drain was closed before the tub fully emptied, there would be water left in it. This is the case with insufficient sleep time resulting in residual sleep drive. Now, if this was repeated every time the tub was drained, then the water level would get even higher just as repeated nights of insufficient sleep result in ever greater sleep drive. Eventually, the tub would overflow causing water damage, just as the ever-increasing sleep drive causes various behavioral and physiological decrements.

Superimposed on this is the approximately 90 min ultradian cycle of NREMS and REMS during sleep. In Chap. 4, you will see even more complexity as normal variations on this pattern are presented.

References

Adler, T. (1993). Speed of sleep's arrival signals sleep deprivation. *American Psychological Association Monitor, 24*, 20.

Anderson, C., & Horne, J. A. (2006). Sleepiness enhances distraction during a monotonous task. *Sleep, 29*, 573–576.

Cartwright, R. C. (2010). *The twenty-four hour mind*. New York: Oxford University Press.

Center for Disease Control and Prevention. (2011). Unhealthy sleep-related behaviors—12 States, 2009. Weekly Report, pp. 233–238.

Coren, S. (1998). Sleep deprivation, psychosis and mental efficiency. *Psychiatric Times, 15*, 1–3. Retrieved from http://www.psychiatrictimes.com/display/article/10168/54471?pageNumber=1.

Dement, W. C., & Carskadon, M. A. (1981). Cumulative effects of sleep restriction on daytime sleepiness. *Psychophysiology, 18*, 107–113.

Dijk, D. J., & Czeisler, C. A. (1994). Paradoxical timing of the circadian rhythm of sleep propensity serves to consolidate sleep and wakefulness in humans. *Neuroscience Letters, 166*, 63–68.

Eastman, C. I., & Burgess, H. J. (2009). How to travel the world without jet lag. *Sleep Medicine Clinics, 4*, 241–255.

Harrison, Y., & Horne, J. A. (1995). Should we be taking more sleep? *Sleep, 18*, 901–907.

Haslam, D. R. (1983). The incentive effect and sleep deprivation. *Sleep, 6*, 362–368.

Hensley, S. (2011). Wake up to your sleep deficit, America! Retrieved from http://m.npr.org/story/134257508.

Horne, J. (2006). *Sleepfaring*. New York: Oxford University Press.

Horne, J. (2010). Sleepiness as a need for sleep: When is enough, enough? *Neuroscience and Biobehavioral Reviews, 34*, 108–118.

Horne, J. (2011). The end of sleep: 'Sleep debt' versus biological adaptation of human sleep to waking needs. *Biological Psychology, 87*, 1–14.

Horne, J. A. (1988). *Why we sleep*. New York: Oxford University Press.

Horne, J. A., & Pettit, A. N. (1985). High incentive effects on vigilance performance during 72 hours of total sleep deprivation. *Acta Psychologica, 58*, 123–139.

Kryger, M. H., Roth, T. R., & Dement, W. C. (Eds.). (2011). *Principles and practice of sleep medicine* (5th ed.). St. Louis: Elsevier.

Kryger, M. H., Roth, T., & Dement, W. C. (1989). *Principles and practice of sleep medicine*. Philadelphia: Elsevier.

Lee-Chiong, T. (2009). Polysomnography. In T. Lee-Chiong (Ed.), *Somnology* (pp. 72–80). Seattle: Amazon.

Leproult, R., & Van Cauter, E. (2010). Role of sleep and sleep loss in hormonal release and metabolism. *Endocrinology Developments, 17*, 11–21.

Moorcroft, W. H. (1993). *Sleep, dreaming, and sleep disorders: An introduction* (2nd ed.). Lanham: University Press of America.

Mullaney, D. J., Johnson, L. C., Naitoh, P., Friedmann, J. K., & Globus, G. G. (1977). Sleep during and after gradual sleep reduction. *Psychophysiology, 14*, 237–244.

National Sleep Foundation. (2011). Annual sleep in America poll exploring connections with communications technology use and sleep. Retrieved from http://www.sleepfoundation.org/article/press-release/annual-sleep-america-poll-exploring-connections-communications-technology-use.

National Sleep Foundation web-site: http://www.sleepfoundation.org/.

Pilcher, J. J., & Huffcutt, A. L. (1996). Effects of sleep deprivation on performance: A meta-analysis. *Sleep, 19*, 318–326.

Pleban, R. J., Valentine, P. J., Penetar, D. M., Redmond, D. P., & Belenky, G. (1990). Characterization of sleep and body composition changes during ranger training. *Military Psychology, 2*, 145–156.

Sadeh, A. (2007). Consequences of sleep loss or sleep disruption in children. *Sleep Medicine Clinics, 2*, 513–520.

Van Dongen, H. P., Maislin, G., Mullington, J. M., & Dinges, D. F. (2003). The cumulative cost of additional wakefulness: Dose-response effects on neurobehavioral functions and sleep physiology from chronic sleep restriction and total sleep deprivation. *Sleep, 26*, 117–126.

Youngstedt, S. D., Kline, C. E., Zielinski, M. R., Kripke, D. F., Devlin, T. M., & Bogan, R. K. (2009). Tolerance of chronic 90-minute time-in-bed restriction in older long sleepers. *Sleep, 32*, 1467–1479 YourSleep.aasmnet.org.

Chapter 4
Normal Variations of Sleep

Contents

4.1 Sleepiness and Tiredness

We all have used the terms sleepy and tired and alert and awake and have a notion of what these terms mean. But in science, we need to be precise in the terms we use. Otherwise, we may find that we are really confusing somewhat different things. Bill Dement, MD/PhD renowned pioneer sleep researcher and retired Director of the Stanford University Sleep Disorders Center, suggests the following continuum:

Specific references to statements in this chapter that can be found in multiple, widely available sources are not included in the text. A selection of these sources is listed below and can also be consulted for verification or more detail. (Kryger et al. 2011; Lee-Chiong 2009; National Sleep Foundation web-site http://www.sleepfoundation.org/;American Academy of Sleep Medicine information web-site YourSleep.aasmnet.org).

W. H. Moorcroft, *Understanding Sleep and Dreaming*,
DOI: 10.1007/978-1-4614-6467-9_4,
© Springer Science+Business Media New York 2013

Awake ⇔ Sleepiness ⇔ Drowsiness ⇔ Sleep

He uses this continuum to distinguish ordinary sleepiness from what precedes sleep. *Drowsiness* is the period of awake with heavy eyelids that occurs just prior to sleep and is accompanied by a strong urge to sleep. Conscious effort is needed during drowsiness to stay awake and keep eyes open. Additionally, he points out that alertness is an antonym to sleepiness. Tiredness is not sleepiness; rather, it is fatigue from muscular or mental exertion. Fatigue may also result from tedium, boredom, apathy, and general lack of interest. Sleepiness is felt in the head but tiredness in the whole body. While there is on overlap—people who are fatigued may feel some sleepiness—they are really different. Sleepiness can lead to sleep, fatigue alone does not.

Dave Dinges, research psychologist specializing in sleep at the University of Pennsylvania School of Medicine, has summarized the factors that can lead to a subjective sense of sleepiness (many of these points are elaborated on in other parts of this book):

1. *Prior Sleep.* Both too little and too much recent sleep can cause a person to feel sleepy.
2. *Amount of Wakefulness.* The greater the time awake since prior sleep, the greater the likeliness of feeling sleepy.
3. *Circadian Phase.* The current time of our circadian clock influences sleepiness.
4. *Health Status.* Illness usually causes sleepiness.
5. *Age.* Beginning with middle age, people generally sleep less well and, thus, often feel sleepier.
6. *Drugs.* Some drugs influence sleepiness.
7. *Surroundings.* Stimulating, novel, exciting situations can reduce the sense of sleepiness. In contrast, situations that are warm, boring, and quiet may heighten the sense of sleepiness. Such situations do not cause sleepiness as commonly believed. Rather, as the bodily need for sleep increases, the influence of environmental factors increases. An exciting situation, such as a football game, may keep a sleep-deprived person from feeling sleepy, while a boring lecture will not put a fully rested person to sleep but can unmask sleepiness in a sleep-deprived individual.
8. *Individual Differences.* Some people are inherently sleepier than other people regardless of these other factors.

Box 4.1 How Much Sleep Do You Really Need?
Given the research that strongly suggests that many people are not getting enough sleep and the negative effects of this (see Sects. 3.1.2 and 3.1.3), what is the bottom line for you? In my opinion, the evidence is strong that most people, very likely including you, are not getting enough sleep and the resulting sleep debt is having serious negative consequences. For most of us,

Table 4.1 Sleep need at different ages

Age	Sleep need per nychthemeron
0–2 months	12–18 hours
3–12 months	14–16 hours
1–3 years	12–14
3–5 years	11–13
5–13 years	9–11
Adolescents	9–10
Adults	7–8
Elderly	6–9

getting more sleep would be better. Imagine right now, how much better off you would be with more sleep and then think about how you can get it.

The problem is that the amount of sleep you or any other individual needs is not simple or easy to accurately determine. There is no known test to give a precise answer. There are charts, such as shown in Table 4.1, that can tell us what the approximate sleep need is by age, but there is now general agreement that an individual's sleep need can vary greatly from such norms because it is influenced by many factors such as genetic inheritance.

These numbers are a good starting place but do not solely rely on them. Rather, do an individual experiment. Start by asking some questions. "How am I functioning during the day?" "Is it hard to get up in the morning?" "Do I experience strong sleep inertia every morning after awakening for the day?" "Do I wake up feeling refreshed and in a good mood?" "Do I struggle to stay awake?" "Do I sleep 2 or 3 h more on weekends and vacations?" "Do I fall asleep in class, when reading, or in quiet situations?" Remember, it is not dull, monotonous lectures or warm, dim classrooms, or boring books that put you to sleep. It is only your own individual sleep drive at the moment that does so. If your answers to these questions are affirmative and you do not have a sleep disorder (see Part V), you need to get more sleep and possibly more regular sleep. For a week, try increasing your nightly sleep by 15 min but getting up at about the same time every day, including weekends. After a few days of this, increase again. Repeat until you are no longer sleepy during the day.

But you also need to be sure that you are not trying to get too much sleep. If you find that your nighttime sleep is not very efficient, that is you are lying in bed a lot wanting to sleep but are awake, and you are not usually sleepy during the day, you may need to spend less time in bed. After first eliminating the possibility that you may have insomnia (see Sect. 13.8), try decreasing your nightly sleep by 15 min but getting up at about the same time every day, including weekends. After about a week of this, decrease again. Repeat until you are sleeping more efficiently but also are not sleepy and are not suffering the effects of sleep deprivation most of the day.

You may have to do a little of both—trying more sleep per night then less per night until you find the happy medium that is right for you. When you are at the point where you still find that you feel a bit sleepy in boring, unstimulating situations, yet your sleep is good but may not be perfectly efficient, you probably have found out the amount of sleep that is right for you. Once you have determined this, try as best you can to stick with it. Notice how much better you feel and how much more productive and successful you are. Congratulations!

4.2 Good Sleep

Some mornings we may awaken eager and ready to get going. On such mornings, we may think, "That was a good night of sleep. I feel great." But on other mornings, our experience may be quite different. We find it hard to awaken, may hit the snooze button a few times, and finally have to drag ourselves out of bed. Such experiences may cause us to wonder just what constitutes good sleep and how we can get more.

Unfortunately, only some of the factors that contribute to a good night of sleep are known at this time. Quality of sleep is primarily a subjective thing. While we can distinguish some poor sleepers by the polysomnogram, others who say they slept poorly show nothing unique in their record. One factor is amount of sleep experienced both most recently and for the last few days. If we have not allowed our brains to get the sleep they need on a given night or series of nights, then we will tend to awaken feeling unrefreshed.

But total sleep time alone is not enough. Sleep continuity has also been found to be important. When our sleep is fragmented by multiple arousals[1] then our sleep is less satisfying and effective. Michael Bonnet, Professor of Neurology at Wright State University, director of the sleep center at the Dayton Department of Veterans Affairs Medical Center, and on the staff at the Wallace Kettering Neuroscience Institute, has done excellent research on this topic (e.g., Bonnet 1986; Downey and Bonnet 1987). He noted a common factor in people with several different types of sleep disorders (to be more fully discussed in Chap. 13). Their sleep was punctuated with brief arousals. He tested his hypothesis by stimulating sleepers in his laboratory just enough to change their EEG briefly at various intervals throughout the night. He then tested their levels of sleepiness and performance the next day. He found that arousals spaced greater than 20 min apart had little effect on subsequent sleepiness and performance, but people aroused every minute tested the same as people who were totally sleep deprived. Partial effects were seen with intervals between 1 and 20 min, with greater intensity of effects the closer the

---

[1] Changes in our EEGs toward lighter stages of sleep or awakening.

interval was to one minute. The conclusion: an important component of good sleep is sleep continuity, and anything that fragments sleep such as noise, pain and other discomforts, stress or anticipated stress, a room that is too warm or too cold, a snoring or restless sleeping partner, and stormy weather can lead to poor sleep.

As can be seen in Fig. 3.8, there are times of the nychthemeron that we are able to sleep more easily and other times when sleep is more difficult to obtain and sustain. Sleep obtained during our subjective night and our mid-afternoon dip is much more likely to be good sleep than sleep obtained at other times. As we shall see in Sect. 12.2.3, the experiences of shift workers demonstrate the problem of getting good sleep during the day.

Regular wake-up times, and to a lesser extent, bedtimes, have also been shown to be important for obtaining good sleep. When we get up at greatly different times, such as staying up late on weekends and sleeping in the next morning, we tend to disrupt the phase of our circadian rhythms. First, this causes us to try to sleep when our circadian rhythm urges us to be awake, which can make sleep less efficient. Second, when we try to return to our weekday schedule and go to bed at our regular time, we may find that it is difficult to fall asleep for a few hours. This experience has even been given a special name—"Sunday night insomnia." The end result is a day or two of poor sleep resulting in daytime sleepiness and impaired performance.

Note that we have said nothing about the different stages of sleep. While we know from Fig. 2.8 and Table 2.1 that typical sleep contains specific proportions of each stage and that a pressure occurs when sufficient amounts of either REMS or N3 are not obtained, it has not been demonstrated that the typical proportions and cycling of NREMS and REMS are related to good sleep. Recent research suggests that inadequate REMS can worsen mood the next day, while inadequate N3 produces lethargy and daytime sleepiness. Yet, good sleep seems more related to the quantity of uninterrupted sleep than the amounts or continuity of the specific stages.

Peter Hauri, clinical psychologist and retired director of the Mayo Clinic Sleep Disorders Center, has talked about good sleep in terms of the balance of the sleep and wake systems in the brain (see Sect. 5.3). Typically, one becomes active while the other becomes inactive, but not always. They are not like ends of a teeter-totter, such that as one goes up, the other necessarily goes down; rather, they are somewhat independent. If the wake system remains active—higher heart rate and other physiological measures sometimes show this—while the sleep system becomes active, then we may not be able to get to sleep easily, and, if we do get to sleep, we do not have quality sleep (called non-restorative sleep insomnia in Sect. 13.8).

4.3 Long and Short Sleepers

Section 2.2 discusses sleep in the average young adult and Sect. 2.3 the amount of sleep people need at other ages. The average young adult needs about 8 h of sleep per nychthemeron, and 68 % of people report they average between 6½ and 8½ h of sleep. Therefore, quite a few people are getting considerably more or less than an average amount of sleep. Many of those getting less sleep are sleep deprived, but others may not need any more sleep than they are getting. Likewise, some people getting more than the average amount of sleep may biologically need it. Evidence is accumulating that genetic inheritance may influence the degree of sleep need in an individual (Allebrandt et al. 2011), just as most people are close to average height but some are much shorter and others much taller for inherited biological reasons. Identical twins raised together or apart have more similar sleep characteristics, including length, than non-twins siblings. There are a few documented individuals who do perfectly well with 3 h of sleep and are otherwise normal and healthy. Reports of people who never slept have been shown to be untrue or caused by very rare diseases that disrupted more than sleep. (See Box 4.1 for how to determine your sleep need.).

The first 5 h of sleep in people who regularly get 9 h is very similar to those who consistently get only 5 h with a lot of N3 interspersed with some N2 and a bit of REMS (Horne 2006). The additional sleep in the 9 hour sleepers is made up of mostly N1, N2 and REMS. It is as if the short sleepers have lost the last few hours of longer sleep. If 8 hour sleepers are allowed to stay in bed in the morning they typically will sleep an additional hour or two. However, after a few nights of this, they took longer to fall asleep and were more likely to be awake longer during toward the end of their sleep.

Box 4.2 Awakening Without an Alarm (Part 1)

What determines when we awaken from sleep? Many of us rely on an alarm clock or some other external means such as a radio, another person shaking us or throwing water in our face, or a cat kneading our stomach. But alarm clocks are a relatively recent phenomenon in the history of human existence. Prior to their invention and widespread use, many people, we might imagine, used to wake up on their own after their body had had enough sleep. But circumstances, such as the need to tend to some chore or social obligation, may have necessitated arising at a particular time regardless of whether enough sleep had been obtained or not.

Is it possible to awaken oneself at a time determined prior to going to sleep? Anecdotally, there are people who say they can accomplish this task. Occasionally, over the last century, there has even been research directed at determining the extent of this ability with usually positive results. However, the existence of this ability has not been widely recognized, and the extent of the ability is not clear.

In the 1990s, several of my students and I undertook to do new research on this question (Moorcroft et al. 1997). We first did a random telephone survey of 269 adults in the upper Midwest of the United States. To our surprise, we found that approximately one-fourth of those surveyed never used an alarm clock or other external means to awaken. Another one-fourth set their alarm but regularly awakened before it; they just did not trust their ability to self-awaken. There was one-fourth who needed their alarm, and often other things, to awaken on time. The remaining one-fourth expressed no consistent pattern. We asked those who said that they self-awakened without or before their alarm how they did so, but no consistent model emerged. Prior to going to bed, some visualized a clock set to the desired time, and others repeated the time to themselves. Many said that they did nothing special; it just happened. We next selected 15 people who said they regularly self-awaken, and then objectively tested for this ability in their own beds for three consecutive nights while choosing their own wake-up times. Each subject wore an actigraph[2] to bed for three consecutive nights. From the data the actigraph provided, we were able to compare intended awakening time, which each subject recorded in a journal before going to bed, to actual awakening time. The mean difference between actual and intended awakening time was +4.61 min. That is, after hundreds of minutes asleep, they were able to self-awaken within an average of 5 min of their target. Five individuals awakened within 10 min of their target time, mostly before it, on each night, five did so on two of the three nights, and of the remaining five, four did so on one night. Choice of target times varied considerably within subjects but more so for those who were more successful. Taken together, these results show that many people have the ability to regularly awaken themselves from sleep at a desired time.

What is known about people who genuinely need much more or much less sleep than the average person? Ernest Hartmann (1973), psychiatrist at a sleep disorders center in Newton, Massachusetts, did research on groups of sleepers who either needed less sleep than average, (the short sleepers) and those who needed more than average (the long sleepers). He was careful to include only people who really needed less than 5½ h or those who needed more than 8 h, with 9 h spent in bed to feel rested. He excluded insomniacs and people who were sleep depriving themselves or willfully oversleeping. Then, using clinical interviews supplemented by psychological tests, he looked for characteristic profiles of people in the two extremes. While no individuals necessarily displayed all of the characteristics, collectively the short sleepers differed from the long sleepers.

In the sleep laboratory, the sleep stages and NREM—REM sleep cycle were not unusual, but the long sleepers got more REMS and N2 sleep than the average young adult—commonly used as the comparison for all sleep parameters—and the short sleepers got less. The long sleepers had twice as much REMS as the short sleepers, and the sleep efficiency of the long sleepers was poorer than that of the short sleepers. Also, in other experiments, long sleepers have been shown to recover more quickly from sleep deprivation.

---

[2] A wrist-watch size device that is able to store data that can be used to determine if a person is asleep or awake on a minute by minute basis.

The main differences Hartmann found were psychological. In many ways, short sleepers seemed to be the opposite of long sleepers. Short sleepers were more likely to report that they were generally self-content, full of energy and proficient, and desired to be productive. Short sleepers were also more socially sophisticated. Long sleepers tended to be more introverted and to worry about things, yet some were very creative. They often were active politically in a critical and non-conformist way.

Psychological tests revealed additional differences between long and short sleepers. Long sleepers tended, as a group, to show mild to moderate neurotic traits. Some of them were not very self-confident and others anxious, inhibited, and depressed. They manifested more bodily aches. Short sleepers were more conforming and had a tendency to deny problems. They also tended to have a lot of ambition, be decisive, and were out-going.

Their attitudes toward sleep differed also. Short sleepers tended to view sleep as a waste of time while long sleepers reported they liked sleep and felt it was necessary to get a sufficient amount. Aeschbach and colleagues (Aeschbach et al. 2001) report that short sleepers tolerated being sleep deprived better than long sleepers.

When awakened near the end of each REMS period, long sleepers showed a change as the sleep period progressed. Early on, they reported that they felt quiet and passive, but this turned to active and energetic by the end of the night. The short sleepers demonstrated no such change. Hartmann interpreted these results to mean that the long sleepers were experiencing psychological change during the night that the short sleepers were not.

These data are intriguing but are correlational, making it impossible to determine whether the personality/lifestyle determined the sleep characteristics or vice versa. In an effort to determine causality, Hartmann (1973) also studied a very rare group of sleepers. These people are like short sleepers in terms of sleep and personality/lifestyle for weeks or months at a time and then are like long sleepers for weeks or months at a time. When things were going well in their lives, they were short sleepers, but when experiencing stress, job uncertainty, physical demands, or emotional strife, most resembled long sleepers. Importantly, Hartmann found that the personality/lifestyle changes preceded the changes in sleep, suggesting that longer sleep serves a psychological function. Hartmann believes that what happens to variable length sleepers is an exaggeration of what happens in most people. He points out that during emotional tumult, average sleepers increase their REMS to a modest, but significant, degree.

Other researchers have not supported Hartmann's findings regarding long and short sleepers. However, some of these researchers (e.g., Webb 1975) used college students as their subjects, which may have influenced the results, since college students have atypical sleep patterns to begin with. Another set of researchers (Stuss and Broughton 1978) only weakly supported Hartmann's findings in six adult, very short sleepers. A different criticism of Hartmann's research on long, short, and variable length sleepers is that he did not directly determine whether the length of sleep was what the sleepers actually needed or was self-imposed sleep deprivation or over-sleeping. Measures like the MSLT were not available at the time to assess these factors. This research needs to be replicated using newer techniques.

Increasingly a lot of attention has been paid to the duration of sleep and mortality and health problems—for a review and analysis, see Gallicchio and Kalesan (2009). Some of these studies have included hundreds or even thousands of people who are typically asked "How many hours do you usually sleep each night?" The answer people give to this question is later correlated with subsequent mortality and detrimental health effects such as diabetes, heart problems, high blood pressure, obesity, cancer, psychiatric problems, neurological disorders, and strokes. Most of the studies conclude that sleeping less than 6–7 h or more than 8–9 h result in an increase in mortality and these problems.

More recent studies have begun to refine these findings. These relationships were not seen until people were 60 years or older (Gangwisch et al. 2008) and the frequency of both long and short sleep durations seemed to increase a few years prior to death which, the authors stated, could be because of inflammations or undiagnosed problems. Another study (Hublin et al. 2007) showed that people who initially slept for around 7–8 h but were sleeping more or less than this by the end of the study, 12 or 17 years later, had greater mortality than those who did not change their sleeping duration. In contrast, those who increased from initially a short duration or decreased from initially a long duration had mortality rates of the consistent 7–8 hour sleepers.

However, this research has critics. Several, such as Lavie (2009) note that most of the studies rely on a single, one-sentence subjective response from participants to determine their sleep duration, ignoring whether it was daytime or nighttime sleep and if weekends were different. Additionally, it is not clear that the participants were reporting actual sleep or time-in-bed that could include wake as well as sleep time. Furthermore, the direction of the reputed causal relationship is not always clear: is the reported sleep duration always responsible for the health problems or vice versa? Horne (2010) points out that some of the studies grouped everyone sleeping less than 7 h together, yet it has been shown that the people getting less than 5 h of sleep are the ones with higher mortality but not those in the 5 to 7 h range. Further, he points out that it is not clear from the evidence the higher mortality in the very short sleepers is primarily due to their short sleep.

4.4 Morning Larks and Night Owls

Some people's sleep is *phase shifted*. By this term, we mean that the shape of the curve showing the likelihood to be awake or asleep (see Fig. 3.9) is the same, but is shifted to the left for *phase advance* and to the right for *phase delay*. The degree of the shift is usually less than an hour in either direction, but this is enough to make a noticeable difference.

You may have noticed that older people tend to go to bed earlier than younger people, but they also get up much earlier. It is not just that they are party poopers; rather, their circadian rhythms are phase advanced. In contrast, the circadian rhythms of teenagers tend to be phase delayed. They stay up later but also sleep later in the morning when they can. Many other people, regardless of age, may also be phase shifted. We commonly call those who are phase advanced "morning larks" and those who are phase delayed "night owls," although the technical terms are *morning types* (*MTs*) and *evening types* (*ETs*), respectively. Most of us are between these extremes and are referred to as *NTs* for *neither types*.

It is important for research, as well as for other uses, to have a simple and fast way to identify people who have certain characteristics, such as being MTs and ETs. Fortunately, there are several valid questionnaires that distinguish between ETs, MTs, and NTs. The best known is by Horne and Östberg (1976). It consists of questions such as the time of day that you typically get up, what time of the day you feel at your best, and how you would feel if you had to sleep at different times. You can take a version of this type of questionnaire at http://www.cet-surveys.org/Dialogix/servlet/Dialogix?schedule=3&DIRECTIVE=START.

Research has shown that in addition to being more alert in the morning and sleepy in the evening, MTs generally fall asleep more easily than ETs and have better moods after awakening but awaken more during sleep than NTs and ETs. The circadian temperature of MTs peaks about 1 hour earlier in the nychthemeron than ETs. ETs feel more alert and believe that they perform better later in the day and on into the evening. The difference between ETs and MTs is typically a two-hour phase shift. However, when this shift interacts with process S (see Sect. 3.3), the result is a possible difference of 4 h in time of peak alertness (Van Dongen and Dinges 2001). Not only do ETs tend to go to bed later and get up later, they tend to be more irregular in their bedtime habits, especially on non-work nights from nychthemeron to nychthemeron but average the same amounts and patterns of sleep as ETs and NTs. ETs also experience less jet lag and tolerate shift work better. More women tend to be MTs than men.

There are some noticeable changes in the circadian rhythm that occur in the elderly that supplement the discussion of sleep changes with age in Sect. 2.3.3. Most elderly people are morning larks, tending to arise early and go to bed early. In older elderly persons, this tendency is more noticeable in women than men. Additionally, the amplitude of the circadian rhythm for sleep/wake is lower in the elderly, and there appears to be an attenuation of response to zeitgebers. Some research also suggests that the period of the circadian rhythm for sleep is shorter in the elderly, but other studies have failed to confirm this.

What causes some people to be MTs and others ETs? There is evidence for a genetic propensity and it is not easy for either group to adopt the sleep habits of the other type. Yet, of people the same age, more with fulltime jobs compared to students are MTs, suggesting that there is some flexibility given demands of work. Still, many of these workers expressed the desire to be able to go to bed later and get up later, so maybe they are going against their internal or other dispositions. Also, as just indicated, age plays an important role in that younger people who tend to be ETs gradually become NTs and then MTs as they get older. Although it is often the elderly who are notorious MTs, recent evidence suggests MT characteristics begin to be noticeable by middle age.

Box 4.3 Yawning

Beware: reading this may cause you to yawn.

Yawning, an involuntary, slow, deep breath accompanied by wide gaping of the mouth, is found in all mammals, maybe all vertebrates. Even human fetuses yawn. Once started it cannot be stopped, but it can be stifled. However, stifled yawns are not satisfying—only a fully realized, gaping yawn is. (Try this: when you feel like yawning, force it through your nose or clench your teeth and note how you felt about this yawn compared to the full blown variety.) The functions of yawning are not conclusively known but seem related to respiration, heightening alertness, and non-verbal communication. A common notion is that yawning serves to increase the oxygen in the blood. It is true that yawning does include extra expansion of the lungs resulting in more oxygen intake and carbon dioxide being expelled. It also increases return of blood to the heart and more blood going to the cortex of the brain. However, breathing pure oxygen does not decrease yawning, nor does breathing a higher concentration of carbon dioxide increase it. Neither does increasing respiration rate affect yawning. Thus, the reason for yawning cannot be to increase oxygen in the blood.

It is also common knowledge that yawning is related to sleepiness and alertness. Yawning is common before going to sleep or after awakening, but not during sleep. It is noticeable when feeling drowsy. Its lowest occurrence is mid-afternoon. Stretching sometimes accompanies yawning. The need to be vigilant in a non-stimulation situation will also increase yawning. Yawning does cause a temporary increase in heart rate, may restore tone to the muscles involved, and may cause reflexive stimulation of the arousal centers in the brain. Yet yawning also occurs before and after eating, after drinking alcohol, and in the midst of a stressful situation.

Yawning is also a form of non-verbal communication. Animals communicate threat and aggression with a teeth-showing, eyes-wide-open yawn. It also can signal dominance or the readiness for sleep, but, in this case, the eyes are shut. In humans, yawning most often signals boredom or the readiness for sleep.

Yawning among humans is also highly contagious. Seeing others yawn greatly increases yawning or the urge to yawn. Even if the face of the yawner is rotated 90 or 180°, it still has this effect. Surprisingly, the gaping mouth is not the most important facial feature to cause this contagion. A gaping mouth alone will have no effect, but viewing the facial features of someone who is covering a yawning mouth is sufficient. But that is not all. Hearing a yawn will produce contagion. And hearing about yawning will also cause this effect. A colleague says she never lectures about yawning until near the end of the class period for just this reason. Reading about yawning will cause yawning, too. (Are you yawning yet?) It is speculated that yawning is contagious in humans because it helped synchronize bedtimes in our early ancestors.

4.5 A Problem Teens Experience with Sleep

A great deal of focus has been directed toward the sleep of teenagers in the United States and other countries such as Italy and Brazil. As mentioned, teens tend to be strongly phase delayed, which can present problems when they have to be in school early in the morning. Because of this, many high school students exist in what has been described as perpetual jet lag. In the United States, many teenagers have to be in class before 8 a.m., requiring arising an hour or two before this time. Yet, their bodies do not want to fall asleep until around 11 p.m. Adding to this problem are the demands of work and the desire to socialize that may make bedtimes even later. The result of late bedtimes and early wakeup times is all too often chronic sleep deprivation in teenagers (Eaton et al. 2010). "It is not unusual to see students sleep in class, especially in the morning," say both high school students and their teachers. Even when awake, they are so "out of it" that paying attention and learning suffer.

There appear to be several reasons for adolescent sleep phase delay (Jenni and Carskadon 2007). First, puberty is associated with circadian phase delay. Melatonin secretion in the brain that influences the setting of the circadian clock (see Sect. 5.1) occurs later. Second, there are suggestions that the length of the circadian nychthemeron is a bit longer compared to that of adults. Third, there may be a greater sensitivity to evening light or less of a sensitivity to morning light, either of which would tend to push the setting of the clock later. Fourth, adolescents may be exposed to light, from TV or computers, into the late evening, which also tends to delay the clock setting. Fifth, the rate of buildup of homeostatic sleep drive is slower and the sensitivity to sleep loss is less while the tolerance to sleep drive is greater.

But all of the sleepiness of teens cannot be explained by the phase delay in their circadian rhythms and remedied by delaying school start times. There are also social demands, and with the increasing number of teens having part-time jobs, the demands of work. It is the opinion of researchers in this area that parents and teens themselves could do more in getting to bed earlier, especially on weekends, and recognizing the importance of adequate amounts of sleep taken at regular times.

At about 20 years of age, an abrupt reversal of this phase delay occurs and sleep times become more and more early (Roennberg et al. 2004).

Many high schools start between 7 and 7:30 a.m. Delaying school start times to 8:30 or 9:00 can help to greatly reduce the chronic sleepiness in teens. Starting in the mid-1990s, a number of studies have been conducted in public and private high schools that have tried a later start time. This includes urban and rural schools in many different parts of the US. The results show an extra hour of sleep per nychthemeron is obtained resulting in reports of better attendance and less tardiness, school counselors and nurses reporting fewer students seeking help for emotional and physical complaints, more homework getting done, better grades, less difficulty staying awake in school, improvements in mood, better student behavior such as quieter hallways, better lunchroom behavior, and fewer car accidents. Interestingly, a number of parents of teens with later school start times report that their teens were "easier to live with" and that they now had "connection time" with their teens over breakfast.

Yet in spite of these demonstrated, beneficial improvements with delaying high school start times, many are skeptical or see problems. Some administrators have said there would be problems with changing bus schedules because the buses would have to take grade school children to their schools earlier in order to have the buses available for high school students at a later time. Many parents similarly complained that this would affect childcare and carpools as well as their work schedules. Coaches worried that there would be difficulties in scheduling practices, yet participation in after-school sports and extracurricular activities has not been negatively affected in schools that have delayed start times. There may be less time for after-school jobs. But overall, the results show that the benefits outweigh these and other problems.

Box 4.4 Communications Technology Use Is Causing Sleep Loss

Communications technology is negatively affecting a lot of people's sleep (National Sleep Foundation 2011). Almost 95 % of people in the United States said they use television, a computer, a video game, or a cell phone within the hour before bedtime several nights a week. However, the type of technology used varies with age. Older adults are more likely to watch TV close to bedtime, but more of younger adults and teens commonly surf the internet, play video games, or use their cell phones during this time. However, for about three out of four children, TV watching is a part of their "bedtime routine" and about one out of four children have a TV in their bedroom (Owens 2008). Nine percent of teens say they are awakened from sleep by their cell phone almost every night while one out of five young and middle age adults say this happens to them a few nights per week.

These uses of communication technology close to bedtime can hinder getting enough good quality sleep because they are too arousing. Light-emitting screens suppress melatonin in the brain, which in turn reduces sleepiness and can shift circadian rhythms to a later setting—both of which make it more difficult to fall asleep. The internet, cell phones, and video games require active interaction that is arousing and therefore counterproductive to achieving relaxed, sound sleep.

4.6 College Student Sleep

In the 1980s, several of my students and I surveyed the sleep patterns of students at Luther College in Decorah, Iowa, where I was teaching at the time. We found that first-year traditional students, around 18 years of age, were getting over an hour less sleep than they had before they started college. However, things gradually got better during their college years so that by the time they were graduating seniors four years later, they were getting an amount of sleep considered "normal" for their age.

Wolfson, sleep researcher, Professor of Psychology, and Associate Dean at the College of the Holy Cross in Worcester, Massachusetts, wrote an article in 2010 reviewing and updating similar findings. Although not as rigidly bound to early school start times, most college freshman get even less sleep than high school seniors, because they choose to go to bed so much later. Delayed bedtimes not only shorten their average night of sleep but also tend to make them even more phase delayed. Additionally, many college students have irregular bed- and wakeup times that are later on weekends and shorter sleep lengths on week days. And things seem to be getting worse; there has been a dramatic increase in the number of college students who report less stability in their sleep habits and more problems with their sleep as well as less average sleep than in the past. However, as in the past, things improve with third and fourth-year students getting to bed and rising earlier than first-year students.

The typical first-year traditional college student is considerably sleepy during the day, causing significant impairment such as academic and emotional stress. To partially compensate, and because a less rigid schedule allows it, napping becomes common. As students continue their college careers, their sleep deprivation gradually reverses, apparently because of earlier bedtimes and needing less sleep. Seniors typically are much less sleepy than freshmen.

Sleepy college students experience consequences. In a study done by Thacher and colleagues that was reported at SLEEP 2011, the Associated Professional Sleep Societies meeting in Minneapolis (Dallas 2011), college students who got to bed later and rise later average poorer grades. Why? Students who tend to select classes that start later do not receive the benefits that later school start times provide for high school students who start school later. Although they sleep longer, they also drink more alcohol which diminishes their sleep quality (see Box 6.4 and Sect. 6.2.7.2) resulting in greater daytime sleepiness and not feeling as well rested. That in turn probably diminishes their cognitive ability to do coursework.

A recent update on sleep in college students can be found in Galambos et al. 2013.

4.7 Sleep in Children

Sections 2.3.1 and 2.3.2 began to review the ways in which sleep in children differs from that of adults. The sleep of children is influenced by both homeostatic and circadian processes just as it is in adults. However, the characteristics of both of these processes differ in children, which are key to fully understanding sleep changes across development (Jenni and Carskadon 2007). Keep in mind that there is little agreement about the development of sleep behaviors that should be viewed as typical and the range of sleep patterns considered within a normal range for a given age. There is agreement, however, that there is large variability in normal sleep in children, and that children's sleep can be affected by cultural values, beliefs of parents, daily activities of parents (such as feeding), and influence of social systems.

Irregular circadian sleep-wake rhythms are evident immediately after birth becoming regular by 2–4 months. Waking homeostatic sleep drive builds faster early in life but also dissipates faster during sleep (Jenni and Carskadon 2007). Additionally, the tolerance for sleep loss in newborns is very low; thus, they are not able to maintain consolidated wakefulness periods. This is why younger children need to nap. Gradually, these things change during development allowing ever greater ability to sustain wakefulness and eventually a consolidated period of sleep at night.

In infancy, the difference between individuals in sleep duration is as great as it will ever be. By preschool age, an individual's relative typical sleep duration, high, moderate, or low, becomes stable and is maintained throughout their life. Preference for MT, ET, or NT first appears between 6 and 12 years and then remains stable for the remainder of life.

Box 4.5 Co-Sleeping/Bed-sharing[3]

In the modern Western industrialized world, the typical infant sleeps in their own bed located in their own separate bedroom. It is assumed that this is natural, necessary, and healthy. However, in most other areas of the world, and even more so in earlier times, co-sleeping[4] is the norm.

A specific form of co-sleeping is bed-sharing where the infant sleeps in the same bed as the caregiver, usually the mother. In places like Japan, India, and Africa, it is usual for families to sleep together in one family bed. It is well accepted among Pacific and other Asian cultures, also. However, the Catholic Church outlawed bed-sharing in the 13th century because of reports that many infants had been smothered when a sleeping adult rolled over.

---

[3] Most of the details presented here can be found in Owens (2008) and McKenna and McDade (2005).

[4] When the infant sleeps in the same room or area with one or more caregivers.

(Actually the incidences most likely were intentional infanticide.) This fear is expressed by many in the Western world who look aghast at bed-sharing. But Anthropologist James J. McKenna, director of the Mother-Baby Behavioral Sleep Laboratory at the University of Notre Dame, maintains that there is no evidence that co-sleeping is detrimental and may even be beneficial if done correctly with the infant laying on its back on a firm mattress, not over wrapped, and its head not covered by blankets. However, he cautions, since specific circumstances may vary, co-sleeping cannot be generally recommended but room-sharing can. His research shows that the sleep of the bed-sharing infant is longer but lighter with more arousals and movements; also the heart rate, respiration, and sleep stages of bed-sharing infant and mother become synchronized. Furthermore, bed-sharing mothers and babies tend to wake each other up during the night, which may prevent long breathing pauses in babies that contribute to sudden infant death syndrome. There is also some suggestion that bed-sharing might be more soothing to infants as well as be stimulatory for their brain development. Bed-sharing provides advantages and convenience for both breast-feeding mother and baby. (More information about bed-sharing from Dr. McKenna can be found on his website: http://www.nd.edu/~jmckenn1/lab/index.html.) Co-sleeping occurs more frequently in the United States than is commonly believed. From a low of around 10 % in the late 1950s to early 1960s, mothers who co-sleep with their infant for part or all of the night may now be over 50 %. Anywhere from 35 to 55 % of preschoolers and up to 23 % of school-aged children co-sleep with their parents. Co-sleeping is more common among Hispanics (90 %) and African-Americans (70 %). Co-sleeping is more common if the child is breast-feeding or having a problem sleeping, a parent is doing shift work, the family is of low socio-economic status, there is a single parent, and there is a history in the family of co-sleeping.

Cultural differences in co-sleeping seem to be related to cultural attitudes toward raising children. Many Asian cultures emphasize fostering mutual dependence rather than independence which leads to helping the child sleep rather than encouraging them to fall asleep and return to sleep on their own. More traditional societies view sleep in the context of social activities rather than a solitary activity. It is not unusual for children in such societies to sleep in the midst of group activities. Mayan mothers would be stunned by the practice of having babies sleep in a separate room and even view this as an example of Western mothers evading parental duties.

Studies have led to the conclusion that co-sleeping is neither detrimental nor beneficial to achievement of developmental milestones or has any effects on psychological health. Bed-sharing that occurs around the world suggests that it can be safe. But, McKenna emphasizes that it needs to be done correctly, such as always sleeping in a bed with a firm, flat surface; always placing the baby on its back; not using wedges and cushions to position the baby; and not using fluffy pillows or loose bedding.

It should be noted that the American Academy of Pediatrics takes a different position on bed-sharing (American Academy of Pediatrics 2005). "Although electrophysiologic and behavioral studies offer a strong case for its effect in facilitating breast-feeding and the enhancement of maternal-infant bonding, epidemiologic studies of bed-sharing have shown that it can be hazardous under certain conditions." The article points to international studies that conclude that the risk of bed-sharing is greatest with young infants (8–11 weeks), when there are multiple people sharing the bed with the baby, when the person sharing the bed with the baby is overtired or has consumed alcohol, when the bed-sharing occurs on a couch, and when there has been a longer duration of the bed-sharing. On the other hand, the article suggests that room-sharing can be beneficial.

Also, the U.S. Consumer Product Safety Commission (Nakamura et al. 1999) has stated, "Children younger than 2 years should sleep in cribs." However, this and similar conclusions have been severely challenged as being based on weak or misinterpreted evidence while ignoring the positive evidence for bed-sharing (McAfee 2000; Rosenberg 2000; McKenna and Gartner 2000).

4.8 How the Sleep of Women Differs

Until now we have said nothing about the differences in sleep between men and women for two reasons. First, the sleep of men and women is nearly identical, especially the nature of the stages, the homeostatic and rhythmic components, and most changes with age. Second, when sleep research was emerging in the mid-20th century, researchers were faced with many questions and wanted to answer the most basic ones first, such as what sleep is like in general in humans. For this reason, they controlled for the menstrual cycle by mostly doing research with men as subjects and, if using women as subjects, only looking at their sleep during their follicular phase. We can suspect that they assumed that someone would get back to questions about how sleep might differ between men and women and how the reproductive hormones influence women's sleep. Surprisingly, with a few notable exceptions, it was not until the late 1980s that researchers finally focus on how the sleep of women might differ from that of men.

For example, Reyner and Horne (1995) found some differences between the sleep of men and women previously unrecognized. They learned that women tend to go to bed earlier than men and fall asleep sooner. As a result, the sleep period tends to be much longer for women. However, women do not sleep as well, with more awakenings and time spent awake during the sleep period. More recent studies have begun to look at how sleep differs in "working women" (e.g., Maume et al. 2010), differences in sleep problems and disorders in women (see Part 5), how female hormones affect the sleep of women, and changes in women's sleep with advancing age.

Sleep differences in women become greater with advancing age. The main difference is that the fraying of sleep in the elderly tends to occur about 10 years later in females. For example, some elderly females still show classical N3, but few elderly males do. Additionally, women have twice as many sleep spindles then do men and a slower decline in delta waves with age. However, older women tend to take longer to fall asleep, report poorer sleep quality, and nap more than older men.

Even greater attention has been paid to conditions distinctive in women, notably changes in their reproductive hormones and related developmental status. The menstrual cycle, pregnancy, and menopause all have been found to have effects on sleep quality and quantity. Much of this research has been spearheaded by Kathryn Lee, PhD, professor at the Department of Family Health Care Nursing, School of Nursing, University of California, San Francisco, for example, chapters in Principles and Practice of Sleep Medicine (Kryger et al. 2011) on menopause and sleep disturbances and sleep-related disorders in pregnancy.

The effects on sleep of the first time that a girl or young woman menstruates have not specifically been studied, but the menstrual cycle has been. First, we must realize the considerable difficulty in investigating this question. For example, there are great differences both within and between women in the length of each menstrual cycle, but the results have to be coordinated by cycle phase, menstrual ⇨ follicular ⇨ ovulation ⇨ luteal ⇨ menstrual and so on. Second, not all women have the same changes in their sleep during the menstrual cycle. Third, ovulation may not occur with each cycle, changing subsequent hormone production. Fourth, the use of oral contraceptives changes hormone levels and thus sleep. Fifth, data from research using retrospective methods are easier to obtain but much less reliable than data obtained using prospective designs.

Progesterone can produce sleepiness, decrease the amount of wakefulness during sleep, decrease the amount of REMS, and reduce the latency to sleep onset and NREMS. Estrogen decreases REMS. Both probably also influence the circadian clock. Thus, changes in the levels of these hormones during menstruation, pregnancy, and menopause have a noticeable effect on sleep.

Although polysomnographic studies show no changes in sleep during the menstrual cycle (Moline et al. 2006), significant subjective sleep disturbance is reported by about 15 % of cycling women, but even more report milder disturbance. While the increase in progesterone after ovulation can improve sleep, later, when the level of progesterone is falling just prior to menstruation, some women experience more problems with sleep, either insomnia or hypersomnia, and recall more dreams that are more vivid. Up to half of menstruating women report that bloating disturbs their sleep quality for two or three days leaving them feeling less refreshed. Women who experience premenstrual syndrome and premenstrual

---

[5] Pain during menstruation.

dysphoric disorder have been reported as experiencing even greater difficulties with their sleep throughout their entire menstrual. Dysmenorrhea[5] causes decreased sleep quality resulting in daytime sleepiness. Oral contraceptives, containing estrogen and/or progesterone, often increase mean levels melatonin, increase body temperature during sleep, decrease or have no effect on N3, and decrease REMS latency.

Sleep and sleepiness also change during the course of pregnancy. Overall, upwards of 75 % of women report their sleep was more disturbed during pregnancy than at any other time in their lives. The most noticeable change during the first trimester is a conspicuous increase in sleepiness and sleeping but disturbed sleep (Moline et al. 2006), both at night and in napping. Probable causes include a decrease in both N3 and sleep efficiency with some insomnia. Things seem to get back to normal during the second trimester, called the "grace period" (Moline et al. 2006), although there may be an increase in the number of awakenings. Sleep becomes decidedly disrupted during the third trimester. The number of awakenings that started to increase both in frequency and duration by mid-pregnancy reaches four or more by the end of pregnancy, contributing to insomnia, less total sleep time, more daytime sleepiness, and often more napping. However, some women report that their sleep seems to return to normal during the last month of pregnancy.

Studies in the sleep laboratory have also revealed changes within sleep during pregnancy. REMS has been found to either decrease or increase during the middle of pregnancy, but almost always decreases later. Changes in REMS latency seem to vary from woman to woman but often diminish toward the end of pregnancy. The amount of N3 gradually declines during pregnancy, frequently approaching total absence during the third trimester. Sleep efficiency begins a decline during the second trimester that continues during the third trimester. For some women, all of these things tend to come close to normal levels during the last month.

The causes for these changes in sleep include direct effect of hormonal changes on sleep but also indirectly via metabolic changes, physical discomfort, and emotional changes—especially anxiety and depression.

Sleep is also affected following pregnancy. In the first months after giving birth, there is obvious fatigue caused in large part by the irregular sleep schedule primarily because of the needs of the newborn, which also may affect the sleep of the father and other caregivers. But factors like recovery from the delivery, breastfeeding, and postpartum depression complicate the picture. Generally, night sleep is broken up resulting in a decline in total sleep time and sleep efficiency and the latency to REMS is greatly reduced suggesting an attempt to compensate for lost REMS. There are also changes in the sleep that is obtained, especially more N3. The frequency of naps increases. By the third month after delivery, but sometimes up to a year later (Moline et al. 2006), there is a recovery of most aspects of sleep when the infant begins to sleep through the night, but sleep efficiency is still low and the number of awakenings high.

There are some differences depending upon if it is the first pregnancy or a cesarean birth. There are greater sleep disturbances in both of these situations.

Women who breast-feed have more N3. Also, it is interesting to note that it has been estimated that in the first year with a new baby, parents lose a total of 400–750 h of sleep.

The end of the reproductive years in a woman is marked by menopause when the production of progesterone and estrogen begin to fall and eventually remain low. Sleeping is the major problem mentioned by women during this period (Lee 2006). Around 40–60 % of perimenopausal women complain of poor sleep (Moline et al. 2006). Hot flashes during sleep, one of the consequences of menopause, are reported by over a third to two-thirds of women typically for around 1½ years but up to 5 years or more (Misra and Malow 2008). Hot flashes contribute to an increase in brief arousals and outright awakenings during sleep. In extreme cases, severe hot flashes can result in hundreds of awakenings per night. Even a moderate level can result in an increase in stage shifts, more awakenings, and lower sleep efficiency. In addition, during and following menopause, there is a notable increase in insomnia and sleep-disordered breathing (see Chap. 13 for information about these disorders) that contributes to the perception of poor sleep. Following menopause, many women complain of difficulties in getting to sleep and of waking more during sleep. However, not all research agrees with the link between hot flashes and poor sleep (e.g., Lee 2006; Misra and Malow 2008). Some women shown to have hot flashes deny they have them whereas others are greatly bothered by them at night, especially if they value getting sufficient good sleep and believe their functioning during the day will suffer following poor sleep. Further, objective laboratory research is lacking and it is possible that the complaints about poor sleep due to hot flashes existed previously. It may be that psychosocial factors more than menopause are causing sleep problems in older women.

Hormone replacement therapy has been reported to increase sleep quality, sleep continuity, and total sleep time plus shorten the time to get to sleep in postmenopausal women. Yet, other research concludes that women taking HRT complained about their sleep more than those not taking HRT (Lee 2006). Differences in the type and the dose of HRT may be responsible for these divergent findings.

More on menopause and sleep can be found at http://medicalnewstoday.health ology.com/hybrid/hybrid-autodetect.aspx?focus_handle=menopause&Content_ID =2948&brand_name=medicalnewstoday&psv=33.

4.9 Naps

Naps are periods of sleep that are shorter than the typical bouts of sleep taken by the individual or typical of the species. They also have been called sleep without pajamas taken during the day. Most human naps range from 20 min to 2 h; the average is 70 min. Napping is encouraged by many cultures in the world, most typically in the afternoon in warm climates, but tends to be discouraged in adults in Western industrialized nations who view it as slothful. All told, about half of the people in the world take an afternoon nap.

Age has a great influence on napping. As we saw in Sect. 2.3.1, the sleep of newborns can be considered to be a distributed series of naps. Even when infants begin to sleep through the night, they still take naps during the day. Napping in toddlers continues for a few years. Napping reappears in teenagers and young adults, especially those in college. Over half of 13- to 39-year-old people report taking at least one nap during the school or work week compared to about four out of ten 30- to 64-year-olds (National Sleep Foundation 2011). This daytime sleep pattern is due to both changes in biological sleep needs in the teens and too little sleep at night at all ages. Napping reemerges again in the elderly, but the reasons for this are not clear. It may be that the elderly now have the time and opportunity to nap, and/or it may be a change in the regulation of sleep that occurs during the later years of life.

Adults nap for one or a combination of reasons. Many naps are compensatory—making up for sleep debt. Napping, or at least the urge to nap, increases in proportion to the amount of sleep debt. Horn and colleagues (Horne et al. 2008) have demonstrated that a 15-min nap around the time of the afternoon dip in alertness can considerably reduce sleepiness for the rest of the waking day and can be considered as effective as extending the prior night of sleep by an hour. Naps increase during illness and seem to have a recuperative function (see Sect. 6.2.1). Environmental factors, especially hot weather, may promote napping. As we saw in Sect. 3.2.2, there is a natural, biological tendency to become sleepy in mid-afternoon suggesting that napping is normal and can reduce sleepiness for the remainder of the day (Horne 2010). Some napping may be recreational—simply for pleasure. Morning people gain more benefit from short naps than evening people. Finally, prophylactic napping—napping in anticipation of sleep deprivation, long periods of wakefulness, or even being awake during the typical sleeping hours—is thought by some to be highly beneficial, even more beneficial than napping after sleep debt has accumulated. Afternoon naps in the classroom by college students are a good illustration: "frequently compensatory, certainly environmental, influenced by biological rhythms, sometimes prophylactic, and mainly recreational" (Moorcroft 1993).

Naps are usually highly beneficial but can also have negative consequences. A short nap of about 20 min can be refreshing and increase alertness. Even if not perceived as refreshing, naps usually enhance performance such as the ability to pay attention, to respond rapidly, to remember better, and to think more clearly. This performance enhancement usually lasts about 3 h but can extend to as much as 18 h. However, naps, especially longer ones, can cause several minutes or more of sleep inertia upon awakening (see Sect. 4.10). Thus, it has been suggested to limit naps to less than an hour, ideally about 20 min, because naps that are longer bring less additional benefit but greatly increase sleep inertia. Yet, it can be necessary to sleep for longer than 90 min to achieve serious sleep debt recovery.

An example of research on naps is that done by Masaya Takahashi and Heihachiro Arito of the National Institute of Industrial Health in Kawasaki, Japan

(2006). They had 12 young, healthy students limit their sleep to only 4 h for one night, on two occasions. The following day, using a counterbalanced design, each subject had no opportunity to nap on one occasion or 15 min in bed available to nap right after lunch on the other occasion. Both before and after lunch, subjects completed tests of memory and logical reasoning and rated their own subjective sleepiness. When they napped they felt less sleepy and performed better on logical reasoning than they did without a nap.

There is no unique kind of sleep that occurs during naps; naps contain the same kinds of sleep that occur during the night. However, REMS is more likely during morning naps. The amount of REMS obtained during a nap has no effect on the amount of REMS during subsequent night sleep. However, N3 obtained during naps does reduce subsequent N3.

Claudio Stampi, MD, director of the Chronobiology Research Institute in Newton, Massachusetts, has researched management sleep in extreme conditions through the use of napping (for a review see Mason 2000). He has studied and advised solo world sailors who engage in 90 or so days of continuous racing. He found that they can get by on cumulative total of 4½ to 5½ h of nap sleep per nychthemeron, but less than this seems to present problems. For the times when even this limited amount of sleep is not possible, the best strategy appeared to be to get whatever sleep possible in 1-h naps, especially when experiencing a wave of sleepiness.

In Stampi's laboratory studies, where subjects were allowed 3 h of sleep per nychthemeron, three 1-h naps caused less performance detriment than two 1½-h naps or one block of 3 h of sleep. He also found that 50 % of N2 sleep and 50 % of REMS is lost using such a strategy, but only 5 % of N3 is lost. Often, N1 and N2 are all but skipped. ETs do better on such a schedule than MTs. However, Stampi found that relentless training can improve either type's ability to utilize such *polyphasic* sleep.

Box 4.6 Should Commercial Aircraft Pilots Be Allowed to Nap?

In the spring of 2011, there were several news reports of commercial pilots and air traffic controllers napping on the job. This caused a flurry of reaction including that of U.S. Transportation Secretary Ray LaHood saying that the government won't pay air traffic controllers to take naps while on duty (Anonymous 2011). What does research have to say about this issue, as well as napping during other types of employment?

Research done on long-haul flight crews shows that preplanned naps were safe and effective (reviewed in Walsh et al. 2011). The crew members rotated 40 min opportunities to nap during the flight. The result showed that although the accumulated sleep debt was not fully eliminated, there was greater alertness and relief from fatigue in the crew members, especially on night flights.

Similarly multiple studies showing similar positive results have been done both in laboratories and workplace situations (Takahashi and Kaida 2006).

For example, experiments in both the laboratory and at a workplace showed that an afternoon nap increased alertness, performance (well into the evening in the laboratory study), reduced yawning in the afternoon (in the workplace study), and improved job satisfaction (in the workplace study).

Thus, the evidence is clear; a short nap during work is not a waste of time. Rather, it is just the opposite. Following a nap, people more than make up for the time taken to nap with greater productivity, accuracy, and efficiency.

4.10 Sleep Inertia

Sometimes people experience foggy-headedness, bleariness, confusion, awkwardness, and less of an ability to perform even simple tasks immediately after awakening from sleep. These effects, called *sleep inertia*, usually seem to gradually diminish over several minutes although there is now some evidence that some effects are present for hours. It is more severe after awakening from a long nap, following awakening from N3, or if sleep drive remains high because of insufficient sleep. Severe, lengthy occurrences may result in confusions and commission of often impulsive and irrational, socially embarrassing or criminal acts with no memory later for what was said and done during this state of inertia. The more difficult it is to awaken a person, the greater will be their sleep inertia. Awakening from N3 has a greater effect on cognitive tasks, especially those depending on memory, rather than on psychomotor and perceptual tasks. For example, a person might not remember a phone call in the middle of the night or might turn off an alarm clock and return to sleep without awareness of having done so later. It may seem paradoxical that such impairments are greater after sleep than preceding it but can be explained by the way the brain reorganizes its functioning from the sleep state to the wake state (see Sect. 5.3.1). It is easier to return to sleep during sleep inertia.

Extending night sleep beyond typical amounts will result in sleep inertia if there was no prior sleep debt but not when extending sleep to recover from sleep deprivation. On the other hand, uncompensated sleep deprivation seems to worsen sleep inertia. Sleep inertia is less noticeable following gradual morning awakenings after a full night of normal sleep.

4.11 Sleepy Versus Alert People

Peretz Lavie, psychologist at the Sleep Laboratory, Faculty of Medicine, Technion-Israel Institute of Technology, Haifa, Israel, was presented with a problem by the Israeli military a number of years ago: a few soldiers frequently fell asleep when on night guard duty. No amounts or types of sanctions were able to alter the problem. Lavie tested these individuals in several ways and found that they were genuinely sleepier than most people and were just not able to remain awake at night. Further, he found that these people were not only sleepier than most people, but extending the amount of sleep per nychthemeron made no difference in their sleepiness. They fell asleep more quickly at night and when napping, slept more efficiently, but found it hard to stay awake.

Lavie concluded that their sleepiness was a trait[6]; in short, these soldiers were simply chronically sleepy people. He also found some people with the opposite characteristics—alert by day but had trouble getting to sleep at night. He called them "alert." Most of us are somewhere in between. The difference may be in the relative strength of the wake-producing and sleep-producing parts of the brain (see Sects. 5.3.1, 5.3.2, and 5.3.3).

Van Dongen and Dinges (2001) report that people who are alike on the amount of sleep need per night during the identical circadian phase can differ by as much as an order of magnitude in how sleepy they are when sleep deprived. That is, there is a kind of individual trait vulnerability to sleep loss. So, one aspect of good sleep and how to get it is simply to be sure you, as an individual, get enough.

4.12 Conclusion

In the sleep field, it is common to start with sleep in what is called the average young adult then make comparisons to others whose sleep differs yet is considered normal. In this chapter, we have seen how normal sleep can differ with factors such as age, individual differences in sleep need, and gender. We also explored components such as morning larks and night owls, napping, and sleep inertia as normal differences that people may have in their sleep. In part V of this book, we will look at how sleep can differ from what was covered in this chapter in ways that are considered problems.

---

[6] A fixed individual characteristic, in contrast to a state which is a variable characteristic depending on circumstances.

References

Aeschbach, D., Postolache, T. T., Sher, L., Matthews, J. R., Jackson, M. A., & Wehr, T. A. (2001). Evidence from the waking electroencephalogram that short sleepers live under higher homeostatic sleep pressure than long sleepers. *Neuroscience, 102*, 493–502.

Allebrandt, K.V., Amin, N., Müller-Myhsok, B., Esko, B. T., Teder-Laving, M., Azevedo, R. V., et al. (2011). A KATP channel gene effect on sleep duration: from genome-wide association studies to function in drosophila. *Molecular Psychiatry*. (Retrieved August 7, 2012).

American Academy of Pediatrics. (2005). The changing concept of sudden infant death syndrome: diagnostic coding shifts, controversies regarding the sleeping environment, and new variables to consider in reducing risk. *Pediatrics, 116*, 1245–1255.

Anonymous. (2011). Retrieved July 16, 2011, from http://losangeles.cbslocal.com/2011/04/18/lahood-vows-to-stop-air-traffic-controller-napping/.

Bonnet, M. H. (1986). Performance and sleepiness as a function of frequency and placement of sleep disruption. *Psychophysiology, 23*, 263–271.

Dallas, M. E. (2011). College students who sleep in drink more, study less. Retrieved August 22, 2011, from Medline Plus: http://www.nlm.nih.gov/medlineplus/news/fullstory_113180.html.

Downey, R., & Bonnet, M. H. (1987). Performance during frequent sleep disruption. *Sleep, 10*, 354–363.

Eaton, D. K., McKnight-Eily, L. R., Lowry, R., Perry, G. S., Presley-Cantrell, L., & Croft, J. B. (2010). Prevalence of insufficient, borderline, and optimal hours of sleep among high school students – United States, 2007. *Journal of Adolescent Health, 46*, 399–401.

Galambos, N. L., Lascano, D. I. V., Howard, A. L., & Maggs, J.L. (2013). Who sleeps best? Longitudinal patterns and correlates in sleep quality, quantity, and timing across four university years. *Behavioral Sleep Medicine, 11*, 8–22.

Gallicchio, L., & Kalesan, B. (2009). Sleep duration and mortality: A systematic review and meta-analysis. *Journal of Sleep Research, 18*, 148–158.

Gangwisch, J. E., Heymsfield, S. B., Boden-Albala, B., Buijs, R. M., Kreier, F., Opler, M. G., et al. (2008). Sleep duration associated with mortality in elderly, but not middle-aged, adults in a large US sample. *Sleep, 31*, 1087–1096.

Hartmann, E. L. (1973). *The functions of sleep*. New Haven: Yale University Press.

Horne, J. (2006). *Sleepfaring*. New York: Oxford University Press.

Horne, J. (2010). Sleepiness as a need for sleep: When is enough, enough? *Neuroscience and Biobehavioral Reviews, 34*, 108–118.

Horne, J. A., & Östberg, O. (1976). A self-assessment questionnaire to determine morningness-eveningness in human circadian rhythms. *International Journal of Chronobiology, 4*, 97–110.

Horne, J. A., Anderson, C., & Platten, C. (2008). Sleep extension versus nap or coffee, within the context of sleep debt. *Journal of Sleep Research, 17*, 432–436.

Hublin, C., Partinen, M., Koskenvuo, M., & Kaprio, J. (2007). Sleep and mortality: a population-based 22-year follow-up study. *Sleep, 30*, 1245–1253.

Jenni, O. G., & Carskadon, M. A. (2007). Sleep behavior and sleep regulation from infancy through adolescence: Normative aspects. *Sleep Medicine Clinics, 2*(3), 321–329.

Kryger, M. H., Roth, T. R., & Dement, W. C. (Eds.). (2011). *Principles and practice of sleep medicine* (5th ed.). St. Louis: Elsevier.

Lavie, P. (2009). Self-reported sleep duration–what does it mean? *Journal of Sleep Research, 18*, 385–386.

Lee, K. A. (2006). Sleep in midlife women. *Sleep Medicine Clinics, 1*, 197–205.

Lee-Chiong, T. (2009). Polysomnography. In T. Lee-Chiong (Ed.), *Somnology* (pp. 72–80). Seattle: Amazon.

Maume, D. J., Sebastian, R., & Bardo, A. R. (2010) Gender, work-family responsibilities, and sleep. *Gender and Society, 24*, 746–768.

Mason, C. (2000, August). Sleep deprivation: The 24/7 sailor's dilemma. *Sail, 32*, 50–53.

McAfee, T. (2000). Bed Sharing Is Not a Consumer Product. *Archives of Pediatrics and Adolescent Medicine, 154,* 530–531.

McKenna, J. J., McDade T. (2005). Why babies should never sleep alone: A review of the co-sleeping controversy in relation to SIDS, bed sharing and breastfeeding. *Paediatric Respiratory Reviews, 6*(2), 134–152.

McKenna, J. J., & Gartner, L. M. (2000). Sleep location and suffocation: how good is the evidence? [letter] *Pediatrics, 105,* 917–919.

Moorcroft, W. H., Kayser, K. H., & Griggs, A. J. (1997). Subjective and Objective Confirmation of the Ability to Self-Awaken at a Self-Predetermined Time Without Using External Means. *Sleep, 20,* 40–45.

Misra, S., & Malow, B. (2008). Sleep in the older woman. In A. Avidan & C. Alessi (Eds.), *Geriatric sleep medicine* (pp. 219–226). New York: Informa Healthcare.

Moline, M., Brock, L., & Zak, R. (2006). The impact of the life cycle on sleep in women. In H. Attarina, *Current Clinical Neurology: Sleep disorders in women: a guide to practical management* (pp. 29–45). NJ: Humana Press Inc.

Moorcroft, W. H. (1993). *Sleep, dreaming, and sleep disorders: An introduction* (2nd ed.). Maryland: University Press of America.

Nakamura, S., Wind, M., & Danello, M. A. (1999). Review of hazards associated with children placed in adult beds. *Archives of Pediatric and Adolescent Medicine, 153,* 1019–1023.

National Sleep Foundation. (2011, March 7). *Annual Sleep in America Poll Exploring Connections with Communications Technology Use and Sleep.* Retrieved August 17, 2011, from   http://www.sleepfoundation.org/article/press-release/annual-sleep-america-poll-exploring-connections-communications-technology-use-.

Owens, J. (2008). Socio-cultural considerations and sleep practices in the pediatric population. *Sleep Medicine Clinics, 3,* 97–107.

Reyner, A., & Horne, J. A. (1995). Gender- and age-related differences in sleep determined by home-recorded sleep logs and actimetry from 400 adults. *Sleep, 18,* 127–134.

Roennberg, T., Kuehnle, T., Pramstaller, P., Ricken, J., Havel, M., Guth, A., et al. (2004). A marker for the end of adolescence. *Current Biology, 14*(24), R1038–R1039.

Rosenberg, K. D. (2000). Sudden Infant Death Syndrome and Co-sleeping. *Archives of Pediatrics and Adolescent Medicine, 154,* 529–530.

Stuss, D., & Broughton, R. (1978). Extreme short sleep: Personality profiles and a case study of sleep requirement. *Waking and Sleeping, 2,* 101–105.

Takahashi, M., & Kaida, K. (2006). Napping. In T. Lee-Chiong (Ed.), *Sleep: A comprehensive handbook* (pp. 197–201). NJ: Wiley.

Van Dongen, H. P. A., & Dinges, D. F. (2001). Modeling the effects of sleep debt: On the relevance of inter-individual differences. *SRS Bulletin, 7,* 69–72.

Walsh, J. K., Dement, W. C., & Dinges, D. F. (2011). Sleep medicine, public policy, and public health. In M. Kryger, T. Roth, & W. Dement (Eds.), *Principles and Practice of Sleep Medicine.* St. Louis: Elsevier.

Wolfson, A. R. (2010). Adolescents and emerging adults' sleep patterns: New developments. *Journal of Adolescent Health, 46,* 97–99.

Webb, W. B. (1975). *Sleep: The gentle tyrant. Englewood Cliffs,* NJ: Prentice-Hall.

Part II
What Causes us to Sleep?

After reading the first four chapters you may be thinking that sleep is more complicated than you had imagined. Then you may begin to think about what causes us to sleep and what effects the brain has on the body.

Look again at the introduction in Part I. Notice that prior to the twentieth century, notions of what sleep was like and how it was produced were intertwined. Also, it was assumed that sleep was a passive phenomenon. During the twentieth century, it became apparent that sleep was an active phenomenon rather than passive, with considerable complexity. This knowledge of sleep was shown by the discovery of REMS and its regular cycling with NREMS, which could only be accomplished by active control mechanisms. Once this information became apparent, scientists began looking for the mechanisms that control sleep. Table II.I gives an indication of the scope of this endeavor. Some of these points were already covered in the preceding chapters. In this section we shall focus on two major sources: Chap. 5 reveals the basics of what is known about the involvement of the brain in sleep and Chap. 6 does the same for the rest of the body. In addition Chap. 6 explores the effects sleep has on the body.

Table II.I Some of the variables that affect sleep. (Adapted from Krueger et al. 2009)

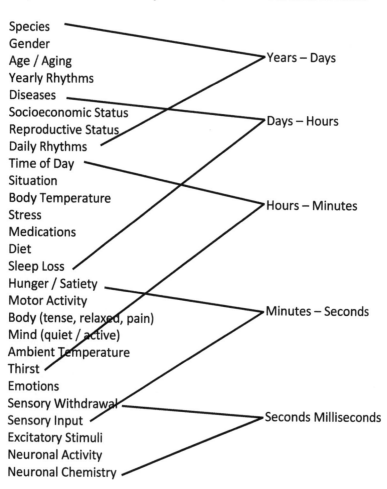

Variables That Affect Sleep   **Duration of Effect**

Species
Gender
Age / Aging   Years – Days
Yearly Rhythms
Diseases
Socioeconomic Status
Reproductive Status   Days – Hours
Daily Rhythms
Time of Day
Situation
Body Temperature
Stress   Hours – Minutes
Medications
Diet
Sleep Loss
Hunger / Satiety
Motor Activity
Body (tense, relaxed, pain)   Minutes – Seconds
Mind (quiet / active)
Ambient Temperature
Thirst
Emotions
Sensory Withdrawal
Sensory Input   Seconds Milliseconds
Excitatory Stimuli
Neuronal Activity
Neuronal Chemistry

References

Krueger, J., Szentirmai, E., & Levente, K. (2009). Biochemistry of sleep function: A paradigm for brain organization of sleep. In C. Amlaner & P. Fuller (Eds.), Basics of Sleep (2nd ed., pp. 69–74). Westchester, Ill.: National Sleep Foundation.

Chapter 5
The Brain in Sleep

Contents

In order to fully understand sleep, it is necessary to understand the brain's role in producing it. It used to be thought that the brain simply reduces its overall level of activity and arousal as the way of producing sleep. This is called a passive mechanism because there is nothing active that the brain has to do. We now know this is not true (see Box 5.1). Rather than a general reduction in activity, as Pittsburgh psychiatrist and sleep and brain researcher, Eric Nofzinger, said (personal communication, June, 2000), "The brain is functioning under a different set of rules during sleep." That is, it functionally reorganizes during sleep such that some areas become more active during sleep, others become less active, and some of the interactions between areas change. In a sense, the night shift takes over as

---

Specific references to statements in this chapter that can be found in multiple, widely available sources are not included in the text. A selection of these sources is listed below and can also be consulted for verification or more detail. (Amlaner and Fuller 2009; Chokroverty 2009; Kryger et al. 2011; Lee-Chiong 2011; Swick 2011).

W. H. Moorcroft, *Understanding Sleep and Dreaming*,
DOI: 10.1007/978-1-4614-6467-9_5,
© Springer Science+Business Media New York 2013

the day shift goes off duty. Even within sleep, there are changes in what the brain is doing as we cycle between NREMS and REMS. Wake, NREMS, and REMS are each produced and sustained by different configurations of neural cells and circuits using specific chemicals as messengers. It is necessary, therefore, to have a basic understanding of brain anatomy and brain functioning to fully understand sleep.

Box 5.1 Discovery of Sleep as an Active Brain Process

For centuries, sleep was assumed to be a passive process, sometimes thought of as "the brother of death." It certainly seems that way to many today. To get to sleep, it seems like you have to allow your brain and body to greatly reduce their activity and arousal. You cannot actively do so; you just have to let it happen. And anything that is activating, whether it is noise, light, pain, discomfort, or thoughts, can prevent sleep. During the twentieth century, several scientific findings changed this notion, at least among scientists, to one of sleep being actively produced in a very structured manner.

The modern story begins with a Viennese psychiatrist and neurologist, Baron Constantine von Economo in the mid-1910s (von Economo 1917). He examined the brains of people who died from viral encephalitis that caused them sleeping problems. Most, who had excessive sleep, had damage in the region where the posterior hypothalamus joins the midbrain (see Fig. 5.1). Von Economo concluded that this area was important to maintain wakefulness. However, some who had insomnia, had damage in the basal forebrain and anterior hypothalamus. This, he suggested, showed that this latter region of the brain is important for the active production of sleep.

Fig. 5.1 A view of the inside of the right side of the brain showing the areas von Economo discovered to be important for sleep

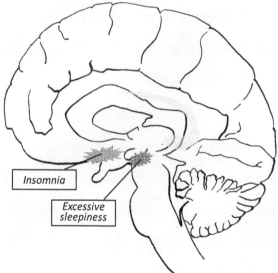
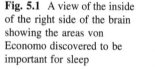

Over the next 50 years, other experiments were gradually done that eventually led to the firm conclusion that sleep was actively produced by the brain rather than a simple passive result of the reduction in sensory stimulation of the brain. Once it became apparent that sleep was active rather than passive, the pace of sleep research quickened as many scientists began to look for how the brain actively produces sleep. The results of these efforts have given us the understanding of the brain's involvement in sleep that we have today. As research continues, our understanding of the mechanisms that produce sleep will become even more detailed and exact.

The key cells for brain functioning are *neurons*. Neurons can become electrically activated via chemical processes. When activated, neurons send electrical impulses, called action potentials, along extensions called axons. When the action potential arrives at the end of an axon, it can increase or decrease the activation level of other neurons situated close to it by the release of chemicals called *neurotransmitters*. Neurons also release *neuromodulators* that have no direct effect on other neurons but can cause the effect of recently released neurotransmitters to be enhanced or diminished. There are many neurotransmitters and neuromodulators, but we shall focus only on those that are known to be most important for sleep and wakefulness. There are also other chemicals found in the blood, in the space between brain cells, and in the cerebral spinal fluid[1] that can influence the sleep/wake systems of the brain.

The cells of the brain are organized in numerous areas and subareas, each with their own names. We will concentrate only on the areas most important for sleep/wake. It is important to realize that these areas do not operate in isolation but influence and are influenced by axons from other neurons in other areas. Importantly, even though these connections via axons are physical, their degree of activity at any time may vary greatly, meaning that some interactions between cells and areas may be functionally more important at one time than at another. The variations in importance are the main determinants of the change in the functional organization of the brain that differentiates wakefulness from REMS and NREMS.

Before looking specifically at how the brain is organized in waking, NREMS, and REMS, we shall overview the chemistry of the brain. It may be necessary to use this section and the next on brain anatomy as a reference to refer back to as you finish the rest of the chapter.

---

[1] Fluid located in canals and spaces around and within the brain and spinal cord.

5.1 The Chemistry of Sleep/Wake

There are several neurochemicals known to be involved in sleep, both NREM and REM, and wake (see Table 5.1).[2] These include neurotransmitters, neuromodulators, hormones, and other types of chemicals. However, no single chemical is absolutely necessary for sleep or wake. Rather it is the complex interaction of chemicals that is important. Some are released at synapses,[3] but others are in the spaces between cells and cerebral spinal fluid in the nervous system. The following discussion focuses on the most important of these chemicals, especially the neurotransmitters.

At this point, you may be asking, "How can the same neurotransmitter be used for different stages of sleep and wake?" The answer is it depends on where it is released in the brain, what other chemicals are also present, and what else is going on.

Acetylcholine is a key neurotransmitter for the low-voltage, high-frequency EEG of waking as well as in REMS. Much is released during waking and REMS, but little during NREMS.

Adenosine progressively builds up during waking. It is a by-product of the use of certain energy-releasing molecules that was shown in the late 1990s to be a strong contributor to sleepiness and sleep need. The greater the duration of wakefulness, the greater the buildup of adenosine and changes in molecules that affect adenosine in the brain. Adenosine levels in the basal forebrain may very well be the cumulative meter of brain activity during waking that influences when and how much sleep is needed. The greater the level of adenosine at sleep onset, the greater the amount of SWS and delta waves during sleep. The levels of adenosine in the brain progressively diminish with sleep. The effects of adenosine on sleep are attenuated for a period of time by caffeine.

Dopamine is believed to contribute to wake and REMS, although the evidence is not as clear as it is for other neurotransmitters.

GABA is short for gamma-aminobutyric acid. It is an inhibitory neurotransmitter that is widely used in the brain during NREMS to damp down neural activity and reduce arousal. It also plays a key role in the production of spindles and delta waves. It is important for the control of sleep by the VLPO (see Sect. 5.3.1), basal forebrain, certain hypothalamic areas, and the suprachiasmatic nucleus (SCN). Many prescription sleeping pills act by enhancing the action of GABA.

Glutamate is a primary excitatory neurotransmitter in the central nervous system, especially in the areas important for arousal, but also plays a role in producing the slow waves and spindles.

Glycine is the main inhibitory neurotransmitter in the spinal cord. It is responsible for the paralysis of the muscles of movement during REMS.

---

[2] The complete list of all substances that influence sleep and wake would be much longer, more complicated, and beyond the scope of this book. Even then, it is recognized that not everything has been discovered.

[3] Synapses are the gaps between the end of one neuron and the beginning of another.

Table 5.1 The major neurotransmitters that influence sleep/wake	Wake	Sleep	NREMS	REMS
Acetylcholine	X	X		X
Adenosine		X		
Dopamine	X			
GABA		X	X	
Glutamate	X			
Glycine		X		
Histamine	X			
Hypocretin/Orexin	X	?		
Norepinephrine	X			
Serotonin	X			

Histamine is another neural transmitter involved in producing wakefulness as demonstrated by the drowsiness produced when it is blocked by antihistamine drugs.

Orexin (aka *hypocretin*) is a more recently discovered excitatory neurotransmitter that promotes wakefulness. It has two names, because it was discovered at about the same time in two different laboratories, each of which gave it a different name (see Box 5.2). It is produced in a small region of the hypothalamus but is widely distributed in the central nervous system via axons. It is primarily produced during waking and is most responsible for the maintenance of wake episodes and, indirectly, the maintenance of sleep.

Box 5.2 Discovery of Orexin/Hypocretin (Hungs and Mignot 2001)
In 1997, two different research teams working on two different research problems discovered a chemical in the brain that is important for waking. One team at University of Texas Southwestern Medical Center at Dallas was working with a newly discovered peptide produced in the lateral hypothalamus that influenced food intake in rats (Sakurai et al. 1998). They named it orexin from the Greek word for appetite. They went on to create a strain of mice that were unable to produce orexin and were studying them for feeding abnormalities by using an infrared camera to record their nighttime feeding. They were surprised to see that these mice would suddenly fall down while doing ordinary things like moving about or grooming. Suspecting that the rats were having seizures, they monitored their brainwaves and discovered instead that they were suddenly falling asleep just as humans with narcolepsy do (see Sect. 13.2).
Meanwhile, a second team working at multiple centers in the United States and Norway discovered a new neurotransmitter in the hypothalamus (De Lecea 1998).. They named it hypocretin, because it was produced in the hypothalamus and chemically resembled another peptide called secretin.
Shortly thereafter, Emmanuel Mignot and colleagues at Stanford University Medical School had been studying a group of Doberman Pinschers that

suffered from narcolepsy and were narrowing the search for the genes responsible for the disorder. They turned their attention to genes responsible for production of receptors for the recently discovered hypocretin. They then published their results that it was indeed hypocretin that was key to the narcolepsy in their dogs. These publications stimulated more research that strengthened the link between orexin/hypocretin and narcolepsy, this time in humans.

In a short time, orexin/hypocretin was shown to be important for the normal control of waking/sleeping. Although only produced in the hypothalamus, it was found to be widely released in many of the areas of the brain important for the control of sleeping/waking. Orexin/hypocretin was shown to be especially involved in regulating REMS. Now, it is confirmed that orexin/ hypocretin is a neurotransmitter important for maintaining normal wakefulness and for preventing REMS during waking.

Norepinephrine enhances arousal but may not be necessary for it. The drugs in the amphetamine family cause heightened arousal through their effects on this, among other, neurotransmitters.

Serotonin, produced mainly by the raphé nuclei, was previously thought to be very important for NREMS but now is thought to promote wakefulness, yet decrease the latency to REMS (see Box 5.3).

Box 5.3 Serotonin and Sleep (Jouvet 1999)
From the late 1950s to the early 1970s, the neurotransmitter serotonin was believed to be the neurotransmitter of sleep, because drugs that interfered with serotonin in the brain caused insomnia, whereas drugs that facilitated serotonin caused stronger and longer SWS. Also, longtime sleep researcher, Michel Jouvet, MD of Claude Bernard University in Lyon, France, showed that damage to the raphé, the area of the brain that is the source of serotonin, produced insomnia in proportion to the degree of damage. Subsequently, restoring serotonin with drugs following damage to the raphé could then reverse this insomnia. In humans, sometimes when brain damage caused insomnia, the damage included the raphé.

During the late 1970s and early 1980s, the notion that serotonin is the neurotransmitter of sleep fell into disfavor, because experiments showed that recovery of sleep eventually occurred following either damage to the raphé or destruction by drugs of the capability of the brain to manufacture serotonin. Also, it was found that both the electrical activation in the raphé and its release of serotonin was high during waking compared to during sleep— just the opposite of what would be required for it to be a "sleep center." Additionally, researchers could not find any areas of the brain where direct application of serotonin resulted in sleep. So, the hypothesis that serotonin was the neurotransmitter for sleep was abandoned.

Then, in the late 1980s, the role of serotonin in sleep was revived. Based on research that showed that stimulation of the raphé by electrodes could quiet behavior and reduce sensory responses, it was hypothesized that rather than being the neurotransmitter of sleep, serotonin is a part of what causes sleep onset. Additionally, Jouvet posited that serotonin is involved with process S (see Sect. 3.3). Indeed, following sleep deprivation, if serotonin is interfered with, the normal rebound of SWS is suppressed. Serotonin was found to influence the ascending reticular activating system and the VLPO to produce its effects on sleep onset. Thus, it now appears that serotonin plays a complex role in both sleep and wakefulness. Yet, the notion persists that you can improve sleep by ingesting foods high in tryptophan because tryptophan is used to make serotonin.

There are several *neuromodulators* involved in wakefulness. A number of immune regulatory molecules have been shown to promote NREMS, some by a direct effect on hypothalamic and brainstem areas. There are also a large number of other chemicals found in the cerebral spinal fluid, the space between brain cells, and the blood that are known to affect sleep/wake. These substances, too numerous to detail here, have been called *sleep regulatory substances* (Krueger et al. 2009). By and large, they affect sleep by affecting neurotransmitters, but specific details about how they do this are often murky. Very often these substances are also involved in other biological functions such as hunger, thirst, digestion, body temperature regulation, hormone regulation, pain attenuation, reproduction, stress, and combating illness.

One substance that deserves special mention is *melatonin*, a hormone secreted and distributed during the night by the pineal gland located within the approximate center of the brain. Melatonin increases in the brain about two hours before habitual bedtime, remaining high until close to the habitual time of awakening. It is a mildly sleep-promoting substance that also acts as a zeitgeber. It is released during the subjective night of the nychthemeron, but sun or room light blocks its release (see Sect. 6.1.7.1).

5.2 Basic Brain Anatomy

All brain areas are involved in sleep/wake, but we shall concentrate on those that are in control of or otherwise particularly important for these states. Think of the brain as being like the planet earth. There are large portions, such as the *brainstem* and *forebrain*, that are like continents (see Fig. 5.2). The brainstem is at the very core of the brain and is like a long tube with bulges here and there. On top and covering the upper sides of the brainstem is the very large forebrain. Within each of these continents, there are areas that are equivalent to countries. Some areas,

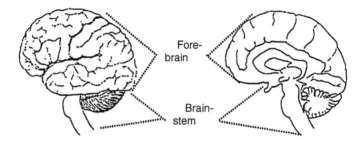

Fig. 5.2 A diagram of the human brain showing the left side (*on the left*) pulled away from the right side revealing the internal surface of the brain (*on the right*)

like some countries, have obvious physical boundaries, but some of the boundaries are not obvious, but are nonetheless real. Within the areas are subareas and sub-subareas, just like there are states, cities, and regions on the earth.

The brainstem can be divided into several regions (see Fig. 5.3). At the very bottom is a long relatively narrow portion, the *medulla*, on top of which is a bulge called the *pons*. Attached to the back of the pons is another bulge known as the cerebellum. On top of the pons is the relatively short and narrow *midbrain*. Above the midbrain is the *diencephalon*. Running up the interior of almost the entire brainstem is a region called the *reticular formation*. Close to the reticular formation is another region that runs up the very middle of the brainstem, the *raphé*. There are areas, equivalent to cities, in the brainstem that are important for sleep/wake. At the very top of the brain stem is a pair of bulbs on the side of the diencephalon, one on the right and one on the left, known as the *thalamus*. Toward each back and side of the top of the thalamus is a *geniculate nucleus*. A small but very important area lies below the thalamus in the diencephalon known as the *hypothalamus*. A very small part of the bottom of the front part of the hypothalamus is the *suprachiasmatic nucleus*.

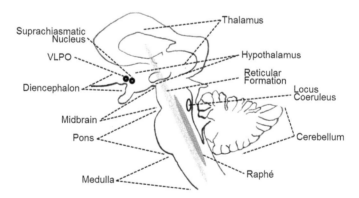

Fig. 5.3 Parts of the brainstem. The geniculates (not shown) are located on the outside of the thalamus

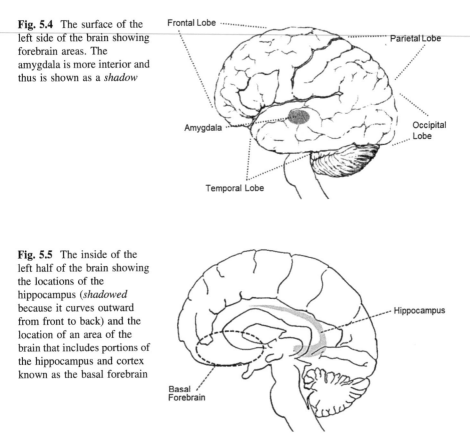

Fig. 5.4 The surface of the left side of the brain showing forebrain areas. The amygdala is more interior and thus is shown as a *shadow*

Fig. 5.5 The inside of the left half of the brain showing the locations of the hippocampus (*shadowed because it curves outward from front to back*) and the location of an area of the brain that includes portions of the hippocampus and cortex known as the basal forebrain

The forebrain is dominated in size by the wrinkled *cerebral cortex* (aka *neocortex*) on its surface. The cerebral cortex is divided into four regions (see Fig. 5.4) on each side known as the *frontal cortex* in the front, *parietal cortex* in the middle, *occipital cortex* at the back, and *temporal cortex* at the side. Below the cerebral cortex are several important forebrain areas. There is an *amygdala* to the left and another to the right toward the back of the thalamus (see Fig. 5.4). A pair of ram's horn-shaped structures, called the *hippocampus*, lay to either side of the thalamus (see Fig. 5.5).

> **Box 5.4** The Executive Function of the Brain (Horne 2006)
> Much of the frontal region of the cerebral cortex is said to exert executive control in the sense that it orchestrates behavior. It is the part of the brain that enables us to decide what we pay attention to and what we decide to do and how we do them. It enables us to quickly switch from one activity to another when we are "multitasking" or enables us to maintain focused

concentration on one detail. It just may be the locus of our self-awareness and consciousness. It exerts control over many other parts of our cortex, recruiting their functions as needed. It is thought to be larger in human beings than in any other animal. It is what makes us human.

Below the cortex but above the brain stem is something like a group of islands called the *limbic system*. To the naked eye, some of these islands appear to be physically connected to one another, while others seem to be isolated but are actually functionally connected by axons. Key components of the limbic system include hippocampus, amygdala, parts of the hypothalamus, and portions of the frontal cortex.

Finally, there is a loosely defined region known as the *basal forebrain area*. It is located on the lower front sides of the forebrain but includes parts of the anterior hypothalamus (see Fig. 5.5).

5.3 Overview of the Brain's Role in Adult, Normal Sleep/Wake

To fully understand sleep, it is necessary to understand the role of the brain in producing it. See http://healthysleep.med.harvard.edu/video/sleep07_scammell_ brainsleep that shows where sleep-controlling areas of the brain are located in an actual human brain.

5.3.1 Overview of Key Brain Areas for Sleep and Wake

The lower brainstem is able to produce wake, NREM-like sleep, and REMS. But damage to higher areas in the brain such as parts of the midbrain, hypothalamus, thalamus, and neocortex cause considerable reductions in the amounts of both NREMS and REMS showing that they play an interacting role in enhancing these sleep states. Likewise, waking is supported by areas in the midbrain, hypothalamus, and basal forebrain via long axons that go to most other areas of the brain, especially the diencephalon, limbic system, and neocortex that serve to keep the brain awake and alert. Active inhibition of these wake-producing areas in the lower brain allows the entire brain to go into sleep mode.

A very small group of cells in a portion of the anterior hypothalamus called the ventrolateral preoptic nucleus (*VLPO*) play a critical role in producing sleep. It can be considered the "sleep switch." It functions by sending inhibitory messages to the arousal systems including those that use orexin to maintain wakefulness. The tiny suprachiasmatic nucleus of the hypothalamus is the master clock that plays an enormous role in determining when sleep and wake occur in the nychthemeron. It does so by influencing other nearby sleep/wake brain regions.

Some of these key areas preferentially use a key neurotransmitter to produce their effects. The *locus coeruleus* uses norepinephrine, the raphé uses serotonin, several sites in the brainstem and basal forebrain use acetylcholine, and the hypothalamus uses histamine and orexin for waking and for suppressing REMS. The accumulation of adenosine in the basal forebrain is a key determinant of sleepiness.

5.3.2   Waking

To remain awake, your brain depends on activation from a few key areas in the brainstem (see Fig. 5.6). This activation[4] puts neurons in your cerebral cortex and other parts of your forebrain in a state of readiness to receive information and to respond to it quickly. Without this level of activation, your brain would drift off into a slow, dull state. The anterior portion of the reticular formation has become known as the *ascending reticular activating system (ARAS)* because of its key activational role. Its output activates the cerebral cortex via two routes using the neurotransmitters glutamate, norepinephrine, and acetylcholine. The dorsal route goes to a portion of the thalamus that in turn projects general excitatory influences widely to the neocortex. The ventral route from the ARAS goes to (1) the neurons active during waking in the posterior hypothalamus, the only place in the brain that produces histamine that then activates the cerebral cortex and (2) the basal forebrain area that uses acetylcholine to excite the cerebral cortex and hippocampus.

The locus coeruleus and the raphé also help produce wakefulness. The locus coeruleus uses norepinephrine to activate the entire forebrain but especially the sensory and integrative areas. The locus coeruleus is a key for controlling what aspects of sensory input are attended to when awake. The raphé uses serotonin to activate the forebrain. There are additional brainstem areas that use dopamine also to help activate the forebrain. Orexin (hypocretin) is produced in the neurons of the upper right and left sides of the hypothalamus. These neurons have axons leading to the cortex and midbrain arousal centers where the excitatory orexin is released into those portions controlling wake to sustained wakefulness.

The role of the thalamus for waking is, first, to generally activate the neocortex and, second, to allow specific information to be passed to and from the neocortex. During REMS, the thalamus also keeps the cortex activated but closes the gate on incoming sensory information. However, during NREMS, it helps maintain the slow EEG in the cortex that is characteristic of this state.

---

[4] An older term for EEG activation is EEG desychronization.

Fig. 5.6 A view of the inside of the right side of the brain showing some key areas important for producing wakefulness and the major neurotransmitter that each uses. The *dotted lines* indicate the dorsal route of the ARAS, and the *dashed lines* indicate much of the ventral route. The path to the hippocampus is not shown. For simplicity, not all areas are labeled, although approximate locations are shown

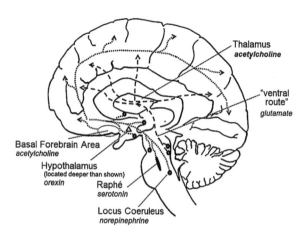

5.3.3 Sleep

What causes the start of sleep? At the turn of the twenty-first century, Dennis McGinty and Ron Szymusiak, sleep and brain researchers in California, summarized their work and integrated it with the work of others directed at this question (McGinty and Szymusiak 2000). The conclusion is that the VLPO (see Fig. 5.7) works with other cells very close by to act as an apparent sleep switch for the brain. These cells are one of the few sleep active areas in the brain. They become active around the onset of sleep, their activity is proportional to the depth of sleep, and they are sensitive to sleep deprivation. Lesions in and around this area result in a reduction of sleep. The VLPO is thought to be activated by numerous sleep

Fig. 5.7 A view of the inside of the right side of the brain indicating how the VLPO initiates sleep using the neurotransmitter GABA. For simplicity, not all areas are labeled, although approximate locations are shown

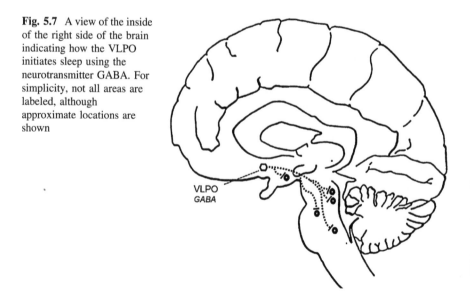

Fig. 5.8 Schematic of the "flip-flop" showing positions for wake (**a**) and sleep (**b**)

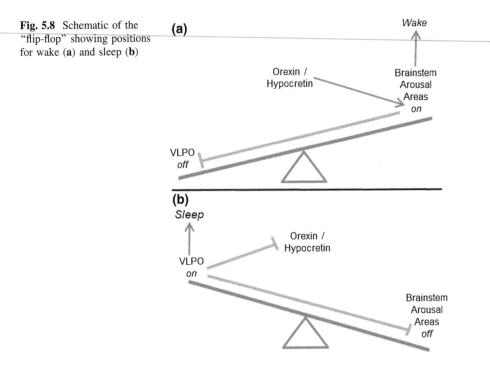

regulatory substances (see Sect. 5.1), especially adenosine. It also is activated by other areas of the brain that promote sleep including nearby warm-sensitive neurons, although details remain to be confirmed. The VLPO was shown to inhibit, using GABA, nearby wake-promoting areas in the ARAS, and posterior hypothalamus. Interestingly, these areas in turn have an inhibitory influence on the VLPO. The levels of activity of the VLPO and wake-promoting areas are negatively correlated.

Why do the sleep-promoting areas and the wake-promoting areas inhibit one another? The answer is stability. When there are influences that cause one area to become activated, it then inhibits the other area thereby reducing the second area's return inhibition. This serves to sustain the activated area's own activity until outside influences are strong enough to inhibit the first area or excite the second area to flip the balance. Such a so-called *flip-flop circuit* [5] (see Fig. 5.8) also avoids in-between states because when one area becomes strong enough to overpower the other, the switch quickly flips to the alternate state. This explains why sleep/wake transitions seem to be relatively rapid. Without this flip-flop sleep/wake circuitry, we would tend to alternate between sleep and wake frequently and have difficulty being fully asleep or fully awake.

---

[5] The switch on the wall that controls the room lights is an example of a flip-flop. It is either on or off.

Box 5.5 Sleep and Wakefulness are not Opposites

We tend to think of sleep and wakefulness as total and complete opposites. More truthfully, they are complementary states that interact with one another (Horne 2006). Each is controlled by different parts of the brain, and in simple terms, each of these parts can be active or not active at any given time. This means there are 4 possible combinations—sleep on, wake off as in NREMS, wake on, sleep off as in alert wakefulness, both on might explain drowsiness, and both off producing REMS which Horne likens to "non-wakefulness" or a wake substitute (see Sect. 11.2).

However, even this is too simple. We talk about falling asleep but actually it is more like going down a staircase to begin sleep and up the staircase to awaken. That is, several brain areas have to change their function for sleep to occur and then do the reverse for sleep to end. These changes usually take place in a quick and coordinated fashion when the areas of the brain-controlling sleep achieve dominance. Thus, we feel like sleep is a unitary process, but in reality, it is a steplike process. The reverse is true when the wake-controlling areas of the brain again achieve control and it coordinates steps to quickly awaken us.

This is known to be true not only from studies of how the brain works in sleep and waking but also from cases when the brain is not fully asleep such as with sleepwalking (see Sect. 12.4.2.1) or automatic behaviors when awake (see Sect. 3.1.3 and Box 12.4).

5.3.4 Response to Sensory Information During Sleep

When we are asleep, our brain's level of awareness of sensory information coming to and from our body is lower (see Fig. 5.9). Cortical responses to such stimuli are reduced to 80 % during N1 and N2, 65 % during N3, and to only 10 % during REMS. Much of this change, especially during NREMS, is due to a decrease in the transfer of such information through the thalamus. Thus, an early event important for sleep onset occurs in the thalamus where there is a reduction in sensory input directed to the cerebral cortex, even though there is no change in the amount of such information arriving at the thalamus. There is, however, some sensory input that facilitates sleep such as general warmth and fullness after a big meal. During REMS, less information arrives at the thalamus itself because of inhibition at the sensory receptors and their transfer points in the spinal cord and brain stem.

5.3.5 NREM Sleep

NREMS occurs at sleep onset. Essentially, two things happen to cause this: directly by an inhibition of forebrain neurons and indirectly by a reduction in

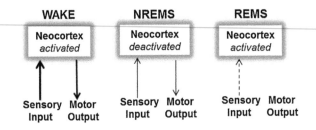

Fig. 5.9 Differences in sensory input and motor output of the neocortex depending on the wake/sleep state of the brain. *Dark line* indicates full communication level, *thin line* represents significantly reduced level, and *dashed line* indicates near absence of communication

arousal influences. The basal forebrain area uses the inhibitory neurotransmitter GABA together with some neuromodulators to directly dampen activation in the forebrain. The cells in the basal forebrain area that perform this function are more active during sleep than during waking.[6] The basal forebrain is sensitive to the accumulation of the sleep-promoting substance adenosine.

Meanwhile, there is a change in the influence of the brainstem arousal mechanisms that influence the thalamus and thus the cerebral cortex. In contrast to waking, during NREMS, the discharge of the thalamus is relatively slow, less than 1 Hz, and comes in bursts. The slow discharge rate of the thalamus sets up a feedback loop with the neocortex resulting in changes in the EEG and less alertness in the neocortex. The results are spindles and K-complexes of N2 and delta EEG waves characteristic of N3. Spindles and K-complexes occur when the thalamus is "gating out" sensory information, thus preventing much of this information from arriving at the neocortex. This is thought to help maintain NREMS. As sleep progresses from N1 to N2 and then to N3, the spindles disappear as delta waves emerge, indicating a general slowing of activity in the neocortex.

Research using brain imaging techniques that enable the study of the functioning brain in humans without surgery shows that overall brain activity is 5–10 % lower during N2 compared to waking but 25–40 % lower during N3. However, these decreases are not uniform throughout the brain. This is consistent with the information already presented that sleep is an active process with specific areas of the brain playing a key role in creating it. Interestingly, during N3, there are small, local wake-like states in various higher portions of the brain.

---

[6] At this point, you may be questioning how an area of the brain that is important for waking is also key to sleeping. The answer is that in the brain, cells that perform one function may exist in the same area with cells that perform the opposite function because their communication with other neurons differs both in where their axons travel and what neurotransmitters they release there.

5.3.6 REM Sleep[7]

During REMS, the overall level of activity in the brain is high as it is in wake; however, the activation pattern of the neocortex is not uniform. That is, some areas are more activated and others less compared to waking. A particularly important finding, as we shall see when considering dreaming later in this book, is that the associative areas of the upper front portion on the sides of the frontal cortex plus a few other portions of the forebrain are much less active.

Additionally, during REMS, the hippocampus is in a different functional state as shown by the presence of high-voltage theta waves. During waking, its waves are faster and more irregular except for the occurrence of theta during body movements. Also, the amygdala in the forebrain area is very intensely activated in human REMS.

Furthermore, there is a dramatic reorganization of the communication between these areas (Fig. 5.10), and the brain is nearly isolated from the rest of the body during REMS (see Fig. 5.9). Little sensory information is arriving at the neocortex, and commands from the brain to the muscles of movement in the body are totally blocked.

The following details about the brain's involvement in REMS are based on the best available information to date plus inferences to fill in the gaps. However, not all scientists who work in this area totally agree with every aspect of this explanation.

While NREMS is a product of the higher parts of the brain, the key areas for generating REMS are lower down in the brainstem, particularly in the pons and nearby portions of the midbrain (see Fig. 5.10). In this sense, REMS seems more "primitive" since the brainstem is an evolutionarily older part of the brain with a simpler organization. In fact, if the cortex were not present REMS would continue, but NREMS as we know it would not occur.

There are three groups of cells in the brainstem that are maximally activated during REMS, collectively called *REM-on* cells. Other cells in a different area are nearly silent during REMS and called *REM-off* cells (see Fig. 5.10). As their names imply, when the REM-on cells are active, REMS occurs, but when the REM-off areas are active during waking and NREMS, then REMS does not occur. Additional areas of the brain may play a modulating role by acting on either the REM-off or REM-on group or on both at the same time.

To initiate REMS, cells near the VLPO are thought to inhibit the REM-off areas, thus releasing the REM-on areas from inhibition (see Fig. 5.10). This starts a sequence of influences that go to both higher and lower areas of the brain. The downstream influence arrives at brainstem and spinal cord mechanisms to inhibit nerves that produce muscle movements. Motor impulses from higher portions of the brain still occur, but any movements they command are blocked in this way. However, muscle twitches may occur when strong impulses break through the

---

[7] The primary source for this section is Chokroverty 2009.

Fig. 5.10 The inside of the right side of the brain showing the major areas and the neurotransmitters they use that are important for the production of REMS

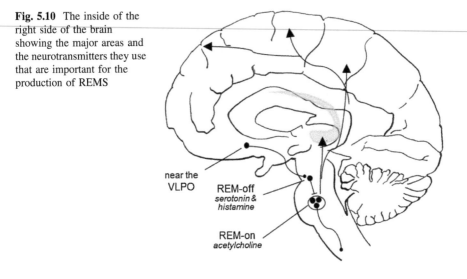

near the
VLPO   REM-off
          serotonin &
          histamine

REM-on
acetylcholine

inhibition. This happens more in animals and human infants than in adult humans. Similar inhibition of sensory input to the brain occurs at the same time in these areas of the brain.

The upstream influence comes from other neurons in the REM-on areas that are active only during REMS and communicate with three nearby areas of the brain. One of these areas is responsible for the activated EEG of REMS in the hippocampus and neocortex, another for PGO waves characteristic of REMS, and the third for rapid eye movements. These areas when released from inhibition by the REM-off area, begin to become active about 30–60 s before full-blown REMS begins. Some REM-on cells manifest high and steady activity during REMS. Collectively, they are the source of the tonic aspects of REMS. Other REM-on cells show bursts of activity during REMS and seem to be responsible for phasic REMS activity such as PGO waves.[8]

As stated in Sect. 2.1.1, NREMS alternates with REMS in a predictable time course averaging about every 100 min and resulting in about 4–5 cycles per sleep period. Robert McCarley and Alan Hobson (Professors of Psychiatry, Harvard Medical School) in 1975 first published the *reciprocal interaction* model as a description of how this is accomplished. During sleep, the REM-off neurons gradually weaken, allowing the REM-on areas to become active, thus resulting in REMS.

---

[8] PGO waves were discovered in animals but are thought to occur also in humans. These waves are phasic clusters of up to 6 sharp electrical peaks closely related to the occurrence and direction of rapid eye movements. They originate in the pons, then travel to the lateral geniculate nucleus in one side or the other of the thalamus, and from there to the cerebral cortex, especially the occipital cortex, on the same side. Since their discovery, they have been found to involve more portions of the brainstem, cerebellum, and cortex than their name implies. They are probably triggered by the hypothalamus and forebrain during REMS when the cortex has few sensory inputs.

Then, the REM-on areas are thought to gradually stimulate the REM-off neurons, so that they eventually become active enough to inhibit REM-on and cause the return to NREMS. This cycle repeats itself several times until the end of sleep.

One factor not as clearly explained is why the REMS periods get longer as the sleep period progresses. There are mathematical models that suggest it might have to do with the high demand for N3 early in the night that leaves little time for REMS. Then, as the homeostatic demand for N3 gradually weakens, there is increasing opportunity for REMS to occur. However, the neurological mechanisms that underlie this are not apparent.

5.3.7 Circadian Rhythms

As presented in Sects. 3.2, 3.3, 4.2, 4.4, and Sect. 5.3.7, sleep is also governed by a nychthermal rhythm called the circadian clock (see Fig. 5.11).

5.3.7.1 How the Circadian Clock Functions

Although it has been known since the 1970s that the *suprachiasmatic nucleus* (SCN) is the location of the circadian clock (see Fig. 5.11), only recently have details of how this clock functions have begun to be understood. If the SCN area is damaged, many circadian rhythms, including that of sleep/wake, cease; sleep becomes essentially randomly distributed throughout the nychthemeron.

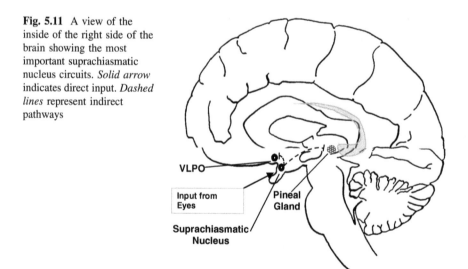

Fig. 5.11 A view of the inside of the right side of the brain showing the most important suprachiasmatic nucleus circuits. *Solid arrow* indicates direct input. *Dashed lines* represent indirect pathways

Individual cells in the SCN have their own circadian firing patterns that coordinate with one another resulting in the circadian rhythms of the entire animal. If a SCN from another animal is subsequently implanted in the brain, the circadian rhythms largely return but with the characteristics of the rhythm, such as the length of the period of the donor!

The SCN is like a microchip for timekeeping (Moore 1999). Within the cells of the SCN, protein synthesis controlled by at least eight clock genes with names like "timeless" and "period" are turned on approximately once per day. This is accomplished because these genes are organized in a net of interrelated negative feedback loops that some time after their activation eventually inhibits their own activity. Essentially, the clock genes cause specific proteins to be produced that in turn slowly inhibit the genes. Then, when the proteins are gradually altered, the genes are released from inhibition and the sequence begins again. Each of the steps takes time that cumulatively has a duration of about a nychthemeron. Separate cells in SCN may have slightly different individual cycle times but when associated with one another, they "couple" to create a single-phased output.

There is some malleability in this whole process that enables the clock to be entrained to the local environmental light/dark cycle. This is possible because information sent to the SCN by a special pathway from the eye via the optic nerve (see Fig. 5.11) is able to modify the coupling interaction. Thus, the output of the SCN responds to decreasing light at dusk by shifting its setting of the clock a bit later, while the light at dawn shifts the setting of the clock a bit earlier. This enables the clock, which left to its own devises tends to run a bit longer than 24 h, to coordinate with the light/dark cycle while giving the clock flexibility to adjust to seasonal changes in the timing of light/dark.

The main zeitgeber is light. Information on this pathway has nothing to do with visual perception or visual reflexes, because some animals like the blind mole rat and some, but not all (see Sect. 3.2.2), blind humans are able to respond to light as a zeitgeber. But the SCN also responds to regulatory input not involved with light, including input from some of the hormones it causes to be released. Although controversial, weaker zeitgebers are thought to include things like the sleep/wake cycle itself, bodily activity, feeding, and melatonin level.

The output from the SCN influences four other nearby areas of the brain (see Fig. 5.11). It does so via its axons and chemicals that it causes to be released in those areas. This output affects many rhythmic physiological and hormonal activities in addition to sleep/wake. It may cause these effects directly by itself or indirectly by being a zeitgeber for other local clocks in the body. These causes are suggested by the fact that the sleep/wake cycle and body temperatures can become desynchronized during forced desynchrony experiments (see Sect. 3.2.1). Importantly, the SCN indirectly sends inhibitory signals into the VLPO sleep switch to help maintain wakefulness during the subjective day portion of the circadian rhythm.

Among the glands influenced by the SCN is the pineal gland that produces melatonin during the subjective night portion of the circadian cycle. However, the production of melatonin can be inhibited by light arriving at the eye. Melatonin, in turn, acts as a zeitgeber on the SCN.

5.3.8 Local Cell Control of Sleep

Traditionally, the emphasis on discerning what controls sleep and waking has focused on specific brain areas and neurotransmitters that impose sleep on the rest of the brain and body—often referred to as top-down control. More recently, it has become apparent that much smaller assemblies of neurons can also be important in regulating sleep—called bottom-up influence. For example, the neurons in the cerebral cortex are organized in columns of cells that serve a coordinated function. These columns can fluctuate between wake-like and sleep-like states because when individual cells in a column are active, there is an accumulation of chemicals that then compel sleep in the column to which they belong. The more columns in the neocortex that are in a sleep-like state, the greater the need for whole body sleep, especially N3. In mammals, it is thought that sleep is the result of the interaction between bottom-up influences and top-down control mechanisms (Vassalli and Dijk 2009). Bottom-up influences help determine the probability of sleep, while the top-down control causes the necessary orchestration for the coordination of sleep.

Greater activity in brain areas responsible for physical and mental efforts during waking produce substances that can modify the effects of neurotransmitters, neuromodulators, and receptor sites on nearby neurons to produce these local "sleep-like" states. As these local sleep-like states accumulate, they exert greater and greater influences on the brain areas and neurotransmitters known to regulate sleep in the brain and body. As such, these local sleep-like states are a major part of the homeostatic, sleep-drive regulation sleep. The number and variety of these local sleep-influencing substances are great, and their interactions are complex (see Krueger et al. 2009; Clinton et al. 2011 for details).

This local cell model of sleep is based on deductions from research. For example, it has been demonstrated that analysis of the EEG during NREMS shows greater sleep debt in the left somatosensory cortex when the hand that sends sensory impulses to that brain area is extensively stimulated before the onset of sleep (Kattler et al. 1994). Similar results have been found in several other experiments in a variety of animals. Additional research has shown that there can be simultaneous differences is local sleep-like states in the neocortex. For example, in a sleeping animal, most neocortical columns are in a sleep-like state, but some others can be in the wake-like state (Recotor et al. 2005). The local control of sleep is discussed further in Sect. 10.4.1 and 10.4.2.3

5.4 Conclusion

Waking, NREMS, and REMS are each governed by different brain cells and networks situated in particular areas of the brain that utilize distinctive neuro-transmitters. Waking is governed by several areas in the brainstem that activate the rest of the brain, especially the forebrain. Orexin/hypocretin is especially important in maintaining wakefulness. Sleep begins when the VLPO in the pons inhibits the wake-producing activation of the brainstem. The VLPO is influenced by chemicals (sleep factors) and other areas of the brain, especially local cells in the neocortex that have recently been active, and the circadian clock in the suprachiasmatic nucleus of the hypothalamus. It is a chemical clock that is synchronized with the environmental light/dark cycle that promotes alertness during the daylight portion but allows sleep at night. An important sleep factor is adenosine. Its build-up in the basal ganglia during waking is a major contributor to the homeostatic regulation of sleep. The wake-producing and sleep-producing areas of the brain inhibit one another resulting in a "flip-flop" relationship, so that only one or the other is active at a time. Additionally, both arousal-promoting and sleep-promoting neuronal groups are regulated by a number of other influences, including sensory, hormonal, metabolic, and behavioral influences. The alternation between NREMS and REMS is controlled by the alternating activity in the REM-off and REM-on areas in the brainstem.

References

Amlaner, C. J., & Fuller, P. M. (Eds.). (2009). *Basics of sleep* (2nd ed.). Westchester: Sleep Research Society.

Chokroverty, S. (Ed.). (2009). *Sleep disorders medicine* (3rd ed.). Philadelphia: Saunders.

Clinton, J. M., Davis, C. J., Zielinski, M. R., Jewett, K. A., & Krueger, J. M. (2011). Biochemical regulation of sleep and sleep biomarkers. *Journal of Clinical Sleep Medicine, 7*(Supplement), S38–S42.

De Lecea, L., Kilduff, T. S., Peyron, C., Gao, X.-B., Foye, P. E., Danielson, P. E., et al. (1998). The hypocretins: hypothalamus-specific peptides with neuroexcitatory activity. *Proc Natl Acad Sci USA, 95,* 322–327.

Horne, J. (2006). *Sleepfaring.* New York: Oxford University Press.

Hungs, M., & Mignot, E. (2001). Hypocretin/orexin, sleep and narcolepsy. *BioEssays, 23,* 397–408.

Jouvet, M. (1999). Sleep and serotonin: an unfinished story. *Neuropsychopharmacology, 21,* 24S–27S.

Kattler, H., Kijk, D. J., & Borbely, A. A. (1994). Effect of unilateral somatosensory stimulation prior to sleep on the sleep EEG in humans. *Journal of Sleep Research, 3,* 159–164.

Krueger, J. M., Szentirmai, E., & Levente, K. (2009). Biochemistry of sleep function: a paradigm for brain organization of sleep. In C. Amlaner & P. Fuller (Eds.), *Basics of sleep* (2nd ed., pp. 69–74). Westchester, III: National Sleep Foundation.

Kryger, M. H., Roth, T. R., & Dement, W. C. (Eds.). (2011). *Principles and practice of sleep medicine* (5th ed.). St. Louis: Elsevier.

Lee-Chiong, T. (2011). *Somnology 2.* Seattle: Amazon.

McGinty, D., & Szymusiak, R. (2000). The sleep-wake switch: a neuronal alarm clock. *Nature Medicine, 6,* 510–511.

Moore, R. Y. (1999). A clock for the ages. *Science, 284,* 2102–2103.

Recotor, D. M., Topchiy, I. A., Carter, K. M., & Rojas, M. J. (2005). Local functional state differences between rat cortical columns. *Brain Research, 1047,* 45–55.

Sakurai, T., Amemiya, A., Ishii, M., Matsuzaki, I., Chemelli, R. M., Tanaka, H., et al. (1998). Orexins and orexin receptors: a family of hypothalamic neuropeptides and G protein-coupled receptors that regulate feeding behavior. *Cell, 92,* 573–585.

Swick, T. J. (2011). The neurology of sleep. *Sleep Medicine Clinics, 6,* 1–14.

Vassalli, A., & Dijk, D.-J. (2009). Sleep function: current questions and new approaches. *European Journal of Neuroscience, 19,* 1830–1841.

von Economo, K. (1917). Encephalitis lethargica. *Wiener Klinische Wochenschrift, 30,* 581–585.

Chapter 6
The Body During Sleep

Contents

Specific references to statements in this chapter that can be found in multiple, widely available sources are not included in the text. A selection of these sources is listed below and can also be consulted for verification or more detail. (Amlaner and Fuller 2009; Chokroverty 2009; Horne 2006; Kryger et al. 2011; Lee-Chiong 2011).

W. H. Moorcroft, *Understanding Sleep and Dreaming*,
DOI: 10.1007/978-1-4614-6467-9_6,
© Springer Science+Business Media New York 2013

If we are going to understand sleep completely, we need to understand what effects sleep has on the body and vice versa. Prior to the latter half of the twentieth century, it was assumed that the physiology of the body was the same when asleep as it was when awake. Since it is generally easier to study the body during waking, little attempt was made to investigate physiology during sleep. As mentioned in earlier chapters, the discovery of REMS prompted scientists to view sleep differently and look for things in sleep that they never thought of looking for earlier. As a result, they soon began to discover that in many ways we are physiologically different during sleep. Some of these changes are large, involving whole organ systems, but others are more subtle. Yet, all of the differences are important. Additionally, contrary to common belief, we do not sleep simply because our body wears out while awake and needs sleep to reverse this effect. It is now realized that changes in any of several physiological processes may either facilitate or impede sleep.

6.1 The Normal Physiology of Sleep

Generally, what happens in the body during NREMS is what we all think sleep ought to be. Things are quiet and at a generally low level as it would be for the body to rest and recuperate. The feedback systems of the various organ systems are working well but maintaining steady levels somewhat lower than during quiet waking when resting. Any internal or external disturbances are quietly compensated for by these feedback mechanisms.

In contrast, REMS is everything we would imagine sleep should not be. It is a time of irregular activation of many bodily processes. Local reflexes are operating the organ systems of the body, but their control is frequently being overridden by lower parts of the brain. What is more, the brainstem controls this operation with a general unresponsiveness to feedback about what is going on in the body. As a result, REMS is anything but restful and recuperative. In fact, REMS entails a bit of a risk to the welfare of the body, since things are a bit out of control and can fluctuate wildly.

6.1.1 Central Nervous System

The central nervous system is composed of the entire brain plus the spinal cord. During NREMS, many neurons in the central nervous system have a lower rate of activity than they do during waking, and the overall metabolic rate in the brain is lower than during waking. It is as if most of the brain is just active enough to keep things going at a basic, low level, much like a car idling. Yet, as we shall see in Chaps. 7, 10, and 11, there is still a lot of mental processing going on. There are a few areas that are more active than they are during waking. These are the areas that assume control in order to actively produce NREMS.

During tonic REMS, the cells in several areas in the brain are actually more metabolically active than they are during NREMS or waking. Not only are these areas active because they are causing REMS, but there is quite a lot of mental activity going on in REMS. Additionally, during phasic REMS, the cells in some regions of the brain, especially the visual areas, are sporadically wildly active.

6.1.2 Autonomic Nervous System

The autonomic nervous system, ANS, is responsible for controlling many of our internal physiological processes such as the heart, lungs, stomach, intestines, and many glands. The ANS is composed of two parts. One part, the sympathetic nervous system, SNS, prepares our body to deal with emergencies and threats. When awake and faced with a perceived emergency or threat, the SNS increases heart rate, blood pressure, and the speed and depth of respiration, but diminishes digestion.

The other part of the ANS, the parasympathetic nervous system, PNS, primarily does the opposite of what the SNS does. It functions to conserve and maintain the body resources in the absence of any perceived emergencies or threats by slowing the heart, decreasing blood pressure, slowing respiration, but facilitating digestion. It is important to note that seldom is the only SNS or only the PNS completely in control. Typically, the *entire* SNS is relatively more or less active, while *individual portions* of the PNS are more or less active.

During sleep the PNS generally increases in activity while the SNS generally decreases in activity. However, the relative balance is more related to the stage of sleep than any real or perceived threats or stresses. NREMS is characterized by an active PNS with a relatively quiet and stable SNS. During tonic REMS, the PNS is at the same level as in NREMS, but the SNS operates at an even lower level than during NREMS. However, during phasic REMS, the PNS is more active, and the activity of the SNS has been described as a storm—variable but with intense activity. Not surprisingly, the result is dramatic and irregular surges of activation of many of the internal organs during REMS.

6.1.3 Cardiovascular

During NREMS heart rate is slower and blood pressure is at a slightly lower than when awake. During tonic REMS (see Sect. 2.1.1), blood pressure and heart rate are even lower than during NREMS. During phasic REMS (see Sect. 2.1.1), heart rate has noticeable surges and pauses and average blood pressure is generally higher but more variable with considerable peaks than resting level.

When in NREMS, most areas of the brain have relatively less blood flow. However, there are few areas that are actively in control of sleep (see Sect. 5.5.3

that have slightly to significantly increased blood flow. When in tonic REMS, unlike other organs of the body most brain areas have a substantial increase in blood flow over what is present during waking, with some brain areas getting as much as 200 % of waking levels. During phasic REMS, there are even greater transient increases in blood flow in the brain.

(Website http://medicalnewstoday.healthology.com/hybrid/hybrid-autodetect. aspx?content_id=2940&focus_handle=heart-disease&brand_name=medicalnews today features a related topic—sleep and heart disease).

6.1.4 Respiration

We breathe for many reasons. Primarily, breathing brings oxygen into the body and expels carbon dioxide. Much of our respiration is under automatic control for this purpose but can be overridden or captured by conscious control, such as when talking or holding breath to dive underwater, or by other automatic control mechanisms, such as when sneezing. There are separate but partially overlapping mechanisms for automatic and behavioral breathing.

Throughout NREMS the control of breathing is entirely automatic, functioning to mainly maintain the level of carbon dioxide in the blood but at a slightly higher level than when awake and to a lesser extent oxygen at a slightly lower level than when awake. There is a moderate decrease in air volume entering and leaving the lungs per minute during NREMS. On the other hand, breathing rate and breathing volume are automatically varied as the levels of carbon dioxide or oxygen vary. Overall, breathing, especially during N3, is regular and slightly deeper.

Breathing during REMS is another story. Breathing rate and depth are very irregular with a rapid and shallow pattern tending to prevail. Pauses in breathing may occur. The average air intake is about the same or less than that of NREMS. The control is much more behavioral with levels of blood carbon dioxide and oxygen having little, if any, influence. As a result, the level of oxygen in the blood may be about the same or lower than that in NREMS and lower than during wakefulness.

During all sleep, the cough response is suppressed. If the irritation in the air passages is great enough, you will awaken to cough. Additionally, because of the changes in breathing regulation, many people, especially the elderly, when falling asleep alternate several deep breaths with several shallow breaths even to the point of stopping breathing for a few seconds. This pattern continues for 10 or 20 or even 60 min until the person is solidly asleep.

6.1.5 Sex Organs

The penis is erect in REMS and sometimes during NREMS in adolescents. The percent of REMS accompanied by erections reaches a peak in the mid-teen years and declines after that. Vaginal enlargement and lubrication also occur during REMS in females though not to the extent that penis erections do in males.

6.1.6 Body/Brain Temperature

While 98.6 °F is your average body temperature, it varies by about a degree warmer or cooler depending on the time of nychthemeron and whether or not you are sleeping. Normally the peak temperature occurs between 6 and 8 pm and the lowest temperature around 4–5 a.m. It would seem that the lower body temperature is due to the immobility during sleep, but people who are paralyzed, bed ridden, or just inactive in bed for the entire nychthemeron still have about half of the average body temperature drop during night sleep. Also, people who remain awake and active during their regular night bedtime also experience about half of the average nightly body temperature drop. Maybe you have noticed becoming cold during the night when you were pulling an all-nighter. Thus the nightly body temperature drop during sleep is due to both a circadian body temperature fluctuation plus reduced heat producing muscle movement.

During NREMS, your body continues to regulate its temperature using the same several methods as it does when you are awake. A portion of the hypothalamus functions as a thermostat, receiving temperature input from sensors throughout the body as well as monitoring its own temperature. It has outputs to the parts of the brain that control temperature regulation mechanisms in the body. If you are too warm, more blood is sent to the surface of the body where it can be radiated to the air. If really hot, you will sweat. When you are cool, less blood is sent to the body surface to avoid losing heat. If really cold, you may shiver. The only difference between sleep and wake is during NREMS when your body temperature set-point, like a thermostat setting, is a bit lower than when awake and your metabolic rate decreases. When you first fall asleep, blood may be sent to the surface of your body to help bring your temperature down to the sleeping set-point. If you are too warm at sleep onset, you may sweat for a while. Whether you realize it or not you sweat a lot when asleep, even if your bedroom is cool. Total sweat may be half a quart or more on a typical night.

Body temperature during REMS is another matter. Your metabolic rate is the same or greater than when in NREMS. However, there is no regulation of your body temperature. It's the difference between having a room with a thermostat that turns on the heater or air conditioner to keep the room temperature steady versus having an unregulated fireplace with a nice fire going in it. With only the fireplace going when it is warm outside, the room will tend to get warmer, but when it is very cold outside, the room may tend to get cooler. The same thing happens during REMS; if you are in a warm room, your body temperature may go up a bit, but the opposite can happen in a cool room. The body makes little, if any, attempt to regulate its temperature, such as by sweating or shivering during REMS. In point of fact we are functioning almost as cold-blooded animals, such as snakes, during

REM sleep. However, if your body gets too cold or too warm, you will wake up and begin regulating again.

Your brain temperature, like your body temperature, will decline a bit in NREMS, but it tends to warm up during REMS because of the high amount of neuronal activity and increased blood flow during that state, which burns so much energy. It may even get warmer than it typically is when awake.

The relationship between sleep and body temperature has yet another level of complexity. Our tendency to sleep and to sleep well depends on our body temperature. We have a propensity to sleep when body temperature is low or dropping but to be awake when body temperature is high or rising. Typically, sleep onset is 6 h before our core body temperature low point, about 6 a.m in the average young adult, and sleep offset follows about 2 h after the temperature low point when body temperature is rising. Interestingly, in the lab, heating the head by blowing warm air on the face increases N3 sleep. A 20 min warm bath a couple of hours before bed for a couple of weeks can do the same thing (Cartwright 2010) and is much more practical. It is not only relaxing but also increases body temperature a bit requiring the body to cool itself down more rapidly, promoting sleep (see Box 6.1). On the other hand if the bed is too warm, such as having an electric blanket set to the maximum, the body has more difficulty cooling down making falling asleep more difficult. An alternative to using too many warm blankets is to wear socks to bed; footwear can be comforting yet not increase body temperature too much.

Box 6.1 Body Temperature at Sleep Onset

The temperature of your body when you begin sleep has an effect on your sleep. Consider the following experiment, which is actually a combination of several research projects done by Jim Horne and colleagues in the mid-1980s (Horne 1988). You and some of your physically fit friends show up at the sleep research lab *during the evening*. Some of your friends have to run hard on a treadmill in a warm room with little air movement until their body temperature increases 2 °C. Others of your friends are luckier, because while they have to run as long as the first group, they can have a fan blowing on them, and they only gain 1 °C of body temperature. But you and a few others are luckiest of all, because you get to soak in a hot tub until your temperature goes up 2 °C. Finally, another group of friends are not so lucky; they get in a different tub only to discover that the water is not hot. They have to stay in it as long as you stay in yours.

After a bit, all of you are prepared for a night of sleep recording in the lab. Before going to sleep, all of you are asked how sleepy you feel. The results are that you and the other hot tubbers and the hot exercisers felt sleepier, slept a bit longer, and got more N3 than the cool exercisers and cool tubbers. The next week, you all come in *during the day* for the same exercise or tub experience. Then you return later that night to sleep in the lab. By the time you go to bed, there are no differences in sleepiness or actual sleep because by this time the increase in body temperature has dissipated. Conclusion: if your body temperature is a bit elevated when you go to bed you may fall asleep more quickly and easily.

Actually heating up just the brain works as well. Jim Horne (personal communication 2004) placed a hood that had warm air blowing through it on volunteer's heads in his lab. The duration of the head warming was thought to be sufficiently long to heat up the brain a bit. They subsequently had deeper and longer sleep. Outside of the lab, warming up the brain to obtain better sleep is impractical. However, brain activity can have the same effect on sleep, but it is the type of brain activity that is important. As Jim Horne has well stated (Horne 2011):

> 'Brain exercise' leading to deeper sleep comes not so much from crosswords or Sudoku but from spending a few hours walking in a changing, interesting environment, looking around and absorbing what is going on. Window shopping, sightseeing; anything new and different enough to hold your attention will do. Having conversations and meeting new people add the important ingredient of novelty, putting further agreeable demands on one's mind and brain. All this new stimulation makes the brain work harder than staying indoors surrounded by familiarity. Reading or watching TV only engages relatively small parts of the brain, unlike getting out and about. Similarly, seeing an exciting film is still too passive—one has to be moving purposely, interacting with your surroundings. In contrast, jogging, while staring at the ground in front and listening to an iPod, is quite a repetitive and boring activity for the brain.

When we try to sleep during a different phase of our temperature rhythm, we may encounter difficulties. If we go to bed later than usual, we can fall asleep easily but may awaken too early or find our sleep fragmented as our body temperature does its typical circadian rise. There is a bit of a mid-afternoon drop in body temperature corresponding to the mid-afternoon dip described in Sect. 3.2.2 during which a brief nap can be beneficial. However, if we try to get all of our nycthemeral sleep during the day when our body temperature is high, we may find that we have trouble falling asleep, remaining satisfactorily asleep, or getting enough sleep.

Finally, REMS and rapid eye movements are more likely when circadian body temperature is low and less likely when it is high. Thus, we have more REMS in the early morning hours.

Room temperature also affects both sleep quantity and quality (Parmeggiani 2000). REMS is generally more sensitive to room temperature than NREMS. As a rule of thumb, people sleep best when the room is about 29 °C (84 °F) but without covers or clothes. When protected by pajamas and covers, a lower room temperature is best. Sleep is still quite good when the room temperature is in the range of slightly above the ideal to several degrees below the ideal. However, the further room temperature gets from this range, the more sleep deteriorates. Also, people show long-term adaptation to air temperature, so during the winter, a lower room temperature would be best compared to the summer.

6.1.7 Hormones

Hormones and sleep have a complex relationship (Leproult 2009). Some hormones can affect sleep and sleep can affect some hormones. Some hormones are affected by specific stages of sleep or affect specific stages. Here are some examples.

Several hormones can enhance sleep such as progesterone, melatonin, neuro-peptide γ, and growth hormone releasing hormone. Adrenalin and cortisol can inhibit sleep or make it more restless. Somatostatin, corticotropin-releasing hormone, and ghrelin can reduce N3 sleep while prolactin, estrogen, and vasoactive intestinal peptide are thought to increase REMS.

Some hormones increase during sleep, such as parathormone, aldosterone, and antidiuretic hormone, while others decrease during sleep, including thyrotropin, insulin, and aldosterone. N3 increases growth hormone in young males and prolactin in everyone, while REMS decreases prolactin. Renin increases during NREMS but decreases during REMS, and insulin levels are higher during NREMS than during REMS. There are further nuances such as during the first half of the sleep period there is an increase in growth hormone but decreases in cortisol and adrenal cortical tropic hormone, but these relationships reverse during the second half of the sleep period.

Some hormones are tied to rhythms. Those tied to the circadian rhythm take several days to adapt to a change in the sleep schedule, such as following jet lag, including cortisol, melatonin, prolactin, and thyrotropin. Cortisol release primarily follows a circadian rhythm beginning to rise about 2 h prior to intended awakening time (Born et al. 1999) with highest levels a few hours later. Sleep, especially N3, does seem to have an attenuating effect on its release, because when sleep is delayed a bit, the low point of cortisol release is also slightly delayed and the peak level mildly attenuated. In women, levels of follicle stimulating hormone and estradiol show a circadian pattern. Other hormones, growth hormone and possibly aldosterone, are more tied to process S and are immediately affected by changes in sleep schedule. Leptin and insulin are affected by both process C and process S, as is thyrotropin. For example, there is an elevation in insulin during the typical sleep period that occurs even when awake, although it is attenuated. And there is an elevation of insulin when sleep occurs during the typical waking period. In adult men, release of luteinizing hormone may be related to the ultradian NREM-REM cycle, but in women it depends on sleep and the phase of the menstrual cycle.

Sleep influences hormones involved in appetite regulation. During sleep elevation of levels of leptin, which reduces appetite, and decreasing levels of the hormone that increases hunger, ghrelin, result in less hunger. Further, glucose regulation, a combination of glucose production by the liver and insulin levels, shows a circadian pattern of a reduction during the typical sleep period, but it is also reduced whenever sleep occurs.

Sleep deprivation adversely affects glucose regulation and decreases the levels of leptin, thyrotropin, and to some extent growth hormone, while increasing the levels of ghrelin. Sleep deprivation or sleep fragmentation diminishes levels of leptin and increases levels of ghrelin. The result of all of these changes is an increase in appetite and unhealthy food choices with the potential for weight gain. (See http://medicalnewstoday.healthology.com/hybrid/hybrid-autodetect.aspx? content_id=2933&focus_handle=sleep-disorders&brand_name=medicalnewstoday for information on sleep loss, hormones, and general health featuring Dr. Eve Van Cauter.)

Box 6.2 Awakening Without an Alarm (Part 2)

In Box 4.2, I reviewed my research on the ability of people to awaken at their desired time without using an alarm clock. A question that followed from this work was just how can people do this? Part of the answer was discovered in subsequent research by Born and colleagues at the University of Lübeck in Germany (Born et al. 1999). They found that the level of the hormone adrenocorticotropin increased during the hour before people were told they would be awakened the next morning. Perhaps this change in this hormone level helps awaken a person.

To further try to understand the mechanism for this ability, Born and colleagues wondered if the expectation of awakening at a certain time influences the secretion of adrenocorticotropin, which tells the adrenal glands to release cortisol. They monitored 15 people during three nights of sleep starting at midnight. For one of the nights, these people were told they could sleep till 6 a.m. For the other two nights, they were told they could sleep until 9 a.m., but on one of those nights were surprised by being awakened earlier at 6 a.m. The amount of adrenocorticotropin in the blood was sampled frequently during their sleep. It began to rise sharply the hour before the early-expected awakening time but not in those expecting the later awakening time but actually were awakened earlier. Born and colleagues conclude that the increase in adrenocorticotropin is a part of the preparation by the body for awakening at a predetermined time.

Still unanswered is how the brain keeps track of time during sleep to be able to cause this release of adrenocorticotropin prior to the anticipated time of awakening. Polysomnographic study of their sleep revealed no difference, including brief arousals, in any of the three conditions. So it was not a change in their pattern of sleep that made a difference in adrenocorticotropin levels. But just what keeps track of time during sleep remains a mystery.

6.1.7.1 Melatonin

Melatonin can facilitate sleep and has been shown to act as a zeitgeber (see Sect. 3.2.2). It is released by the pineal gland located in the middle of the brain about 14 h after awakening. This is normally two hours before sleep onset. Melatonin reaches its peak near the middle of the sleep period, returning to its low waking levels by the end of sleep. Its release is strongly controlled by process C and light. Light striking the eyes inhibits its release (see Sect. 5.1), but if there is an advance or delay in the schedule of light and dark, it will take several days before the release of melatonin follows.

Melatonin has been shown to mildly cause sleepiness, speed sleep onset, and facilitate sleep maintenance. When ingested in pill form, it may have some sleep promoting effects depending on the time of day when it is taken. It promotes sleep when taken several hours before typical sleep time. However, it seems to have little effect on sleep in normal sleepers when taken near or during the typical time of nocturnal sleep. This is perhaps because the pineal gland is already releasing it. Also, depending on time of day, melatonin ingestion may increase REMS or decrease NREMS.

Melatonin also has mild zeitgeber properties and can cause phase changes of the circadian rhythm for sleep/wake (see Sects. 5.1 and 5.3.7.1). However, it has a weaker effect than light as a zeitgeber. See the cautions in Sect. 13.6 about using melatonin as a sleeping pill or to reset the circadian clock because of jet lag or shift work.

6.1.7.2 Age Changes

As we age, there appear to be two phases during which the relationship between sleep and hormones changes. The gradual decline of N3 correlates with the decline in growth hormone through about 50 years of age. After age 50, correlated with what some researchers see as a decline in REMS, cortisol levels increase. These changes in endocrinology with age may be the cause of some aging effects such as memory impairments and reduced response to insulin.

6.1.8 GI Tract

Generally, digestive processes are slower during sleep. Gastric acid production is decreased in the latter sleep period except in those with duodenal ulcers. They produce 3 to 20 times the levels of gastric acid produced in people without ulcers. Swallowing rate decreases in sleep, and the swallowing reflex is absent. Saliva is not produced during sleep. Generally, there is a decrease in the speed at which food and waste move through the GI tract during sleep, but some of this process may be circadian rather than a direct sleep effect.

6.1.9 Renal

Smaller quantities of urine are produced during NREMS, but it is more concentrated. Production is further decreased and concentration further increased during REMS.

6.1.10 Endogenous Sleep Factors

There is evidence for several substances in the body that influence sleep such as cytokines (see Sect. 6.2.1) and adenosine (see Sect. 5.1), and other substances that are thought to also affect sleep. Some of these substances are found primarily in the cerebral-spinal fluid, while others can be found in the blood. This idea is a derivative of a very old "hypnotoxin" notion about what causes sleep. This notion held that during wakefulness a chemical builds up that eventually poisons the brain, resulting in sleep. During sleep, this chemical is degraded or eliminated allowing the return of waking.

Some of the earliest experiments in the twentieth century on sleep occurred when Papenheimer removed cerebral-spinal fluid from a sleepy animal and injected it into the ventricles[1] of an awake animal. The recipient appeared to fall asleep. However, relatively little research attention was directed toward such substances until the last two decades of the twentieth century. It turned out to be not all that is easy to do. Often, when techniques were available to isolate components of the fluid from the donor and inject only that into the ventricles of the recipient, the result was not genuine sleep but a kind of coma. However, some substances did seem to produce genuine sleep, yet none seemed to be necessary and sufficient for sleep. Rather, they appear to be one of many things that facilitate sleep. As of this time, adenosine is the only substance that satisfactorily meets all the criteria for a "hypnogenic" substance.

6.1.11 Genetic

Since the 1980s, evidence has been accumulating that there is a genetic basis for normal and abnormal sleep (see Chaps. 12 and 13). The most convincing data comes from the studies of twins. Identical twins, even if not raised together, have more similar sleep patterns and characteristics than non-identical twins. However, these same studies also show that environment plays a large role in some sleep/wake variables.

More extensive genetic studies of sleep in animals reinforce these findings. Species-specific sleep patterns have been shown to be highly stable, strongly suggesting a genetic basis. Some studies have included using genetically similar versus genetically dissimilar animals. Other studies used selective breeding techniques to show a genetic basis for sleep characteristics, especially total sleep, total REMS, and aspects of circadian rhythms of sleep/wake. Studies in rats show that the amounts of N3 and REMS are inherited via different genes. Studies involving direct genetic manipulation of certain genes in mice resulting in consequences for their sleep are noteworthy.

---

[1] The ventricles are large fluid filled spaces within the brain.

More recently research has shown the genetic basis of the effects of circadian rhythms on sleep. Specific genes with interesting names, such as clock, period, and timeless have been identified. Whether a person tends to be a lark or an owl has, in part, been shown to have a genetic basis.

Box 6.3 Effects of Sleep Deprivation on the Body

Eve Van Cauter, PhD, research associate and professor at the Department of Medicine of the University of Chicago, and her colleagues have shown the negative physiological effects of chronic sleep deprivation on the physiology of the body. Prior to her work, it was shown that the release of growth hormone is severely reduced during sleep deprivation but rebounds when sleep is subsequently obtained. Her studies looked at sleep deprivation effects involving other hormones, especially insulin.

In one study (Spiegel et al. 1999), 11 young adult males were allowed to sleep for only four hours per night for six nights, and then as much as they wanted while in bed for 12 h for the subsequent six nights. Naps were not allowed. They found that during the sleep deprivation, it took 40 % longer to regulate blood sugar levels after a high-carbohydrate meal, a 30 % decrease in insulin secretion ability, and 30 % drop in ability to respond to insulin—all characteristics of early diabetes. Since similar changes are found during normal, non-sleep deprived aging, Van Cauter and colleagues concluded from these and other observations that sleep deprivation mimics human aging and can speed it up.

Van Cauter's studies of people who maintained that they had adapted to chronic shortened sleep again showed a 40 % decrease in insulin sensitivity, unusual cortisol release, a decrease in leptin, a hormone that reduces hunger, and greater sympathetic nervous system activity. There is also an increase in insulin secretion causing more storage of fat that then causes more secretion of insulin that causes more storage of fat and on and on. Chronic shortening of sleep also results in elevated evening cortisol levels and increases sympathetic nervous system activity. The long-term results of chronic partial sleep deprivation are obesity, high blood pressure, diabetes, and memory impairments.

A growing body of studies are showing that sleep is important for other aspects of optimal health (Irwin 2012). Examples include studies showing that insufficient sleep reduces the functioning of the immune system, increases susceptibility to the common cold, and renders vaccinations less effective.

(Website http://medicalnewstoday.healthology.com/hybrid/hybrid-autodetect. aspx?content_id=2957&focus_handle=diet-news&brand_name=medicalnews today features sleep and weight control).

6.2 Effects of the Body on Sleep

Just as sleep can affect the body, so too can the body affect sleep.

6.2.1 Health and Illness

No research is needed to confirm that sleep and sleepiness often increase when illness strikes. It has been assumed by mothers and doctors that this increase in sleep is beneficial, but little research has actually been done to confirm this assumption. In contrast, the common belief that sleep deprivation can increase susceptibility to illness has research support. Little research was directed at these questions until the late 1980s, but continuing efforts since then have begun to provide answers.

It is now well established that bacterial infections lead to changes in sleepiness, N3, REMS, and sleep maintenance. An increase in sleepiness is an early and enduring symptom of infections involving the whole body. N3 time and the amount of delta waves typically increase for a day or two following infection, followed by decreases to below normal levels. In contrast, REMS is decreased for the duration of the infection. Sleep maintenance is disrupted, but other aspects of sleep, such as the NREM-REMS circadian cycles, appear to remain unchanged. It has been shown that this occurs because of increases of certain biochemicals, especially the cytokines, that impact the sleep controlling areas in the brain. A moderate level of these biochemicals is ever-present in our bodies. Their source comes from our body constantly fighting off bacteria in our GI tract. During illness, their quantities are increased, resulting in exaggerated effects on sleep. The degree and timing of these effects depends on the nature of the bacteria, how it got into the body, and the state of the immune system at the time. For example, drugs that increase or decrease the immune system also change sleep during an infection.

Fungal, viral, and protozoan-induced illnesses have effects on sleep that are similar to those of bacterial infections.

There is some research that supports the notion that sleep during illness aids recovery (Opp and Toth 2003). It is likely that extra sleep with more N3 enables the body to devote more resources to healing, to the high metabolic demands that fever causes, and to reduce the possibility of spread of a localized infection.

On the other hand, sleep deprivation compromises the immune system (Bryant et al. 2004). Prolonged sleep deprivation decreases host defenses such as natural killer cells and interleukins. Experiments have also shown that sleep deprivation will increase vulnerability to viral illnesses. Even some lost sleep on one night results in a reduction of natural immune responses. Additionally, it has been shown that sleep deprivation significantly decreases the effectiveness of flu vaccine for several weeks.

Complaints of daytime fatigue and sleep problems are among the earliest signs of HIV infection, the agent that causes AIDS, and worsen as the disease progresses.

Early on, it becomes somewhat more difficult to fall asleep and to stay asleep, and there is a slight increase of daytime sleepiness. During this phase, there is an increase in N3 and other changes and the N3 is more evenly distributed during the sleep period. As the infection worsens, the daytime sleepiness gets worse and sleep onset and maintenance problems continue to get worse. N3 now decreases as does sleep efficiency. The NREM-REMS cycles become more and more disorganized. During the advanced stages of the disease, sleep quality is very poor, and fatigue and lethargy are great. N3 is absent or nearly so, and sleep efficiency is very poor. There are no recognizable NREM-REMS cycles. Yet, the need for sleep greatly increases. Those with HIV who show fewer disturbances of N3 survive longer. The exact mechanisms by which HIV causes these sleep changes is unknown, but changes in cytokine levels that occur during HIV infection are suspected.

Box 6.4 Sleep Hygiene (Moorcroft 2007)

It should be obvious from the material in this and other chapters that our wake time affects our sleep time just as much as our sleep time affects our wake time. There are guidelines to follow when we are awake that can make our sleep come easier and be more effective and less of a problem. All of these suggestions are based on research and have been shown to help many if not all people. People who have difficulties with their sleep should pay special attention to these guidelines.

- It is best to attempt sleep only when you are drowsy. Trying to sleep when you are not ready for sleep may make it more difficult.
- Avoid looking at the clock when in bed. It usually makes people anxious and upset.
- If you are unable to sleep and become upset, get out of bed and go to another room and do something you planned ahead of time that takes your mind off of trying to sleep and that will allow you to relax. Return to bed when you feel drowsy or after about half an hour.
- Get up in the morning at the same time every day, even on weekends and holidays. Going to bed at the same time is a good idea, also. Irregular sleep times can causes changes in your circadian clock that can make future sleep difficult. Choose these times so that you get around 8 h of sleep per night more or less depending on your individual sleep needs (Box 4.1 and Sect. 4.3), leaving you feeling alert after you get up.
- Reserve the use of the bed for sleep. Using it for pleasurable sex is also appropriate, but do not use it to watch TV, read, work, or for other non-sleeping activities. Your conscious and unconscious mind needs to associate bed with being asleep, not awake.

- Avoid excessive napping. A brief, 20 min or so, mid-afternoon nap can be refreshing and natural. More than this amount can cause sleep problems later that night because it can diminish your sleep drive too much.
- Try to relax for an hour before bedtime. Also have a pre-sleep routine close to bedtime that is calming and separates going to sleep from the activities of waking. This routine might include bathing and teeth cleaning, reading, meditating, or praying.
- Regular exercise in the late afternoon or early evening can help you sleep. Morning exercise is alright if it is the only available time. However, avoid rigorous activities and aerobic exercise a couple of hours prior to bedtime. Even better is to get the exercise outdoors in bright sunlight.
- Refrain from consuming caffeine for several hours or more before bedtime if you are especially sensitive to it.
- Do not drink alcohol prior to bedtime and especially do not use it as a sleep aid. While alcohol makes people sleepy, it also causes disturbed sleep, especially later in the sleep period.
- Do not smoke for several hours before bedtime. Reduce or stop smoking if you awaken during the night because you need to smoke.
- If you find yourself worrying after you go to bed, tell yourself that you will worry tomorrow and then think of or imagine something else that is calming and relaxing. If worrying in bed nevertheless occurs, you may want to choose a time earlier in the day to write out potential problems and their possible solutions.
- Arrange the bedroom to make sleeping easier. A comfortable bed in a dark and quiet bedroom with comfortable temperature, humidity, and air circulation can greatly help sleep.

6.2.2 Stress

Stress, whether negative or positive, can affect sleep (Van Reeth et al. 2000). You, like everybody else, have probably noticed this effect at one time or another, although some people are more sensitive to stress. Both acute and chronic stress can disrupt sleep, fragment sleep, and change the amounts of some of the sleep stages. Stress causes an increase of several hormones including adrenal cortical tropic hormone and cortisol that can disrupt sleep continuity and stages. Stress also affects the immune system that, as we have seen, also impacts sleep. Animal studies show that recovery from acute stress includes an increase in both NREM and REMS.

6.2.3 Drugs

Some drugs prescribed for non-sleep related problems, especially those that act on the brain, affect sleep/wake in one way or another. Some drugs may cause insomnia and other problems with sleeping. Others may cause sleepiness, sedation, and/or fatigue. Some drugs prescribed for specific sleep or wake problems may have effects that carry over into the succeeding wake or sleep period, respectively. Other drugs may affect sleep/wake for a period of time after they have been discontinued. Although there are many kinds of drugs that cause some or all of these effects, those drugs used to treat depression, schizophrenia, anxiety, breathing disorders, cardiovascular problems, or those drugs that manipulate histamine or steroid production or response more commonly have significant effects on sleep/wake. Some over-the-counter drugs including nasal decongestants, pain relievers with caffeine, and antihistamines can affect daytime sleepiness and/or nighttime sleep.

Nicotine also affects sleep and sleepiness. It increases alertness and reduces sleepiness. Smokers get these benefits during the day, but one-pack-a-day smokers also have more difficulty getting to sleep and have lighter sleep. Although no differences in amounts of REMS and NREMS are seen in smokers, many have more difficulty staying asleep. Quitting smoking results in the shortening of the amount of time to fall asleep and an increase in N3 and REMS. Some reports also say there is a decrease in waking during sleep, but other reports say there is an increase in arousals for a number of nights.

6.2.4 Pain and Other Sensory Stimuli

In addition to the effects of room temperature on sleep, it is well known that other sensory stimuli can also affect sleep. Pain, either sudden or chronic, affects sleep, but sleep also affects pain. Laboratory studies have confirmed that people in pain may find it more difficult to get to sleep and/or not sleep as well, have less N3 and experience more awakenings. Not sleeping well can make pain worse since it is known that sleep restriction can decrease the pain threshold. (Additional information about pain and sleep is shown at http://medicalnewstoday.healthology.com/hybrid/hybrid-autodetect.aspx?content_id=2949&focus_handle=back-pain&brand_name=medicalnewstoday pain and sleep).

Stimuli such as loud or disturbing noise, including stimulating or annoying music, can make it more difficult to get to sleep and even disturb sleep. Soft and soothing noises or music may facilitate getting to sleep. Likewise, bright or changing light can disrupt sleep onset as can irregular bumping and jarring of the body, like when riding in a car on poor roads. Some people report that some smells can cause problems with sleep, while other smells facilitate it. Indigestion, too, can cause fragmentation of sleep.

6.2.5 Exercise

It is not possible to make a blanket statement about the effects of exercise on sleep. Exercise can mean many different things to different people such as aerobic or non-aerobic, mild to intense, and causing sweat or not. Also fitness level and age make a difference in the effects of exercise on sleep. While most exercise is generally recognized as beneficial to the body, it can also cause injury, which in turn can affect sleep. These considerations notwithstanding, the overall experimental evidence shows that exercise four to eight hours before bedtime that is sufficient to raise body temperature can increase total sleep time, slightly delay REMS onset, increase N3, and slightly reduce REMS. Reduced exercise in trained athletes can produce the opposite effects. Many sleep specialists caution against exercise in the evening close to bedtime because it may be too arousing, making falling asleep difficult.

6.2.6 Sexual Activity

Many men report that orgasm aids them in falling asleep. In contrast, sexual activity and orgasm are arousing, not relaxing, for many women. Not only can this difference affect sleeping, it can also affect relationships. Men fall asleep after sex because of biological-based tendencies, not insensitivity. Women do not share the same tendencies and like loving attention, not sleep, following sexual activity.

6.2.7 Nutrition

Throughout recorded history, sleepiness has been thought to be a consequence of eating a big meal. Not only how much you eat, but also what you eat has been thought to contribute to sleepiness and influence subsequent sleep. Scientific research has confirmed some but not all of these relationships.

William C. Orr, Ph.D., Director and CEO of The Lynn Health Sciences Institute at the University of Oklahoma Health Sciences Center, has reviewed the published reports covering the influence of eating on sleep (Orr, personal communication 2011). He concludes that many people report experiencing sleepiness after eating. They also report that this is true after an especially large meal. Studies by others in animals show that larger meals result in longer N3 and REMS periods. Excess food intake increases sleepiness because of increased absorption of bacteria and bacteria products into the blood (see Sect. 6.2.1).

Orr also concluded that sleepiness is greatest after an hour and a half to two hours after a meal. However, when lipids are consumed, the maximal sleepiness is delayed by three to three and one half hours. On the other hand a study published in 2011 concluded that, while more research is needed, late dinner or snacking correlated with poorer sleep (Crispim et al. 2011).

> While there have been numerous articles in the popular press about what types of foods to eat to improve sleep they do not back up their claims with research. To my knowledge, there have been no studies of the sleep/wake effects of specific foods like carrots, spinach, hamburgers, and rice. (Many of us have also looked in vain for a sleep study confirming the benefits of eating oatmeal raison cookies!) Most studied have been the effects of caffeine, alcohol, nicotine, and tryptophan in food. (Orr, personal communication 2011)

Even the little research that has been done—much of it on specific foods and how they effect sleep—is very controversial and poorly replicated (Orr, personal communication 2011). There is one study that was well done (Orr et al. 1997). Orr and colleagues investigated sleep onset times following different types of meals. They had 10 male subjects take five polysomnographically recorded naps over a period of more than four hours. Between the first and second nap, they ate a meal that was either high-fat, or high-carbohydrate, or a mixture of the two. For another group of 10 males, the meals were either solid, liquid, or an equivalent amount of water. There were no significant differences in sleep latencies as a result of consuming the high-fat, high-carbohydrate, or mixed meals, but the solid meals, unlike the liquid meal or plain water, resulted in shorter sleep onset times.

Weight loss as a result of malnutrition or dieting has the opposite effect on sleep than weight gain. When losing weight, there is an increase in the time it takes to get to sleep, less time spent asleep, and a decrease in N3. Additionally, there is more fragmentation of sleep when losing weight. During the time a person is gaining weight, total sleep time increases because of increases in both N3 and REMS as well as less fragmentation of sleep. Skipping a single meal or several meals prior to bedtime increases the amount of N3 but also increases sleep fragmentation. A light snack such as cereal and milk, yogurt, or crackers prior to bedtime tends to increase sleep duration and reduce the amount of wake time during the sleep period. However, a large meal or eating something that results in indigestion before bedtime may disturb sleep. For example it is now well established that nighttime heartburn can cause significant sleep disruption and subsequent daytime sleepiness (Orr et al. 2004).

In some very interesting studies, Iraki and associates (see for example Iraki et al. 1997) have found that Moslems experience decreases in daytime alertness resulting from changes in sleep habits during the month of Ramadan, when they give up eating and drinking between sunrise and sunset.

Although sleep is typically a long period of fasting, glucose levels in the blood do not decrease. They do decrease during a similar period of fasting while quietly lying down awake. This difference occurs because glucose is used more slowly during night sleep. A minimum of glucose usage occurs during mid-sleep but begins to increase as morning approaches. Two-thirds of the decrease in glucose usage occurs because of the lower metabolic rate of N3, but other factors also play a role, such as a decrease in muscle tone and changes in hormone levels during sleep. The gradual increase later in sleep occurs because of less N3 during that time.

6.2.7.1 Caffeine

Caffeine has been confirmed to combat the effects of sleep deprivation but also to disrupt sleep. It works by reducing the effects of adenosine in the brain (see Sect. 5.1). Although it has little effect on people who are not sleep deprived or not dependent on it, caffeine can increase arousal and decrease sleepiness in sleep-deprived people. It can make performance more efficient and more accurate in people who are sleep-deprived. The degree of the effects depends upon the amount of caffeine consumed. Generally, good effects are seen with 100 mg, although its effects can vary with individual sensitivity, the type of task, and the level of sleepiness. Consumption of caffeine every few hours has improved alertness and performance over that of a placebo for 40 to 48 continuous hours without sleep. Notice carefully what this statement says; caffeine did not restore alertness and performance to the level it would have been with normal sleep, but it did make things better.

Caffeine consumed before bed, even several hours before bed in some people, will disrupt sleep. This disruption can occur even in people who have no awareness of the effects caffeine is having on them. It increases the time it takes to get to sleep, sleep fragmentation, and the frequency and duration of wakefulness during the sleep period.

Considerable caffeine is found in many popular drinks but is also in many foods and medicines (see Table 6.1). It reaches its peak concentration in the body about ½–1 h after consumption, with half still present after an additional 2–6 h. It may not be totally cleared out of the body for 8–14 h. In some individuals, children, pregnant women, and the elderly, it stays active even longer, sometimes much longer. Regular consumption of caffeine can lead to tolerance and dependence. That is, it becomes less effective, yet the person experiences negative withdrawal effects such as headaches, lethargy, sleepiness, fatigue, and performance decreases for a few days without it. Some people may continue to consume caffeine to avoid these withdrawal effects.

6.2.7.2 Alcohol (e.g., Roehrs and Roth 2001)

Like caffeine, alcohol affects waking, daytime sleepiness and nighttime sleep. During waking, the effects of alcohol can be described as having two phases; it is initially arousing followed by a sedating effect. The higher the alcohol level in the blood, the shorter the MSLT sleep onset times. But its effects on sleepiness also depend on the degree of prior sleep deprivation and the circadian time of the nychthemeron. It has been calculated that three drinks (drink = 1 oz of 80 proof liquor, 12 oz of beer, or 4 oz of wine) are the equivalent of six drinks in a person who has had five successive nights of only five hours of sleep. In contrast, people who have extra prior sleep are made less sleepy by alcohol than a person who has averaged eight hours of sleep per night. Alcohol produces a greater sleepiness when consumed during the night or mid to late afternoon, such as during happy hour, when the body's circadian rhythm for sleepiness is higher. Blood alcohol levels as little as one-fifth of the legal limit in the United States have been found to impair

Table 6.1 Amount of caffeine in some common products	Coffee, brewed	100–150 mg
	Tea, cup	60–75 mg
	Cola soft drinks, 12 oz	40–75 mg
	Chocolate, 1 oz	36–47 mg
	Pain medicines, over the counter	32–65 mg
	Cold remedies	15–60 mg
	Stimulants, over the counter	100–200 mg
	Energy drinks	0–2352.9 mg/oz (most of them 5–100 mg/oz)

driving in sleepy people in the early morning hours. Surprisingly, the sleepiness produced by alcohol has been shown to outlast the presence of alcohol in the blood for several hours or until sleep is obtained. It is as if alcohol flips a sleepiness switch in the brain that stays that way until it is switched off again. Thus, experiments have shown that a sleepy person who has a few drinks during happy hour can be a dangerous driver long after their blood alcohol level returns to zero.

Since alcohol causes relaxation and sleepiness, it is widely used by people to help them sleep at night. Unfortunately, this practice, too, is a problem because of the two-phased effect. After drinking moderate amounts of alcohol that brings the blood concentration to 0.05 at bedtime, the time to get to sleep is much shorter, and N3 time often is initially increased. However, there is a delay in getting to the first REMS period, and total REMS in the first half of the night is reduced. By the second half of the night, blood alcohol level is at or close to zero, since the body clears about one drink per hour. At this point there is a rebound effect. Sleep is generally disturbed and restless, there is more wakefulness or N1, and REMS is increased. The net effect can be a relatively poor night of sleep. After several consecutive nights of going to bed following moderate drinking, the first-half-of-the-night effects are diminished but not the second-half-of-the-night effects. Subsequently, the night or nights of sleep not preceded by drinking alcohol may contain excessive amounts of REMS.

6.2.7.3 Tryptophan

Tryptophan is an amino acid prevalent in foods like dairy products, fowl, beans, some nuts, and bananas. It is also the raw material used in the brain to manufacture the neurotransmitter serotonin. Since early research implicated serotonin with sleep (see Box 5.3) and anecdotes prevail about the sleep inducing properties of foods like turkey and a warm glass of milk, it was thought that ingestion of tryptophan could promote sleep onset. While research was being conducted to test this hypothesis, many people tried taking easily available, unregulated tryptophan pills during the 1980s as an alternative to other sleeping pills. But a serious side effect, possibly from contaminants in the unregulated tryptophan pills, quickly caused them to be removed from availability in the United States in 1991. This ban was loosened in 2001 but only for tryptophan manufactured in the US. Meanwhile, the research was equivocal about tryptophan's ability to promote sleep. It was suggested that some of the research used too low of a dose or that it was tested on normal sleepers in whom it would be hard to show an improvement in sleep. Later studies suggested that it could help about half of insomniacs get and stay asleep if they took doses of one to two grams.

Since there are problems with the pill form of tryptophan, can eating foods rich in it before going to bed help your sleep? The answer is unclear. It is not all that simple for tryptophan in food to get to your brain, and often there simply may not be enough of it that gets there to make a significant difference. It has to go through the digestive process that may be too slow when a lot of other food is also being digested. Additionally you cannot be sure that the food you eat contains a sufficient amount of tryptophan to make a difference. Finally, it competes with other amino acids to get into the brain; if there are many competitors, little gets in. At best, it takes about an hour for the brain to manufacture serotonin from newly arrived tryptophan. In the end, it seems that even if all goes well, the effect of consuming tryptophan rich food is a mild one that does not always work. So consume something like milk or bananas an hour or more before bedtime if you like. It might help you sleep simply because having a little something in the stomach can be relaxing, but do not count on it simply because of the extra tryptophan you take in.

6.2.7.4   Herbs and Supplements

The use of herbs and supplements to obtain better sleep has become very popular with many "natural substance experts" offering advice on what is effective. However, the information provided is too often conflicting, actual scientific evidence from well-designed research studies to back up the claims is sparse, and sometimes dangerous interactions of these herbs with one another or with drugs are becoming apparent. The most frequently mentioned herbs are passionflower for temporary insomnia, the aroma of lavender for calming, and valerian or kava for promoting sleep. Also others such as catnip, chamomile, lime flowers, gotu kola, cowslip flowers, hops, lemon balm, lady's slipper, and skullcap have been recommended for sleep disorders. Supplements suggested for sleep include melatonin, GBL, and magnesium for sleep disorders, and serotonin for good sleep.

Valerian has been used for centuries for its reputed relaxing and calming effects as a way to relieve insomnia. There has been some good research done on it, but the results are equivocal (Fernández-San-Martín et al. 2010). For example, Donath et al. (2000) had 16 people with insomnia, 4 males and 12 females, take valerian extract for 1 day or 14 consecutive days preceded or followed by a look-alike placebo for another 1 day or 14 consecutive days. Neither the subjects nor the researchers knew when the subjects were taking the valerian extract or placebo until the experiment was completed. Polysomnographic recordings were made before and after taking the course of valerian or placebo, and subjective ratings of sleep and daytime performance were also obtained at these times. The one-day dose of valerian extract had no effect on any of the measures. The 14-day use of valerian extract resulted in no difference in sleep efficiency, but a more rapid onset of N3 and an increase in the amount of N3 were seen. Subjects reported they fell asleep more quickly. They also noted few side effects from taking valerian extract. The authors concluded that valerian extract might be useful for the treatment of mild insomnia. However, other studies have not shown such clear-cut or even positive results (Cauffield and Forbes 1999).

Yet there are potential problems with available valerian extract in purity and actual strength as well as with its stability. A study (ConsumerLab.com 2001) by an independent lab that evaluates nutrition products and dietary supplements and independently confirmed by a second lab showed that 4 of 17 products claiming to contain valerian actually had none, and another 4 contained about half of what was stated on the label. Cautions about the use of other herbs and supplements have been issued because of preliminary or inconclusive research data on their effectiveness and the potential for bad side effects (Cauffield and Forbes 1999).

Kava has also received research attention. It has been shown to reduce the time to get to sleep and promote deeper sleep. However, cautions about liver damage following use of Kava have been issued (FDA 2002). Studies of the long-term effects of taking valerian and kava are needed. There have been few published studies using good scientific methods on the other herbs.

Other folk and natural remedies for improved sleep have included rubbing garlic on your soles, putting a cut raw onion under your pillow, or sleeping on a small pillow filled with hops flowers. There are suggestions to avoid foods with a lot of tyramine, the raw material the brain uses to make norepinephrine, before bedtime. This list includes cheese, sauerkraut, wine, cured meats, eggplant, spinach, and tomatoes. There appears to be little if any scientific research to back up the use of any of these remedies.

6.3 Effects of the Weather on Sleep

Except for the effect of air temperature (see Sect. 6.1.6), there has been little research done on the effects of weather on normal sleep. It is thought that weather extremes or obvious changes in the weather can have effects, generally negative, on sleep. But there is also some evidence that more subtle differences in things like barometric pressure, ionic fields, lunar phase, and solar disturbances also affect sleep.

6.4 Conclusion

Sleep affects the body. Many of the physiological systems of the body such as the autonomic nervous system, the cardiovascular system, the respiratory system, hormonal system, and the control of body temperature function differently to some or a great extent during sleep. This provides many benefits. But the health of the body and what is put into it such as food, drugs, caffeine, and alcohol also affects sleep timing and quality. Depending on the choices made by an individual these effects can be beneficial or detrimental.

References

Amlaner, C. J., & Fuller, P. M. (Eds.). (2009). *Basics of sleep* (2nd ed.). Westchester, Illinois: Sleep Research Society.

Born, J., Hansen, K., Marshall, L., Molle, M., & Fehm, H. (1999). Timing the end of nocturnal sleep. *Nature, 397,* 29–30.

Bryant, P. A., Trinder, J., & Curtis, N. (2004). Sick and tired: does sleep have a vital role in the immune system? *Nature Reviews Immunology, 4,* 457–467.

Cartwright, R. C. (2010). *The twenty-four hour mind.* New York: Oxford University Press.

Cauffield, J. S., & Forbes, H. J. (1999). Dietary supplements used in the treatment of depression anxiety and sleep disorders. *Lippincotts Primary Care Practice, 3,* 290–304.

Chokroverty, S. (Ed.). (2009). *Sleep Disorders Medicine* (3rd ed.). Philadelphia: Saunders.

ConsumerLab.com. (2001). *Many herbal sleep products lack key claimed ingredient.* Retrieved from http://www.consumerlab.com/news/Valerian_Tests/7_9_2001/.

Crispim, C. A., Zimberg, I. Z., dos Reis, B. G., Diniz, R. M., Tufik, S., & de Mello, M. T. (2011). Relationship between food intake and sleep pattern in healthy individuals. *Journal of Clinical Sleep Medicine, 7,* 659–664.

Donath, F., Quispe, S., Diefenbach, K., Maurer, A., Fietze, I., & Roots, I. (2000). Critical evaluation of the effect of valerian extract on sleep structure and sleep quality 47–53. *Pharmacopsychiatry, 33,* 47–53.

FDA. (2002). *Consumer advisory: Kava-containing dietary supplements may be associated with severe liver injury,* 25 March 2002. Retrieved from http://www.fda.gov/Food/ResourcesForYou/Consumers/ucm085482.htm.

Fernández-San-Martín, M. I., Masa-Font, R., Palacios-Soler, L., Sancho-Gómez, P., Calbó-Caldentey, C., & Flores-Mateo, G. (2010). Effectiveness of Valerian on insomnia: a meta-analysis of randomized placebo-controlled trials. *Sleep Medicine, 11,* 505–511.

Horne, J. (2006). *Sleepfaring.* New York: Oxford University Press.

Horne, J. (2011). Walking to a good night's sleep. *The Telegraph,* 18 Nov 2011.

Horne, J. A. (1988). *Why We Sleep.* New York: Oxford University Press.

Iraki, L. B., Hakkou, F., Amrani, N., Abkari, A., & Touitou, Y. (1997). Ramadon diet restrictions modify the circadian time structure in humans a study on plasma grastrin, insulin, glucose, and calcium and on gastric pH. *The Journal of Clinical Endrorinology & Metabolism, 82,* 1261–1273.

Irwin, M. R. (2012). Sleep and infectious disease risk. *Sleep, 35,* 1025–1026.

Kryger, M. H., Roth, T. R., & Dement, W. C. (Eds.). (2011). *Principles and Practice of Sleep Medicine* (5th ed.). St. Louis: Elsevier.

Lee-Chiong, T. (2011). *Somnology 2.* Seattle: Amazon.

Leproult, R. S. (2009). Sleep and endocrinology. In C. F. Amlander (Ed.), *Basics of sleep guide* (2nd ed., pp. 157–167). Westchester: The Sleep Research Society.

Moorcroft, W. H. (2007). Sleep hygiene. In L.-C. T. Burkov N. (Ed.), *Fundamentals of Sleep Technology* (pp. 515–520). Philadelphia: Lippincott Williams & Wilkins.

Opp, M. R., & Toth, L. A. (2003). Neural-immune interactions in the regulation of sleep. *Frontiers in Bioscience, 8,* d768–d779.

Orr, W. C. (2011). Personal communication.

Orr, W. C., Shadid, G., Harnish, M. J., & Elsenbruch, S. (1997). Meal composition and its effect on postprandial sleepiness. *Physiology & Behavior, 62,* 709–712.

Orr, W. C., Heading, R. L., Johnson, F., & Kryger, M. (2004). Review article: sleep and its relationship to gastro-oesophageal reflux. *Alimentary Pharmacology & Therapeutics, 20,* 39–46.

Parmeggiani, P. L. (2000). Influence of the temperature signal on sleep in mammals. *Biolgical Signals and Receptors, 9,* 279–282.

Spiegel, K., Leproult, R., & Van Cauter, E. (1999). Impact of sleep debt on metabolic and endocrine function. *Lancet, 354,* 1435–1439.

Van Reeth, O., Weibel, L., Spiegel, K., Leproult, R., Dugovic, C., & Maccari, S. (2000). Interactions between stress and sleep: from basic research to clinical situations. *Sleep Medicine Reviews, 4,* 201–219.

Part III

Dreams and Dreaming

Humans have been curious about dreams throughout recorded history, and most probably well before then. Typical questions about dreams include:

What are they about?

Where do they come from?

What are their functions?

How can people use them?

There have been a variety of different answers

Part of the problem with finding answers is that dreams are so very private. We are the only ones who can experience our dreams. People have endeavored to share their dreams with others when awake by describing their recall of them verbally or even by drawing them, acting them out, or dancing them. Sometimes this recall occurs the next morning but it can be hours, days, or even years later. And almost always people report that they cannot completely and adequately do justice to their dream experiences in their dream reports. They are just not easy to recall and relate. Often we know we have had a dream but only can recall wisps of it or even nothing at all. This inability to remember causes a problem of representativeness (Domhoff 1996). We cannot be sure that the dream recalls we are able to collect for study are an unbiased sample of all dreams in all people.

Also, there is not much that can be done to influence the content of dreams (Domhoff 1996). This difficulty severely limits the experimental possibilities for manipulating dreams to see what they are all about. And it is not possible to independently check the accuracy of the dream recall, which constrains the ability to be certain of the findings about the contents of dreams (Domhoff 1996).

For centuries, these problems have limited the ability to study and understand what dreams are all about. That limitation did not stop people from trying to study and understand them, but until recently there was only a smattering of scientific research done on dreams and dreaming. The late nineteenth century marks the beginning of systematic dream research, for this period is when a few psychologists began to write down their own dreams and then to study the nature of these recalls. But it was during the twentieth century that there was an increase in interest within the scientific community in dreams. Starting with Freud's Interpretation of Dreams published in 1900 (see Chaps. 8, 9), there was great psychological interest that continues today.

Just as important, there was another transition point in the mid-1950s with the discovery of REMS and its apparent association with dreaming that stimulated broader interest in dreams and the process of dreaming. People sleeping in the lab could be awakened during or right after a period of REMS and immediately asked what was going through their mind before they were awakened. Eighty to ninety percent of the time, they responded with a recalled dream. As a result, it was believed that scientists could get a greater number of dream reports, and since they were recalled immediately after they were experienced, much more accurate ones.

This awakened interest in dreams and dreaming led to an explosion of research. Today, people in various academic areas including clinical psychology, cognitive psychology, biopsychology, anthropology, brain research, religious studies, and literary criticism are doing research on dreams and dreaming for the purpose of trying to understand these things themselves (Bulkeley 1996). Because of these efforts, we now have a greater and better understanding of dreams and the process of dreaming. But, as we shall see, there is still considerable disagreement about the nature of dreams and dreaming.

Chapter 7 describes what is known about the content of dreams based on the study of people's recall of their dreams. Chapter 8 looks at the process of dreaming. Chapter 9 summarizes many of the major theories about dreams and dreaming.

References

Bulkeley, K. (1996). *Among all these dreamers*. Albany, NY: State University of New York Press.

Domhoff, G. (1996). *Finding meaning in dreams: A quantitative approach*. New York: Plenum.

Freud, S. (1900). *Interpretation of dreams*. New York: Modern Library.

Chapter 7
Dreams

Contents

In this chapter, we will focus on the characteristics and content of dreams as gleaned from studies of what people recall of their dreams. But first I have to clarify several issues related to this endeavor.

Specific references to statements in this chapter that can be found in multiple, widely available sources are not included in the text. A selection of these sources is listed below and can also be consulted for verification or more detail. (Carskadon 1993; Domhoff 1996; Kryger et al. 2011; Lee-Chiong 2006; Moorcroft 1993).

W. H. Moorcroft, *Understanding Sleep and Dreaming*,
DOI: 10.1007/978-1-4614-6467-9_7,
© Springer Science+Business Media New York 2013

7.1 Discovery of REMS and Its Relationship to Dreaming

Discovery of REMS was one of those serendipitous discoveries that are surprisingly important in the history of science. Graduate student Eugene Aserinsky was working with physiologist and pioneer sleep researcher Nathaniel Kleitman in the sleep laboratory at the University of Chicago early in the 1950s, looking for slow eye movements throughout sleep like those that had previously been observed when people fell asleep (Aserinsky and Kleitman 1953). But watching the eyes move under the eyelids during the wee hours of the morning was tedious. Therefore, they decided to record them electrically using EOG. To their surprise, they found periodic occurrences of rapid eye movements during sleep. When they turned their focus on these periods of rapid eye movements, they soon found the movements were associated with dreaming.

Shortly thereafter, medical student Bill Dement joined Kleitman's lab and took over the study of these rapid eye movements. The team noted the apparent association of dreaming with rapid eye movement sleep that occurred every 90–100 min during the course of sleep (Dement and Kleitman 1957). It took several years for these observations to become recognized by the scientific community, but once they were, many researchers were waking people up during REMS to intensively study dreams.

At first, it was eagerly anticipated that the study of dreaming during REMS would lead to an understanding of the unconscious mind, but that hope has not been borne out. Other researchers investigated the effects of REMS deprivation, thinking that they were investigating the effects of dream deprivation, which at that time was thought to be potentially psychologically devastating. Although it was found that this hypothesis also was wrong, much interest in sleep and dreams and good information about REMS came out of these misdirected experiments.

Videos of Drs. Kleitman and Dement using older equipment but featuring their ground breaking discoveries can be found at http://www.youtube.com/watch?v= 9nmVzXxdUeU&NR=1&feature=endscreen from 3:00 to 4:30 and all of http:// www.youtube.com/watch?v=GidiLjnbNGc&feature=related.

7.1.1 Lab Versus "Home" Dreams

Once it was possible to collect dreams in the lab by awakening people from REMS, the question was soon asked, "Yes, but what is the effect of the lab on the dreams?" It was noted that images and references to the lab environment were present in 20–30 % of lab dream recalls. Could the lab have other effects on the content of recalled dreams? Research was undertaken to answer this question.

It was reasoned that the lab dream recalls were *sampled*, but home dream recalls were *selected*, which could make a difference in content. That is, *lab dream recalls* were similar to having you wear a beeper during the day and recording what was happening to you every time the beeper went off. *Home dream recalls* were like asking you at the end of the day, or even days later, to describe what you experienced during the day. The "beeper technique" would probably produce a lot of bland, ordinary content, but the "asking later technique" would more likely return the notable or unusual. It was hypothesized that obtaining dream recalls in the lab was similar to the "beeper technique" whereas home dream recalls were like the "asking later technique". Another hypothesis was that people would feel more inhibited in what they reported in the lab because it is a more public venue than recalls privately recorded at home.

Research in the 1960s found those very differences predicted by both hypotheses (Domhoff and Schnelder 1999). Lab dream recalls are blander such as containing less aggression, less sex, and fewer misfortunes. Yet, in other ways, lab and home recalls were very similar in details like types of characters and the presence of at least one bizarre element.

Researchers in the 1970s endeavored to make the conditions for dream collection in the lab and at home more similar by using the same procedures in each. For example, in both situations, an alarm clock would randomly awaken people from sleep, then tape record any dream recall. The result was the virtual elimination of the differences in dream recall content from the lab compared to the home. Also, reanalysis of some of the key 1960s data showed that the differences reported earlier were actually quite small except that there were less hostility and aggression in the lab dream recalls.

More recently, comparisons have been made of sleep-awakening recalls with what was recalled of those same dreams the next morning. Contrary to expectations, saliency of dream content did not appear to be a factor influencing which dreams were recalled in the morning. However, there was a greater likelihood to (1) recall the dreams from the end of the night; (2) recall those that were longer; and (3) recall those with more emotional intensity (Domhoff 2003).

Today, it is realized that the setting of dream recall collection and the techniques can affect dream content, but the more similar the collection conditions are the less the difference. It can be concluded that while setting can have a bit of an effect on what is recalled about the dream, the essential dreaming process is the same. Also, the few effects of the laboratory on dream content appear now to be known. The major advantage of the laboratory has been the ability to sample dreaming across the night and in specific stages.

It is important to note that there is another useful method of studying the nature of dreams—namely to study dream journals kept by individuals for long periods of time. Such studies show that while there may be great differences in what is dreamed about among individuals, there is a great deal of consistency in dream content within an individual beginning in the late teens and continuing to old age. Day to day experiences seem to have little influence on dream content. In contrast, dream reports collected in the context of psychotherapy have not been used very much in scientific studies of dreaming, probably because the reports are often considered to be contaminated by the psychological interpretation of the therapist.

7.2 Problems with Studying Dreams

Before we turn to what has been discovered about dreams and dreaming, we need to address the fact that dream research is difficult.

7.2.1 No Direct Access to Dreams

The main problem with dream research is that there is no direct access to dreams. REMS awakenings are thought to come the closest to accessing dreams because of how close in time the recall is to the experience of the dream. Also REMS awakenings yield more dream recalls and more details per dream.

Yet, even this technique is far from perfect, because the dreamer still needs to awaken in order to relate what the dream was about. But awakening causes a change in the functional organization of the brain (see Chap. 5 especially Sect. 5.4) that may affect what is recalled. Also, dreams are experienced primarily visually, but the typical dream report is verbal. Verbally describing a visual experience is imperfect and incomplete at best. Furthermore, studies have shown that factors such as the gender, age, and status of the person who collects the recall and whether the recall is written down or tape-recorded; affect the content of the recall. In addition, my research has shown that our memories of dreams are highly labile (see Box 7.1). Additionally, people usually report more about what *happened* in a dream than how intense or detailed these experiences were (Strauch and Meier 1996).

Additionally, it has been found that if a dream lasts less than about 15 min then it is possible to recall the entire dream (Horne 2006). However, if it is longer than 15 min the early part seems to be forgotten. This is like reading only the end of novels after skipping the beginning.

7.2.2 No Clear Definition of a Dream

Everybody knows what a dream is from their own experience. Yet, it is surprisingly difficult to develop a clear definition with universal agreement. The lack of a universally accepted definition is another source of problems for dream study.

Part of this problem comes from the wide range of backgrounds among those who study dreams—psychological, medical, anthropological, literary, philosophical, and physiological. For some researchers the definition is very narrow; dreams are only created during sleep and have a narrative quality but with hallucinatory and bizarre elements. For others dreams are more broadly defined; dreams may also occur when awake, such as during meditation, drug influenced states, daydreaming, hallucinating, and during drifting waking thought. Even if the definition is restricted to sleep, there can be wide disagreement. For some, any mental activity (mentation) during sleep should be considered a dream. For others mental activity needs to be restricted "to more elaborate, vivid, and story-like experiences recalled upon awakening" (Kryger et al. 2011).

Jim Pagel, a sleep disorders physician and dream researcher in Colorado, asked college students, sleep disorder patients, and medical professionals with an interest in dreams to select what they thought was the best definition of a dream from a list of widely differing definitions (Pagel et al. 2001; Pagel and Myers 2002). The most commonly selected definition was "a report of mental activity occurring during sleep," but this definition was chosen by only slightly less than one-third of the participants. The selections also differed by group. For example, the most frequent selection by college students, selected by one in three, was "any non-conscious thought, feeling, or emotion," but this choice was the least selected by the medical professionals—less than 1 in 20.

This is an important issue, though. Science means precision and a part of being precise is defining terms carefully. Without doing so, there is a very real danger that misunderstandings and miscommunications will occur, because when people are not talking about the same thing, this results in a muddled understanding of natural phenomena. Without precise definition, the data collected and labeled as dreams may be quite different in different studies, making the conclusions non-comparable.

In spite of these difficulties, it is still beneficial to study dream recall, because it gives us insights into the nature of dreams and dreaming, and the recall itself can be useful for dream interpretation. Nevertheless, the constraints these difficulties pose need to be kept in mind.

Before continuing the discussion of how to define a dream, another important issue first needs to be considered.

7.2.3 Does Dreaming Occur in NREMS?

Right from the start of research on the relationship between REMS and dreaming, researchers noted that they could occasionally get a dream report from awakenings out of NREMS. Nevertheless, the notion that dreaming only occurs in REMS was maintained for many years. However, eventually more attention began to be paid to mental content during NREMS.

One of the early explanations was that these NREMS dreams were not really experienced in NREMS but were memories of a dream left over from the recent REMS period or from bits of REMS brain processes occurring during NREMS. Later, others examined these NREMS dreams and concluded that there was mental content during NREMS, but it was, for the most part, not like that of REMS dreams (see below). But this did not satisfy everyone nor explain all of the data.

Soon it was reported that a good dream report could sometimes be obtained from people in the sleep lab who were awakened before the first REMS period.

Obviously, these recalls were not left over from the prior REMS period, since that was many waking hours ago. Also, when corrected for length, some studies report that naïve judges were unable to determine which reports were from REMS awakenings or NREMS awakenings but other studies find that considerable differences remain. Subsequent studies found that NREM recalls toward the end of the sleep period resemble REM recalls more than NREM recalls from earlier in the sleep period. At this point, the equating of dreaming solely with REMS apparently had broken down. But not entirely, for REMS awakenings continue to result in dream recall more frequently than did NREMS awakenings, and there are often differences in their quality.

Nielsen (2000) extensively reviewed 29 REMS and 33 NREMS studies of dream recall rate. The average REMS recall rate was around 80 % compared to an average recall rate for NREMS of around 40 %. It was not unusual for subjects never to report a recall following NREMS awakenings in spite of multiple tries over several nights. In contrast, it is rare to not obtain several dream recalls during a succession of REMS awakenings. Yet, today there is still no clear consensus about dreams occurring in NREMS (e.g., Hobson et al. 2000; Nielsen 2000).

Much of the controversy over whether dreams occur in NREMS is about what should be considered a dream and what should not. If any kind of mental activity is accepted as a dream, then around 60 % of NREMS awakenings yield dream reports. However, as the criteria for a dream becomes more stringent, the percent of awakenings from NREMS that yield dream reports drops. Using the strictest definition, a dream is a holistic mental experience, some would say hallucination, while asleep. It consists of characters interacting over a period of time in a succession of several organized and apparently real, although often bizarre, vivid images or scenes. Using this strict definition reports of dreams following NREMS awakenings occur less than 10 % of the time.

There is no doubt that some mental processes are occurring during much of NREMS, but using the stricter definition the vast majority of these experiences cannot be called dreams. Most NREMS mentation is shorter, less dramatic, less vivid, not as emotional, not as elaborate, not progressive, and contains less activity. Most of what is recalled from NREMS is more like logical and linear thinking (Cartwright 2010) or like a photograph, often not clearly in focus. These recalls are more often based on autobiographical events, specific times and places. In contrast the experience in REMS contains elaborated story lines clearly presented as in a movie, with story-like sequences that are more perceptual and emotional. They are more like bizarre fantasies with emotional tone. And as long-time sleep researcher Alan Rechtschaffen eloquently put it, there is a "single-mindedness and isolation" by the dreamer in a dream (Rechtschaffen 1978) meaning a total absorption in the dream without an awareness that it is not reality. In contrast to REMS mental processes, those occurring in NREMS have no sense of the dreamer participating in the experience and there are no social interactions.

For the rest of this text, we will assume the following more restricted definition: (1) *dreams are a kind of thinking that occurs during sleep when the brain is activated with little input from our environment, and* (2) *dreams are experienced as a series of events that seem real at the time they are experienced*. Furthermore, the dreamer is often a participant in the dream but always an observer. Other sleep mentation does occur, but is more like an image or a thought, often vague, that lacks the sense of participation and sequential actions. Such mental activity during NREMS should be called *NREMS mentation* to distinguish it from dreams. Furthermore, dreaming only occurs during sleep and not when awake.

The problem is if REMS dreaming and NREMS mentation are truly different but mixed together, then our research and understanding of dreaming and other mental processes become muddled, just as if we were to say that apples and bananas are really the same and mixed them in a bowl to study their attributes. On the other hand, if we treat REMS dreams and NREMS mentation as separate, but later discover that, as some now maintain (e.g., Foulkes 1978), they really are results of the same mental processes, it would be easy to combine our knowledge and understanding of them into a unified theory. So, for the rest of this book, we will consider them as separate. For a more complete analysis of the data leading to the strong conclusion that REMS dreams are indeed different from NREMS mentation, see Hobson et al. (2000). Furthermore, we will assume that when we are in REMS we are dreaming, and that the memory of the dream is "lost" during the 10–20 % of the time that no dream recall occurs when awakened from REMS. In contrast, there may be mentation occurring in only a portion of our NREMS.

Box 7.1 Accuracy of Dream Recalls

There is no denying that dreams are difficult to remember. Almost everyone can report having difficulty completely recalling a dream they had or even remembering anything at all of a dream they know they recently had. But when people report their recall of a dream, whether following a sleep awakening, the next morning, or days, weeks, or even years later, it is tacitly accepted as being a faithful reproduction of that dream as it actually occurred. After finding very little experimental research in the literature about this issue, a number of my students and I set out to test this assumption.

In as yet unpublished research from my sleep lab, my student assistants and I awakened 17 sleepers during an early morning REMS period and tape-recorded their dreams. Upon the participants' final awakening later in the morning, we again tape-recorded their recall of this same dream. We also tape-recorded their recall of this dream a week later and a month later. In all we had four recalls from each of 14 sleepers. Each recall was transcribed and parsed into its "storyboard" components (=any aspect of the dream that was a portion that could be removed or inserted as a unit such as, "He played his harmonica for the people waiting in the line"). From this we composed a composite dream for each dreamer that included every component mentioned in any of the four recalls. Then we compared each individual recall to the composite and to the REMS recall to see which components were present or missing.

We found that any single recall of a dream contained only half the number of components of the composite. There was no statistical difference in the number of components included in any of the four recalls, although many specific components were different. Likewise, each of the later recalls were missing more than half of the components that were present in the REMS awakening recall but also contained 22 % *new* components not found in it. Yet, the changes did not distort the gist of the dream, because several people who had nothing to do with the experiment could correctly group all the recalls.

In a follow up study, we awakened 15 sleepers during an early morning REMS period and immediately had them experience a synthetic dream, namely a 6 min dream-like video taken from a 20 year-old movie they had not seen before. We then proceeded as if this video segment was a dream to be recalled immediately, the next morning, a week later, and a month later. The advantage of using this procedure was that all subjects had the same "dream" which made comparisons between subjects easier. Additionally, we knew the exact content of the synthetic dream and could tell what was included, left out, and added. We had complete recall data from 11 of the sleepers for analysis.

The data were analyzed just as they were in the first experiment, and the results paralleled those of the first experiment except that recall was slightly better for the synthetic dream, and for some measures the morning recall was slightly better than subsequent recalls.

Additional analysis was possible, since we knew the components that were in the synthetic dream. We found that the average recall contained only about one-third of the storyboard components from the entire synthetic dream. We were quite liberal in our comparisons. For example, if the recall contained a component that even partially resembled a component in the synthetic dream, we counted it. However, we also found that about 10 % of the recalled components were not actually present in the synthetic dream. When we excluded the REMS awakening recall done immediately after viewing the video, the average recall contained over 20 % of components not present in the synthetic dream.

In a third experiment, we looked for any rehearsal effect from repeatedly recalling the same dream that may have improved later recalls. Again using the synthetic dream technique, we always obtained an immediate recall but only one subsequent recall per subject, either next morning, next week, or next month, but not all three. There were 10 subjects per group. The results showed a slight but not significant drop off in the number of components recalled with the passage of time. Thus, we concluded that there was not much of a rehearsal effect in the first two experiments.

We conclude from these experiments that although the gist of the dream is present in each recall, many of the components vary depending on the time of recall with many components of the actual dream never recalled, some components only sometimes recalled, and other components added that were never part of the original dream. Furthermore, there is no indication in these data that the REMS awakening recall or the next morning recall is greatly superior to any subsequent recall. These results imply that what we know of dreams and dreaming may be imperfect due to the imperfections of recall. Nevertheless, the study of dreams and dreaming—as well as dream interpretation—utilizing dream recalls is the best we can do for now and is worthy of our efforts as long as we realize that actual dreams may be somewhat different.

Reinforcing this view that dreaming occurs during REMS are studies of brain activity during sleep (see Sect. 5.3). They suggest that much of the cerebral cortex during REMS shows activity levels comparable to that of waking. During NREMS, however, the activity patterns in much of the brain, including the cerebral cortex, are diminished compared to that of waking and REMS. Assuming that the cortex needs to be active to engage in the mental processes necessary to put dreams together, we can conclude that while some mentation can occur during NREMS, it is not of sufficient quality to be called dreaming.

New York cognitive psychologist Antrobus (1983) has a different explanation. He maintains that the generation of REMS dreams and NREMS mentation is identical, but retrieval of the content is more difficult from NREMS than from REMS because of the different state of the cortex in NREMS. However, there is little evidence to support this notion, and it cannot explain the qualitative differences frequently found between REMS dreams and NREMS mentation.

Another dissenting line of evidence comes from the fact that about one-third to three-fourths of awakenings shortly after sleep onset result in reports of NREMS mentation. These reports are short, but otherwise have all the elements of REMS dreams (Strauch and Meier 1996). However, they lack a narrative structure, and the occurrences of the dreamer being an active character are unusually low. Additionally, it has been noted that often when *still awake but about to enter sleep* the mind creates images. These could easily be misidentified as dreams occurring early in sleep. Furthermore, these images are qualitatively different from REMS dreams as they are more related to the dreamer's immediate and recent past and more resemble waking fantasy than do dream recall from REMS (Stickgold et al. 2001).

I should note that it has become standard to ask subjects, "What was going through your mind?" rather than "What were you dreaming about?" Some people may not consider NREMS mentation or fragments of REMS dreams to be dreaming and fail to report them when asked to recall a dream. A loss of valuable data is less likely to occur when asking the more general question about what was going through the person's mind when asleep.

7.2.4 Does the Method of Dream Recording Make a Difference?

Dreams can and have been recorded in a variety ways. They can be written down by the dreamer, verbally recorded on a recording devise, or dictated to a person. Sometimes standardized questionnaires or checklists may be used or the most recent dreams collected in group settings. Who is present at the time of the collection, such as same or opposite gender, peer or experimenter, no one, one person or many others, can have an effect. Increasingly there have been studies comparing the data obtained from these various conditions to see how they might influence the results. This has led to a better understanding of the true nature of dreams and the process of dreaming.

Another difficulty comes from having sufficient "sample size" to adequately detect differences in the aspects of the contents of dreams. The suggestion is that a minimum of 50 words is needed to do adequate analysis of a dream. And at least 20 dreams from an individual are needed to assess that dreamer's pattern of dreaming. It may take over 100 dreams to discern content differences among types of people.

In spite of these difficulties, it is still beneficial to study dreams, because it gives us insights into the nature of dreams and dreaming, and recalled dreams can be used for dream interpretation. Nevertheless, keep in mind the constraints these difficulties pose.

7.3 Who Dreams and How Often

Everybody dreams every night. We know this fact because 80–90 % of the time when people are awakened during REMS in the sleep lab and immediately asked what was going through their mind just before being awakened, they report a dream. Even any of the 6 % of people who adamantly profess that they never dream when awakened during REMS frequently, in a groggy manner, begin describing the dream they were just experiencing. Then they would suddenly pause with this look of surprise on their face when they realized that they do dream. So we conclude that everybody dreams every night, but some people do not remember doing so. Not frequently recalling dreams may be an indication of good solid sleep (Horne 2006).

This information brings up a related question. Why is there no recall following 10–20 % of REMS awakenings? One possibility is that there was no dreaming going on then. While there is no direct evidence to refute this statement, there are some indirect indicators. Dreams are not always easy to recall. Most of us have had the experience of being able to recall only a fragment of a dream or of knowing that we dreamed but were unable to recall anything about it. On other occasions, something we experience later in the day may trigger recall of a recent dream previously unrecalled. From these common experiences, it can be inferred that it is likely that we all dream during every REMS period, but sometimes recall of the dream is lost in the transition to waking. Jim Horne draws a different conclusion from the lack of dream recall during some REMS awakenings, and some other data: REMS and dreaming are separable phenomena. That is, REMS can occur without dreaming and dreaming can occur without REMS (Horne 2006).

7.4 Characteristics of Dreams

One of the interesting things about dreams is how typical or universal they can be. Freud noted 23 different typical dreams including death of loved ones, nudity, flying, and taking an exam. The content of such dreams is influenced by the age of the dreamer, such as children's dreams of monsters. Also, there is remarkable similarity across cultures in the frequency of universal dream themes. For example, dreams are more similar than different across cultures in details like the percent of male and female characters, more aggression than friendliness, more misfortune than good fortune, and more negative emotions than positive emotions. Yet in other ways a person's culture will influence their dreams. For example, aggressive content in dreams is highest in the United States of all industrialized nations. Hunter-gatherers often dream of animals but Japanese urbanites seldom do (Mestel 1997). Our personal experiences also influence our dreams. For example musicians have twice as many dreams about music than do non-musicians Uga et al. 2006.

7.4.1 How Much are Dreams Like Waking Experiences?

The majority of dreams are quite realistic and simulate the dreamer's life and general experiences, but not daily events. They are as multifaceted as waking experiences and seem as integrated and as real as waking experiences.

Yet, our dreams resemble but are not exact reproductions and literal reenactments of our waking, real world. Rather, they are a perceptual expression and dramatization of the dreamer's thoughts and ways of seeing the world. Our dreams seem to be self-governing and out of our control. They have been described as "inventive realism" or "realistic-fictional". They are more akin to creative short stories than to factual histories.

In a clever experiment, Rechtschaffen and Buchignani (1983) prepared 129 variations of a single photograph. They varied aspects like the degree of fuzziness in the foreground and in the background, the brightness, and the color intensity. They then awaked 22 subjects from REMS and asked them to choose the photograph that best matched the visual quality of their dream. Four out of ten times, they selected the photo that was most like a typical waking visual experience. The rest of the time, there was less intense color and/or fuzzy background. Early in the night, the selected photos were least like that of typical waking perception.

Antrobus et al. (1987) did a similar experiment but found that images experienced in dreams were at best three-fourths as bright as those experienced during waking, while the clarity was close to that of waking. Yet, some dreams were experienced as having little color and poor clarity. Interestingly, they also found that the clearer the details perceived in a dream, the more likely that they were strange in some way, such as being too large.

When looked at from a waking perspective, dreams often seem bizarre (Hobson et al. 2000). The most common kind of bizarreness in dreams is sudden discontinuities between sequences. These perceptions are often marked by the dreamer's words, "All of a sudden …". But dreams often contain other kinds of bizarreness, such as characters in our dream may be a composite of two or more real people, have something about them that is highly irregular, or may physically change during the course of the dream. The same things can happen with settings, objects, and even time.

Yet, just as it does when awake, our mind attempts to integrate all the experienced elements of our dreams into a unified whole. However, unlike when we are awake, dreaming accomplishes this task by creating a story line attempting to meld everything into a single confabulatory narrative from which self-reflection and critical evaluation are missing. In this regard, dreams have been called "single minded" by Alan Rechtschaffen (1978), a research psychologist and long-time sleep and dream researcher at the University of Chicago. He meant that while dreaming the mind is wholly focused on the dream and less interrupted by other thoughts and images. It does not reflect on the fact that it is dreaming, what it is dreaming about, or that it is actually lying in bed. Likewise, it is much less influenced by external and internal stimuli. This experience contrasts greatly from waking where our attention easily shifts from our thoughts to salient internal or external stimuli and back again; we reflect on our mental processes and current state; and we evaluate our experiences.

Dreams are primarily experienced perceptions. Dreams are almost always primarily visual. Sounds are noted in well over half of dreams, touch is a distant third at 8 %, while the rest of the senses are reported in less than 4 % of dreams. Pain sensation is extremely rare. However, over 40 % of dream report content is more like thinking. The thinking is simple with no complex relations or reflections on questions from multiple points of view. Nor is there any puzzling at length over a problem. Often dreamers are unable to confirm that they actually heard talking; rather, they just knew that it occurred.

Box 7.2 Dreams of People Who Are Blind

I am often asked about the dreams of people who are blind. Since dreams are so visual, do blind people have dreams? If so, what do they dream about? The answers to these questions, as so often happens, are not simple but understandable. They are summarized by Hurovitz et al. (1999).

Blind people dream. Their dream reports are as complex as those of the sighted. Whether or not there is a visual aspect to their dreams depends on when they became blind. If totally blind since birth, they never report visual images in their dreams. If they became totally blind before the age of five, they seldom report visual images in their dreams. Those people who lost their sight after the age of seven continue to report visual aspects to their dreams, but often the clarity and frequency of them diminish with time. Those who lost their sight between the ages of five and seven may or may not report some visual imagery in their dreams. When visual images are absent in the dreams of people who are blind, they are replaced by more taste, smell, touch, and sound.

In other respects, with a few exceptions, their dream report content is much like that of sighted persons. Two notable exceptions involve aggression and moving from one place to another. People who are blind report having more dreams with at least one incidence of aggression. They also have higher numbers of dreams involving moving about, either under their own power or by some means of transportation. These transportation dreams are often linked to misfortune for the dreamer. Two women who were blind reported an unusually high number of dogs in their dreams, mostly their guide dogs.

7.4.2 What People Typically Dream About

Leaving interpretations aside, just what kinds of things do people describe dreaming about? Common folklore and Freud's writings leave the impression that dreams are full of sex and violence, but this assumption is more apparent than real because people remember and tell others more of these types of dreams. It turns out that simply asking or surveying people what they typically dream about does not provide very accurate data when compared to the content of actual dream reports from REMS awakenings, dream diaries, or having people write out their most recent dream.

The best research with dream reports often uses what is called content analysis developed by two psychologists, Calvin Hall and Robert Van de Castle (Hall and Van de Castle 1966). Essentially, this method first categorizes things like the characters, settings, objects, activities, and social interactions that are found in a dream and then counting the number of instances in each category. For example, characters might be grouped according to gender and age, such as male adult, female child, or indeterminate elderly. The categories are carefully developed so that different researchers working with the same dreams will produce nearly the same results. An excellent resource to learn more about the technique of content analysis and how to use it is www.dreamresearch.net. Also www.dreambank.net

contains the initial dream reports used to derive norms together with their codings, which is useful when practicing this method of content analysis.

Results from such objective studies of the content of dreams show that rather than being filled with sex and aggression with lots of emotion, dreams are mostly mundane and ordinary but with some bizarre elements or happenings. The typical dream is best described as a set of novel creations with a theme, using mostly the common and ordinary from the dreamer's waking experiences. They are most akin to a short fiction story or TV program. But neither do dreams precisely reproduce memories and typical waking experiences. For example, there is a noticeable absence of activities such as writing, reading, keyboarding, or calculating. People mostly dream about people, things, and pets that directly influence and interest them during their waking lives. They frequently reflect the individual's life experiences and interests, their combination of preoccupations, interests, and concerns. They often take place in familiar settings and are populated with familiar characters. However, there is more focus on strangers or unrecognizable people and more unknown settings than occur in our waking experiences. They tend to center on everyday concerns and social interactions. The patterns of connections among characters in a person's dreams are very much like their waking relationships. For example, when a character appears in your dream, there is a greater likelihood that certain other characters associated with that character in waking life will also be in it. Only a small number of dreams contain unknown characters and out-of-the-ordinary activities.

An example of modern research showing what people typically dream about can be found at http://www.youtube.com/watch?v=9nmVzXxdUeU&NR=1&feature=endscreen from 28:55 to 33:50.

7.4.2.1 Specific Content

Most notable in the study of the content of dreams are the findings of Bill Domhoff and Inge Strauch. Bill Domhoff, a psychologist and sociologist at the University of California Santa Clara, has been carrying on the Hall-Van de Castle tradition. He summarized the accumulated norms, which have not changed in the last 50 years, in his book *Finding Meaning in Dreams: A Quantitative Approach* (1996). Additionally, Austrian dream researchers, Inge Strauch and Barbara Meier, summarized their findings on 500 REMS awakening reports supplemented by morning follow-up questions from 44 young adult, self-reported good dreamers in their book *In Search of Dreams: Results of Experimental Dream Research* (1996). Here we will summarize some key findings gleaned primarily from both of these sources with a special focus on differences in the dreams of males compared to females, characters, social interactions, activities, emotions, and bizarreness. Consult the references and additional sources for more details.

Overall the typical dream averages 2.6 characters, 4.8 activities, 1.4 social interactions, and 1.3 settings. Three out of four dreams contain emotions and negative aspects, a little less than half have misfortunes, while around one in ten contain failure, success, or good fortune. The events recalled in dreams, with their actions and interactions, are most often the focus of dreams. The setting is usually secondary to the events. Unknown settings are most common (44 %), followed by familiar (26 %), then vague and non-specific (19 %) and distorted (11 %). Only 1 % of settings is fictional or fantasy. In 25 % of the recalls the setting was changed before the end of the dream.

Our dream characters sometimes react to what occurs in our dreams much like when awake, with two very key exceptions—thinking and bizarreness. Thought processes during remembered dreams are simpler than those when we are awake, and we seem to recall uncritically accepting what occurs during our dreams no matter how bizarre. The dreamer as a character focuses almost entirely on the moment to the exclusion of concern for the past or future. We do not wonder who we are or how we impress others.

Differences in Dream Content Based on Gender

In many studies, the gender of the dreamer has more influence on dream content than age, race, marital status, and social class. Men's dreams have fewer characters that are more likely to be less familiar and mostly males. Women's dreams contain more people equally distributed between male and female who are more likely to be familiar. Women also recall how their dream characters looked, including what they wore and how their hair was styled, more than do males. Men more frequently dream about school, work, and politics but less frequently of leisure time activities. Men have greater physical activity and aggressive social exchanges while women have more friendly social interactions. Familiar settings are more common in the dreams of females. Males recall more dreams involving automobiles and weapons, while female dreams contain more household objects.

In contrast, Strauch and Meier (1996) found fewer differences in the content of dreams of males compared to females, and any differences were more in emphasis rather than sharp contrasts. There was no gender differences found in the quality of friendliness and unfriendliness, whether unfriendly actions were physical or verbal. However, male dreams contained a bit less aggressiveness and friendliness and were a bit more realistic. However, in male dreams, males were more frequently the perpetrators rather than the recipients of aggression—just the opposite of female dreams.

Additionally, Strauch and Meier found some other differences. Female dreams had relatively more negative emotions. Women recall dreaming more about babies and children. Overall, males are more active as characters in their dreams, but the activity that women display as characters is generally more verbal than physical. Female dreams contain a greater array of events, but there are no gender differences found when comparing the ratio of everyday events to leisure events.

Characters

It is extremely rare for there to be no characters at all in a dream. Most often dreamers are a character in their own dreams and most often as an active character rather than a passive observer. Yet the dreamer is usually not the central focus. Sometimes strangers are in our dreams by virtue of their role or function such as firemen or teachers. Most characters are adults, and more of them are from our present life rather than from childhood. Acquaintances and colleagues are more common than are family members. Seldom do we populate our dreams with characters from fiction or with prominent persons. Animals are not nearly as common as people. Generally characters are more consistent and less bizarre in dreams than are other features.

Social Interactions

Characters in dreams frequently have neutral interactions with other characters but they tend to be more negative than they are in waking life. When there is interaction it is most likely to vary in the nature of aggressive content. Aggressive or friendly interactions are mainly through words and gestures rather than physical contacts. Overall, people show the most aggression in dreams toward those with whom they most clash during their waking lives.

The dreamer as a character in the dream is as likely to be initiators as recipients of social interactions. Most conversations focus on everyday practical things with few occasions of professional, political, school, or impersonal topics reported. Nor is there much superficial conversation, such as talking about the weather or sports, or much social ritual, such as asking, "How are you?"

Interactions that are sexual are surprisingly low at 12 % for males and 4 % for females, but the dreamer as a character has sexual interactions with familiar characters more often in female dreams than in male dreams. The sex dreams of females have a more romantic quality, whereas the sex dreams of males are more in the nature of conquests.

Activities

Characters usually engage in multiple activities in any one dream. Movement and talking contribute to around three-fourths of the activities in the dream reports. Conversations occur in two-thirds of remembered dreams. Characters often move under their own power but also move in vehicles.

Emotions

Emotions or moods are experienced in about three-fourths of dreams but often are not mentioned in dream reports unless dreamers are specifically prompted to do so. However, when asked, dreamers may report experiencing emotions in the dream that they would have experienced had they been awake. Contrary to what people think they dream about, negative emotions are actually experienced far more often than positive emotions in dreams. Apprehension and confusion are the most frequent emotions experienced. Moderate emotions are experienced much more often than either extremely strong or very weak emotions. Positive emotions turn negative more often than the other way around.

Bizarreness

One of the striking features about dreams is bizarreness. However, this aspect of dreams has been difficult to assess. While in less than one in ten dreams is everything bizarre, a bizarreness aspect is present in about three out of four dreams. It is strongly present in one out of three dreams, otherwise usually only one minor element is bizarre. Bizarreness in both form and content occurs in less than one in five dreams. Bizarreness occurs in actions 43 % of the time, characters 27 %, settings 18 %, objects 13.7 %, experiences 10.3 %, and speech 3.4 %. However, these percents simply parallel the percents of all occurrences of these contents, bizarre plus non-bizarre, so bizarreness seems to be equally spread around.

Other elements

- Overall, over one-half of dreams combine realistic with fictional elements with another one-fourth having only realistic elements. Entirely fictional or fantastic situations account for only one-fifth of all dreams. However, some individuals consistently have more fictional or fantastic elements than do other individuals.
- Dreams contain few crimes, little illness or injury. Likewise war, national catastrophes, severe losses, or deprivation are rare as are outstanding good fortune, unexpected success, and distinctions.
- Some of the content typically reported in dream dictionaries such as transmogrification of objects, losing teeth, flying, and falling are actually not very common.

Those who are more interested in dream interpretation in order to get at the "true or real meaning" of the dream have a different view of what people typically dream about. For example, San Francisco psychologist Gayle Delaney talks about the following common elements in dreams in her book *All About Dreams* (1998): being chased, losing teeth, appearing in public naked, unable to run, sex with an unexpected partner, loss of purse or wallet, finding new rooms in a house, taking exams, dreams of flying, famous actors or actresses, dictators, automobile break-down, drugs or cigarettes or alcohol, clothing, family or another close relative's home, a certain town or state or country, cats, and snakes. However, as already mentioned, many of the things that people say they typically dream about in surveys show up much less often in more objective content analysis of dream reports with the exception of being inappropriately dressed in public and flying (Domhoff 1996). Yet, some things, while not generally common, may be more frequent at certain times in a person's life, such as dreaming of a deceased loved one months or years after the person died.

7.4.3 Categories of Dreams

Other researchers have maintained that we cannot lump all dreams together and then try to discern their essential nature. They maintain there are different cate-gories of dreams including those extremely important, pivotal dreams that do not happen very often. Just as in the study of literature, novels, essays, and poems are usually not mixed together for study, but each category is studied in its own right. For example, Don Kuiken, a psychologist at the University of Alberta, Canada, obtained dreams from 26 women and 10 men of (1) a recent impactful dream which he defines as a dream that influenced how they felt or what they did during subsequent waking, and (2) the first dream that they had after at least 4 days had transpired from the impactful dream (Busink and Kuiken 1996). The subjects also filled out questionnaires about features of these remembered dreams. Both the dream content and the questionnaire data were then statistically analyzed for clusters, such as feelings of discouragement, being weak or unable to move, vivid sounds, and amazement. Five cluster patterns emerged that they labeled Existential Dreams, Anxiety Dreams, Transcendent Dreams, Mundane Dreams, and Alien-ation Dreams. The characteristics of each of these are elaborate and need not concern us here (see Busink and Kuiken 1996 for these details). However, such categorizing of qualitatively different kinds of dream reports may lead to more fruitful ways to study dreams in the future.

Box 7.3 Some Popular Myths About Dreams

1. *People only dream in black and white.* One study found that when awakened from REMS in the lab and asked immediately about the presence of color, the response is affirmative over two-thirds of the time. However, if the color question follows other questions or the complete recall of the dream, then this ratio drops to one-third. In other studies, 75 % to over 80 % of dream reports collected following REMS

awakenings contained color. It thus appears that much, if not all, dreaming is done in color, but this detail like many other dream details is easily forgotten.

2. *Eating spicy or exotic foods will cause us to dream more.* Anything that causes indigestion, such as spicy or exotic foods, will cause us to awaken more frequently from sleep. The more we awaken, the more we are likely to recall the dreaming that has been going on regardless of what we have eaten.

3. *The eye movements of REMS are following or causing the activity of the dream.* When dreaming of looking up at the Eiffel Tower, for example, there would be vertical eye movements, whereas when watching a tennis match, there would be many horizontal eye movements. This intuitive hypothesis has occasionally been explored for over 30 years with generally negative results, mainly because the nature of the eye movements differs from those that occur when awake (Hobson et al. 2000). Also, correlations between reported dream content and recorded eye movements are not always present. Rapid eye movements occur in human fetuses, cats with no cortex, and people blind from birth. None of these have visual experiences, so it is unlikely that they are scanning visual images in their dreams. Nevertheless, some studies find support for this hypothesis (e.g., Hong et al. 1997).

4. *If you dream that you are falling and you hit the ground, then you are really dead.* Whenever I hear this one, I ask the question, "How were the data for this conclusion collected?" Also, there are people who have awakened quite alive from a dream in which they report they were falling and hit the ground.

5. *Sleep talking and hypnosis can be used to find out what people dream about.* Incidents of both of these have been investigated many times but with very little success.

7.5 Developmental Changes in Dreams

The data on common elements in dreams presented above is for young adults. As we saw in Sect. 2.3, sleep changes with age. Does what people dream about likewise change with age?

7.5.1 Children

Careful study of dream reports collected from children has yielded information about the characteristics of children's dreams. Beginning at around 3 years of age it is possible to have children relate what they were dreaming, although there is some question how accurate the reports are until about 5 years of age. Extensive numbers of dream reports have been obtained from children awakened during sleep in a sleep lab (Foulkes 1982, 1999) and from morning recall of the dreams of the night reported at home (Domhoff 1996; Resnick et al. 1994; Strauch and Meier 1996). Several general conclusions can be drawn from these studies although not always with universal agreement.

There are developmental changes in dream content through late adolescence. The frequency of dream recall increases with age until near the end of the first decade of life, then levels off. The length of dream reports increases as children get older, although there is disagreement on whether the dreams themselves become longer or the ability of the children to describe more of what they dreamed about increases. And children's dreams contain more animal characters, especially when younger. The developmental changes in children's dreams seem to parallel their emotional and cognitive development. However, aggression seems to increase gradually with age in the dreams of children, then begins a slight decline during adulthood. Contrary to popular beliefs about children's dreams, there was no emotion reported in the vast majority of their dreams, but Rosalind Cartwright (2010) suggests having the children draw their dreams would have yielded more emotional content. Overall, children create dreams in the same way as adults; both put the components together in unusual yet mostly plausible ways.

Selected details from these studies follow:

Foulkes (1982, 1999):

- At younger ages there was no distortion such as unfamiliar characters or settings, and dreams were seldom reported as frightening.
- Preteen boys' dreams contained more aspects of assertiveness, aggression, venturesomeness, self-reliance, and success orientation.
- The dreams of preteen girls showed more social awareness, interpersonal orientation, munificence, and openness.

Domhoff (1996):

- Generally boys report more boys than girls in their dreams (69–31 %), while girls report equal numbers of boys and girls in their dreams.
- Children more often report dreams with misfortune.
- Although more study of teenagers' dreams is needed, there are suggestions that when compared to males, female teens report more friendliness but are more likely to be victims of aggression. However, a smaller percent of this aggression is physical. Male teenagers report more aggression than do female teenagers, and a higher percent of it is physical.

Resnick et al. (1994):

- The dreamer was reported to be an active character in well over 80 % of the dreams.
- Thirty percent of the characters recalled were identified as family members.

Box 7.4 Do Animals Dream?

If you have been around dogs or cats much, you probably have noticed that they sometimes twitch their feet or face when asleep, and dogs even make sounds. If you are like most people, you probably assumed they were dreaming. Yet, knowing for sure that animals dream is difficult to establish directly. We cannot ask them if they are dreaming like we can people. Reflexes, not dream content, may cause the movements and sounds they make. Yet, there are many indications that they probably do dream.

The strongest arguments in favor of the presence of dreams in animals, at least in other mammals, include the following:

1. There is great similarity in brain structure and functioning, especially among mammals, that includes the areas known to be involved in sleep and dreaming.
2. Animals also show signs that they have mental processes similar to those of humans such as those involving emotions, sensory perceptions, and even cognitions—the very processes that are a part of dreaming.
3. Cats with damage in the brainstem area that causes muscle paralysis during REMS are completely normal whether asleep or awake except for one thing. They move while in REMS in ways that strongly suggest they are reacting to or interacting with something they are experiencing in a dream. Some even walk and seem to be searching or looking at something imaginary, yet they do not react to real stimuli. Similar behaviors occur in humans with damage to this area, and they report having had dream content that matches well with the behaviors they were doing while in REMS (see Sect. 13.7).
4. A gorilla that was taught to communicate to its handlers in sign language spontaneously combined the signs for "sleep" and "pictures".

Arguments against the notion that animals dream include the fact that we cannot ask directly or indirectly what they were dreaming about so that we can make qualitative comparisons of their dreams to the dreams of humans. Until we have direct access to the content of animal dreams, we simply have no way of knowing for sure if they dream. Also the presence of REMS does not unequivocally indicate dreaming because humans with lesions of parietal cortex do not dream although their REMS is normal. Some animals, namely the platypus and the short-nosed echidna, show signs of REMS in the brain stem but not in the forebrain where dreams are constructed. Finally, from a more philosophical point of view, it is argued that only humans can do the symbolic mental processing necessary to dream (Foulkes 1999).

7.5.2 Adults

Studies of people's dream logs, often composed of more than a hundred samples sometimes spanning decades, show that the dreams of each individual remain essentially consistent (Domhoff 1996). Throughout the long period of adulthood there is great consistency in the major categories of what people report they dream about. However, some changes do occur that are consistent with changes in their waking lives. That is, on the whole, the types of characters, social interactions, objects, and activities an individual dreams about changes little during the extent of their adult years—except for possibly a reduction in aggression and negative emotions. Domhoff also found remarkable consistency in what U. S. college students almost 50 years apart dream about. This stability is in spite of much social and political change over that span of time. Especially noteworthy is the consistency in the differences in the dream content between males and females in spite of the change in women's roles during this time span. At all ages there is a general tendency for people's dreams to focus on the present.

At the same time there are great differences among individuals in what they dream about (Domhoff 1996). This is consistent with the notion that an individual's dreams are meaningful to them echoing mostly the individual's gender but also things like age, race, marital status, and social class. For example, working women have more masculine types of dream imagery, featuring more aggression and anxiety, than do women who are homemakers. Additionally, Domhoff notes, there are changes in peoples' dreams that are consistent with changes in their individual lives, such as career upsets and marital changes.

More clinically oriented studies of peoples' dreams as they age (Cartwright 1979) show that young people report that they dream more about guilt and morality; middle-aged people report dreaming more about sexuality and aggression; and elderly persons report dreaming more about death and illness. These differences reflect the changing concerns that typically accompany aging in the United States.

7.6 Dreams Through the Night

In the lab, it is possible to awaken a dreamer several times during the night, usually near the end of REMS and collect a dream each time. This makes it possible to see if all the dreams in a night are related like chapters in a book or installments of a weekly TV series. The results of such studies are equivocal. Based on uninterpreted content alone, the answer is no. The content of what you recall dreaming about during one REMS period and the next, or NREMS periods for that matter, appears unrelated. Each dream usually has different setting, characters, and activities. It is rather like watching a sequence of different half hour programs on TV on a particular night.

Cartwright's (1978) analysis of the dreams in a night leads to some different conclusions. But first she found that the first REMS period yielded only 50 % recall, but this increased to 99 % by the last REMS period. She also observed that as the night goes on, there is more emotion, less distortion, and more drama in the dreams. Even reports of NREMS mentation become more dreamlike as the night wears on. Importantly, she, like some other psychologists and psychiatrists, finds that the dreams obtained by REMS awakenings during a single night are related when looking below the surface content to see what the dream purportedly really means (more on dream interpretation is presented in Box 9.1).

Cartwright sees three phases in the dreams of a single night as the typical pattern. The dream during the first REMS period sets the theme on an emotional level, such as threat to self-esteem. During the second and third REMS periods, past experiences related to that theme are brought to bear. Then during the fourth and fifth REMS periods, the theme is extended into possibilities for the future. The result is a progression, often beneficial to the dreamer, in this emotional concern. But this sequence may not occur if the dreamer is under either a lot or conversely very little stress (Cartwright 1979). If stress is too high, then the single theme is simply repeated without progression and benefit. If the dreamer's stress is low, then the dreams are not ordered and have many themes.

On a related note, there are several factors that are thought to determine which of the several dreams on a single night are most likely to be recalled the next day. The key factors include the most recent dreams, longer dreams, and dreams with more drama.

7.7 Recurrent Dreams

Fifty to eighty percent of college students report having recurrent dreams over a period of a few months to many decades. They may occur a couple of times per week or a couple of times per year. Most begin in childhood, others in adolescence, and a few during the adult years. About two-thirds of the dreams feature negative effect and are experienced as nightmares. Most frequently, the main character in the dream is the dreamer who is being attacked, or chased, by living things or threatened by natural forces such as fires, floods, or storms. For many people, recurrent dreams eventually cease, but not for everyone. They are more frequent during times of waking life stress (see Recurrent Dreams and Repetitive Nightmares in Sect. 12.4.2.2).

7.8 Lucid Dreaming

Lucid dreaming means being aware that you are dreaming while you are dreaming. When people are asked if they have ever experienced a lucid dream, 50 % respond positively and 15 % say that they experience one more frequently than once a month. Many people also report that while having a lucid dream, they have the ability to modify the dream in minor to major ways. For example, a high school student who competed on the track team once told me he dreamed that he came in third in a race. When he realized he was dreaming, he had everyone run backwards to the starting line, then race again, only this time he arranged it so that he came in first.

The legitimacy of lucid dreaming has been scientifically verified in a number of experiments. Self-avowed lucid dreamers are given an instruction before going to sleep in a sleep lab to give a prearranged signal when they are having a lucid dream. Signals used have included a specific sequence of eye movements, an unusual pattern of breathing, or even twitching a finger a number of times. The sleepers may be awakened right after giving the signal, a few minutes later, or at the end of the REMS period for a dream report. Upon awakening, the sleepers verified that they had experienced a lucid dream. Furthermore, the time between the signal and the moment of awakening closely corresponded to the time that the events recalled in the dream would be expected to take if they had occurred in real life.

Some dream researchers maintain that anyone can learn to become a lucid dreamer, but others believe that this ability ranges from easy to hard to acquire. Other dream researchers have cautioned that it may not be advisable to control many of your dreams, because dreams seem to have their own agenda (see Sect. 8.3.5) and controlling them may upset their natural function (see Sect. 11.3).

For more on lucid dreaming go to http://www.youtube.com/watch?v=9nm VzXxdUeU&NR=1&feature=endscreen from 50:23 to 56:03.

7.9 Creativity in Dreams

Every night each of us composes, directs, stages, and usually acts in what is the equivalent of several TV programs—a highly creative endeavor. But we can be creative in other ways in our dreams, creative in the sense that we bring something novel yet useful back to our waking lives. There are numerous historical examples to illustrate this ability.

Ellias Howe had spent years trying to invent a mechanical sewing machine. He was successful only when he had a dream of "natives" throwing spears at him. These spears had holes just below the sharp point at the front and they kept bouncing in and out of the ground. Upon awakening, he realized that he first needed to move the hole for the thread from the blunt end, where it is on a typical hand-sewing needle, to the sharp end. Second, the entire needle should not pass through the cloth, but just the sharp end should penetrate then withdraw over and over again. With these changes suggested to him by the dream, he successfully developed the sewing machine.

James Watt was familiar with how to make lead pellets to be used as shot for the guns of his time. A block of lead was cut into pieces and formed into nearly spherical shapes by hand. However, the shot was not always formed into a perfect sphere, having a negative effect on how it performed. Howe dreamed on three different occasions that he was caught in a rainstorm of molten lead. After the third dream, he realized that this image was the key to making perfect shot, because drops of hot lead, just like drops of water, assume the shape of near perfect spheres while falling. He constructed the first shot tower—a tall structure from which splattered molten lead was dropped. As the drops fell, they assumed a spherical shape and cooled before hitting bottom. The result was nearly perfectly shaped shot.

Notice what happened in both of these examples. Each time, the dreamers were very involved with a problem in their waking life. It was personally important to them, and they were very familiar with it. These facts probably caused them to have the dream, but certainly caused them to attend to the dream and recognize the creative solution to the problem.

There are numerous examples of creative solutions coming from dreams in areas beyond technology. Kekule made the scientific discovery of the nature of the benzene ring when he dreamed of snakes each biting their own tail. Writer Robert Lewis Stevenson got the idea for his famous story of "Dr. Jeckel and Mr. Hyde" from a dream. Composer and violinist Tartini heard the devil playing a beautiful tune on his violin. Upon awakening, Tartini reproduced, as best he could, what he heard in his dream, resulting in his greatest composition "The Devil's Trill Sonata". Beatle Paul McCartney says he got the tune for his song "Yesterday" in a dream that he wrote down upon waking. These examples are not unusual. You, or somebody you know, probably have had some creative insight that came from a dream, even if it was less spectacular than these examples.

Dream researcher Deirdre Barrett (1993), asked students to try for a week to incubate (see Sect. 8.3.2) a dream about a problem that was of personal importance to them and to seek a solution in their dreams. Later, the submitted dream reports were scored independently as to their relevance to the problem and whether or not the dream presented a reasonable solution. The results showed that about one-half of the dreams were about the problem and one-fourth also contained an apparent solution.

Deirdre Barrett can be seen focusing on problem solving during dreaming at http://www.youtube.com/watch?v=9nmVzXxdUeU&NR=1&feature=endscreen from 33:56 to 36:11.

Box 7.5 How to Improve Dream Recall

Often people are frustrated because they cannot remember their dreams, and they want to know how they can remember more of them. It has been estimated that less than 10 % of dreams are recalled and that most people recall about two dreams per week with fewer people recalling either more or less. Research has shown that how often people recall their dreams has very little relationship to their personality except for somewhat greater recall in people with "thin boundaries" (see Sect. 9.3.1), high creativity, a positive approach towards dreams (Blagrove and Akehurst 2000), and openness to experiences. People with better visual memories when awake recall more dreams as do people with greater waking creativity and fantasy (Schredl 2001). Also, people who awaken easily report recalling more dreams. Mood and stress also affect dream recall frequency.

Recall is facilitated by a brief arousal of the brain following the dream or a period of quiet upon awakening. Habitual short-duration sleepers recall fewer dreams (Hicks et al. 1991) but shortening REMS intensifies dreaming (Fiss 1991). Women tend to remember more dreams than men, and it seems like the most vivid and emotional dreams are the most recalled (Strauch and Meier 1996).

While there is no magic formula that works for all, the following have helped many people increase their dream recall:

1. Tell yourself that dreams are important and that you want to remember them. People who take their dreams seriously and attend to them usually remember more dreams.
2. Have a tape recorder or notebook at your bedside so that you can record the dream as soon as you awaken. Memory of dreams tends to fade quickly, so the sooner you record a dream, the better.
3. Before you go to sleep, tell yourself several times, "I will remember a dream tonight."
4. If all else fails do something to awaken you during the early morning such as setting your alarm clock to awaken you or, better yet, have someone else set it to an early morning time you are not aware of or have someone else awaken you then. REMS is more likely to occur early in the morning, and you are more likely to remember a dream when waking from REMS.
5. To improve what you do recall, right after you awaken stay in bed and concentrate on what you were dreaming about from beginning to end.
6. If nothing comes, force yourself to write or voice record a sentence about the first thing that came into your mind when you awoke. This practice gets you into the habit of concentrating on what is mentally occurring to you at awakening. Often, after a week or two of practice, the dream recalls start coming.
7. Get enough sleep. People who awaken sleepy may not be awake enough to recall their dreams.
8. Finally, be aware that alcohol and some drugs may make the recall of dreams more difficult. Make adjustments accordingly.

7.10 Conclusion

Everyone dreams several dreams every night. There is universal agreement that dreaming takes place during REMS. There is also agreement that there is mental content that occurs during NREMS but in many ways does not qualify as dreaming. Typically, dreams simulate the people and animals and their activities and interactions in settings that we are familiar with from our waking lives but are not exact replicas. The content of dreams changes through childhood and late adolescence but then stay reasonably consistent and steady for the rest of our lives. The gender of the dreamer also influences dream content. In the end dreams can be viewed as unique psychological products of our minds that are full of personal meanings.

References

Antrobus, J. S. (1983). REM and NREM sleep reports: comparison of word frequencies by cognitive classes. *Psychophysiology, 20*, 562–568.

Antrobus, J., Hartwig, P., Rosa, D., Reinsel, R., & Fein, G. (1987). Brightness and clarity of REM and NREM imagery: Photo response scale. *Sleep Research, 16*, 240.

Aserinsky, E., & Kleitman, N. (1953). Regularly occurring periods of eye mobility and concomitant phenomena during sleep. *Science, 18*, 273–274.

Barrett, D. (1993). The "committee of sleep": A study of dream incubation for problem solving. *Dreaming, 3*, 115–122.

Blagrove, M., & Akehurst, L. (2000). Personality and dream recall frequency: Further negative findings. *Dreaming, 10*, 139–146.

Businck, R., & Kuiken, D. (1996). Identifying types of impactful dreams: A replication. *Dreaming, 6*, 97–119.

Carskadon, M. A. (Ed.). (1993). *Encyclopedia of sleep and dreaming*. New York: Macmillian.

Cartwright, R. D. (1978). *A primer on sleep and dreaming*. Reading: Addison-Wesley.

Cartwright, R. D. (1979). The nature and function of repetitive dreams: A survey and speculation. *Psychiatry, 42*, 131–137.

Cartwright, R. D. (2010). *The twenty-four hour mind*. New York: Oxford University Press.

Delaney, G. (1998). *All about dreams*. New York: HarperCollins.

Dement, W., & Kleitman, N. (1957). The relation of eye movements during sleep to dream activity. *Journal of Experimental Psychology, 53*, 89–97.

Domhoff, G. W. (1996). *Finding Meaning in Dreams: A quantitative Approach*. New York: Plenum.

Domhoff, G. W. (2003). *The scientific study of dreams: Neural networks, cognitive development, and content analysis*. Washington: American Psychological Association Press.

Domhoff, G. W., & Schnelder, A. (1999). Much ado about very little: the small effect sizes when home and laboratory collected dreams are compared. *Dreaming, 9*, 139–151.

Fiss, H. (1991). Experimental strategies for the study of the function of dreaming. In S. Ellman & J. Antrobus (Eds.), *The mind in sleep: Psychology and psychophysiology* (2nd ed., pp. 265–307). New York: Wiley.

Foulkes, D. (1978). *A Grammar of Dreams*. New York: Basic Books.

Foulkes, D. (1982). *Children's dreams: Longitudinal studies*. New York: Wiley.

Foulkes, D. (1999). *Children's dreams and the development of consciousness*. Cambridge: Harvard University Press.

Hall, C., & Van de Castle, R. (1966). *The content analysis of dreams*. New York: Appleton-Century-Crofts.

Hicks, R., Lucero, K., & Mistry, R. (1991). Dreaming and habitual sleep duration. *Perceptual and Motor Skills, 72,* 1281–1282.

Hobson, J. A., Pace-Schott, E., & Stickgold, R. (2000). Dreaming and the brain: Toward a cognitive neuroscience of conscious states. *Behavioral and Brain Sciences, 23,* 793–842 and 904–1121.

Hong, C. C., Potkin, S. G., Antrobus, J. S., Dow, B. M., Callaghan, G. M., & Gillin, J. C. (1997). REM sleep eye movement counts correlate with visual imagery in dreaming: A pilot study. *Psychophysiology, 34,* 377–381.

Horne, J. (2006). *Sleepfaring*. New York: Oxford University Press.

Hurovitz, C., Dunn, S., Domhoff, G. W., & Fiss, H. (1999). The dreams of blind men and women: A replication and extension of previous findings. *Dreaming, 9,* 183–193.

Kryger, M. H., Roth, T. R., & Dement, W. C. (Eds.). (2011). *Principles and practice of sleep medicine* (5th ed.). St. Louis: Elsevier.

Lee-Chiong, T. (Ed.). (2006). *Sleep: A comprehensive handbook*. Hoboken: Wiley.

Mestel, R. (1997, April 26). *Get real, Siggi*. Retrieved from http://www.newscientist.com/article/mg15420799.700-get-real-siggi–freud-would-have-been-furious–hardnosed-pragmatists-are-invading-the-fabulous-dream-industry-he-founded.html.

Moorcroft, W. H. (1993). *Sleep, dreaming, and sleep disorders: An introduction* (2nd ed.). Lanham: University Press of America.

Nielsen, T. A. (2000). A review of mentation in REM and NREM sleep: "Covert" REM sleep as a possible reconciliation of two opposing models. *Behavioral Brain Science, 23,* 851–866.

Pagel, J. F., & Myers, P. (2002). Definitions of dreaming: A comparison of definitions of dreaming utilized by different study populations (college psychology students, sleep lab patients, and medical professionals. *Sleep, 25,* A299–A300.

Pagel, J. F., Blagrove, M., Levin, R., States, B., Stickgold, B., & White, S. (2001). Defining dreaming—a paradigm for comparing disciplinary specific definitions of dream. *Dreaming, 11,* 195–202.

Rechtschaffen, A. (1978). The single-mindedness and isolation of dreams. *Sleep, 1,* 97–109.

Rechtschaffen, A., & Buchignani, C. (1983). Visual dimensions and correlates of dream images. *Sleep Research, 12,* 189.

Resnick, J., Stickgold, R., Rittenhouse, C. D., & Hobson, J. A. (1994). Self-representation and bizarreness in children's dream reports collected in the home setting. *Consciousness and Cognition, 3,* 30–45.

Schredl, M. (2001, July). Factors of dream recall. Presented at the annual meeting of the Association for the Study of Dreams. Santa Cruz, California.

Stickgold, R., Hobson, J. A., Fosse, R., & Fosse, M. (2001). Sleep, learning, and dreams: Off-line memory reprocessing. *Science, 294,* 1052–1057.

Strauch, I., & Meier, B. (1996). *In search of dreams. Results of experimental dream research*. Albany: State University of New York Press.

Uga, V., Lemut, M. C., Zampi, C., & Salzarulo, P. (2006). Music in dreams. *Consciousness and Cognition, 15,* 351–357.

Chapter 8
Dreaming

Contents

In Chap. 7 we reviewed what people dream about, in other words exploring dreams as objects. We now turn to examining the source of those dreams, that is dreaming as activity. We will need two chapters to do this. In Chap. 9 we will explore the

---

Specific references to statements in this chapter that can be found in multiple, widely available sources are not included in the text. A selection of these sources is listed below and can also be consulted for verification or more detail. (Cartwright 2010; Domhoff 1996; Moorcroft 1993; Strauch and Meier 1996).

W. H. Moorcroft, *Understanding Sleep and Dreaming*,
DOI: 10.1007/978-1-4614-6467-9_8,
© Springer Science+Business Media New York 2013

theories of dreaming from the early twentieth century followed by a look at more recent theories. But first, in this chapter, we will review various elements of dreaming that are not comprehensive enough to be called a theory but nevertheless offer some understanding of the process of creating dreams. We will start with an overview of how people in various cultures throughout recorded history have viewed the process of dreaming, emphasizing current Western views.

8.1 Historical/Cultural Views on the Sources of Dreams

People from different cultures and different historical periods have had varying opinions about what dreams are. These beliefs can be sorted into the following four categories (Webb 1992):

1. During the dream the dreamer exists in a different world.
2. Dreams are omens and other indicators of the future.
3. Dreams are meaningless artifacts of brain activity.
4. The dreamer creates dreams using experiences from their waking life.

8.1.1 Dreams as Visits to a Different World

Various peoples isolated in different parts of the world have independently had some form of the notion that when we dream, our *self*, what we would call soul or spirit, leaves our body in this world and travels to another world where it exists for a while. The dream is an awareness of this other existence. For some peoples, this other existence is totally separate from the waking world. For others, the two are related.

The Pantani Malay people and the unrelated Eskimos of Hudson Bay are two examples of peoples who perceive dreaming as existence in a totally separate world. The Tajal of Luzon so strongly believe this idea that it is taboo to awaken a person who is asleep for fear that the person's "self" that is off in another world will be unable to rejoin the body in this world.

For other people, the dream world and the waking world are connected. People, such as those of the Kamchatka, Zulu, Borneo, and Kurdish cultures believe that a favor received in a dream requires a return favor when awake. Likewise, if the dreamer insults someone in a dream, then an apology must soon be issued when awake. A crime committed in a dream is just as bad as one committed when awake. Other cultures seek to carry useful messages from the dream world back to the waking world. In many cultures, recalled dreams are used in collective decision making such as waging war and choosing political leaders.

Another variation of this category comes from some of the ancient Greeks who did not believe that persons went somewhere in their dreams; rather they were visited by dreams. Hypnos, the god of sleep, had a son Morpheus who was the god of dreams and who oversaw this process.

Box 8.1 Senoi Dream Theory

During the 1960s, the Senoi dream theory became very popular and influential. This theory is said to derive from a small tribal group by that name that lived in the mountains of what is now central Malaysia. Senoi dream theory was described by Kilton R. Stewart, most notably in his widely reprinted 1951 journal article (Stewart 1951). Stewart reported that the Senoi greatly valued dreams which in turn gave them better creativity, superior mental health, and a peaceful, cooperative culture.

In fact, Stewart reported that the Senoi had exemplary health and happiness. Mental illness was unknown among the Senoi and violence among them was nonexistent. All these traits were true, Stewart claimed, because the Senoi daily shared and discussed their dreams with others in their communities, encouraged and guided their children in sharing and using their dreams, and even were able to control and shape their dreams. Furthermore, they acted upon what happened in their dreams. For example, he reported that if a Senoi man dreamed that he hurt another person in a dream, then the dreamer would try to be especially friendly to that person during subsequent waking life. Or if another person injured the dreamer in a dream, then the dreamer should inform that person when awake in order to reverse the effects in a friendly manner.

Additionally, the Senoi were said to shape their dreams. They would meet threats in their dreams head-on, confronting them and attacking them if necessary. They would continually attempt to allow and even work toward the most pleasurable experiences in their dreams. They endeavored to have positive outcomes to their dreams and to bring to their waking life a message or gift from each dream.

Stewart's reports of Senoi dream theory led a number of people in the United States in the 1960s to try to emulate the Senoi in order to obtain the same kinds of benefits from working with their own dreams. Groups shared and discussed their dreams, and individuals made efforts to control their dreams for better outcomes. Reports of the benefits of the Senoi theory were given at psychological, anthropological, and sleep society meetings. Articles were written and published in both the academic journals and popular magazines. In short, the Senoi dream theory was taken seriously and became popular in the United States.

In 1985 the Stewart study of the Senoi was seriously challenged by psychologist and sociologist William Domhoff, a research professor in psychology and sociology at the University of California at Santa Cruz. He had done his Ph.D. thesis on dreams a couple of decades earlier and had published a number of articles after that. For his book, Domhoff (1985) gathered and read what Stewart had written, some of it unpublished, about the Senoi, especially details Stewart had written prior to his pivotal 1951 article. He also interviewed or corresponded with colleagues and family of Stewart, who was dead by this time, and read accounts by others who had studied the Senoi. His conclusion was that Stewart had over time infused his own notions about the benefits of dream sharing and dream control into idealized notions of Senoi society. The Senoi, by all other accounts, were not as happy, peaceful, and mentally healthy as Stewart described them in 1951. Nor was the sharing and controlling of their dreams a dominant aspect of their daily lives. In fact, the Senoi thought about and used dreams no more than any other native culture. Nothing special was going on. Domhoff speculated that Stewart wrote about the Senoi and their supposed dreaming practices based on Stewart's personality.

Domhoff goes on to say that regardless of the veracity of Stewart's claims regarding the Senoi, there may be benefits of dream sharing and control. Yet, the research evidence covering the application of Senoi dream theory in the United States is not very encouraging. It has not been possible to demonstrate many positive benefits of the type Stewart and contemporary Senoi dream theory practitioners have claimed.

8.1.2 Dreams as Omens

The notion that dreams are a means to guide or forecast the future also has its origins in the ancient world. For example, dreams play an important role in the *Odyssey*, offering guidance and providing omens. Vestiges of this notion remain today in the Western World often joined with other understandings of the psychic role of dreams, such as clairvoyance and telepathy.

Numerous cultures have designated certain individuals to aid people in understanding what their dreams are telling them about the future. Typically these priests, priestesses, elders, and the like were held in high esteem and were often very powerful and influential. The Greeks had hundreds of temples where people could go in order to receive guidance dreams, with the priests interpreting the meanings for them.

The Judeo-Christian world is familiar with this concept because of the many prophetic dreams found in the Bible, especially those of Jacob's ladder, the dreams of Pharaoh that required interpretation by the Hebrew slave Joseph, and the dreams Joseph had about Mary being pregnant with Jesus as reported in the Christian New Testament. These stories reflect the prevalent understanding of the source of dreams at the time the Bible was written and the serious regard that people had for them then.

While this idea can no longer be considered the dominant understanding of the source of dreams in the Western world, the idea that dreams have predictive capabilities is nevertheless prevalent. People still consult dictionary-like books in which they can look up an object or action from a dream to see what it "really means," especially for the future. Great caution should be exercised when using such books. They have never been shown to have any accuracy or validity. Many draw heavily from the Oneirocritica written by the Roman physician Artemidorus in about 150 A.D., using the writer's personal experience and imagination or surveys. None of these books demonstrate any attempt at objective verification. It is better to consider them entertainment rather than taking what they say seriously.

Psychic dreams, a variation of this category, are given serious consideration by some in the Western world today. Reports of dreams that are telepathic (=thought transfer), precognitive (=seeing the future), and clairvoyant (=perception of current events beyond ordinary sensory awareness) are taken seriously by many. The notion of psychic dreams is present even at the annual meetings of the Association for the Study of Dreams in the United States where organized attempts at group dreaming and thought transfer via dreams are interspersed among the scientific sessions.

A number of attempts at scientific verification of such psychic dreams has occurred in the twentieth century and still continue today. However, none of these experiments has been found to be satisfactory when critically scrutinized. In some cases, the designs of the experiments contain flaws or lack appropriate controls. In other cases, minimal effects are exaggeratedly viewed as being significant.

For example, in one experiment (Ullman et al. 1989), pairs of friends participated. One slept in a typical sleep lab, while the other spent the night concentrating on a famous painting randomly selected from a group of 12. During each REMS period, the sleeping friend was awakened for a dream report. Any kind of a similarity between some aspect of the selected painting and any portion of any of the dreams were considered evidence of telepathy. Additionally, the next morning the sleeper was shown the 12 paintings and was asked to rank in order how similar each was to dreams from the night. If the painting selected for the night viewing was in the top six picked out by the sleeper, this result was considered additional evidence for telepathy. Both of these criteria for validation are extremely weak. Directly dreaming about the entire painting and then being able to emphatically pick the painting out from among the 12 would be far more convincing. Additionally, appropriate controls should have been used, such as repeating the experiment with exactly the same procedure except never letting the awake friend view any of the pictures.

Other research has produced decidedly negative results. For example, in the 1930s when the baby of the world famous flyer Charles Lindberg was kidnapped, Murray and Wheeler (1937) placed ads in newspapers asking people to submit their dreams of the location and fate of the baby. Thirteen hundred dream reports were received. Later, after the baby's body was found buried, the dream reports were compared to what actually happened. Only 7 contained content that even partially resembled the truth. Most contained false speculations that were widely reported in the newspapers. This study concluded that there was no support for psychic dreaming.

Box 8.2 Comments on the Apparent Psychic Sources of Dreams

Why, you might ask, have people in various cultures at various times believed that there may be psychic sources of dreams? Why do some people today still hold these views? The answers are simple, while the reasons for rejecting these views are more complex, yet more valid. On one hand, the simple answer is that psychic phenomena are easy explanations for what people have experienced for which they have no other simple explanation. Some people have had "out-of-body" dream experiences. Others have dreamed something that later seemed to come true. Still others dreamed that something was wrong with a distant loved-one only to find out that the individual had been in an accident or had died. Such experiences can be very compelling and seem to offer proof of the psychic source of dreams, or at least some dreams. Yet experience is not proof. Another explanation is that some people find it comforting to feel they have control over or at least simple information about what is happening. Here is where the more complex reasons for rejecting these views enter in.

Our experiencing of the world depends on our brain putting together information from our senses of vision, hearing, touch, taste, and smell in a meaningful way (see Sect. 9.2.1). The brain usually does quite a good job, but not always. We can and do perceive things that are not really there. Visual illusions are a good example. We can perceive things that appear quite real yet are physically impossible. Movies are another good example. We perceive continuous action when we view a movie, yet what we are really seeing is a series of still images. The portions of our brain responsible for perception smooth things over so that we do not perceive jerky transitions between the individual images. Numerous psychological and brain studies have led to a detailed understanding of how our brain/mind creates our reality as well as these illusions.

The brain does the same thing when we are sleeping. It endeavors to make the best perceptions of the sensory information available to it. However, little of the sensory information available to the brain while we are sleeping actually originates in our sensory receptors such as our eyes, ears, and skin (see Sect. 5.3.4). Rather, it is generated from the areas of the brain that normally receive and process the information from our sensory receptors (see Sect. 9.2.1). Perceptions, such as being outside of one's body, often seem as real and as vivid as when we are awake, but they are no more real than are our waking illusions. They have not occurred in a physical, real world sense.

Apparent telepathic, clairvoyant, and precognitive dreams can likewise be explained using scientifically verified knowledge about the workings of the brain/mind, albeit complex, without having to resort to simpler yet hypothetical powers and energies. The experiences of some persons that their dreams have been telepathic, clairvoyant, or precognitive necessarily rely on recall of the contents of these dreams. However, as we have seen in Box 7.1, our memories of our dreams are far from accurate and are subject to change over time. Experiments with waking memories for events likewise show that memories can be influenced by what was experienced later. For example, the memory of a witness to an automobile accident can easily be changed by later seeing a similar accident or even similar vehicles. Thus, it is entirely likely that the memory of a dream that later seemed to come true may have been altered by the later, actual event, giving the strong impression that the dream foretold the future.

An example I have used before (Moorcroft 1993) comes from one of my students. The event:

We were at Grandpa's farm. I went for a walk by myself toward the hill that was part of the pasture. I had new white nail polish on. It was a beautiful spring day. Suddenly, Gramp's new white puppy ran over the hill toward me and wanted to play.

The related dream report:

It was just like the dream I had the week before. In the dream, I was in my backyard putting white polish on my nails. I was sitting on the ground on a bright, warm, sunny day. I looked up and there was a hill covered with wildflowers extending from our backyard, and there was a white puppy running down the hill toward me. It came up to me and playfully kissed me. Both the event and the recall of the dream occurred several days after the dream. It is probable that the event influenced the dream report, especially in its details. It may seem that the dream foretold the event, but it is far more likely that the event altered the memory of the prior dream. More convincing would have been if the dream was recorded very soon after it occurred and there was some objective evidence of the event such as a video recording. Without these, it is likely that the event changed the recall of the dream.

Additionally we tend to focus more on the dreams that seem to be psychic while ignoring all the rest. In the example above, had the event not occurred after the dream, it is doubtful that the student would have paid as much attention to the dream later. Or if there was no dream related to the event, it is likely that the event would have received little attention. It is only in those relatively rare but startling cases where the event seems to relate to a prior dream that we focus on this connection and may attribute it to being a psychic dream.

Another rational explanation for the apparent psychic nature of dreaming includes the fact that we perceive more than we can consciously attend to when we are awake. Sometimes these perceptions become part of a dream that appears to be psychic. For example, we may have subconsciously noticed that a railing is loose and that may be incorporated into a dream. Shortly thereafter, somebody has an accident because the railing broke, making it look like the dream was psychic.

Yet, for the most part, science cannot *prove* the nature of things and especially cannot prove that something is unable to happen. All science can do is show that something is more or less probable. It can show that apparently psychic dreams are much more likely due to known behavioral and brain mechanisms rather than to hypotheticals. Another way of putting it is that the supposed psychic phenomena in dreams suffer from a low fact-to-assumption ratio. There is just no hard data to back them up. Nevertheless, it is possible, but only remotely so, that scientists do not yet have the tools with which to discover the facts of psychic phenomena. We need to leave the door open just a crack on the possibility of the existence of psychic dreams.

8.1.3 Dreams as Meaningless

There are people, including many brain scientists during the twentieth century and continuing through today who view dreams as meaningless. "Träume sind Schäume" (=German for "Dreams are foam," just like that fluffy stuff on the top of the real thing, the beer) was what many of Freud's contemporaries said. According to this view dreams are meaningless accompaniments of random activity of the brain during sleep; or are accidental fabrications of the brain during the period of transition from the state of sleep to the state of wakefulness (see Sect. 5.3.3); or are merely responses of our brain to occasional external stimulation such as a noise; or internal stimulation such as indigestion. In any case, dreams are seen as essentially meaningless whether at an unconscious level or at the level of full awareness. One theory (Crick and Mitchison 1983) even maintains that dreams are the result of the mind clearing out useless memories, and that if we try to recall and analyze our dreams, we are undermining this process. Others, especially non-scientists, simply reject dreams as not being relevant and important to their own waking lives. To them, it is a waste of time to pay any attention to dreams.

8.1.4 Dreams as Related to the Dreamer's Waking Life

According to the viewpoint that dreams are related to the dreamer's waking life, each of us conceives of, writes, directs, casts, creates the scenery, and usually stars in several dreams every night, seven days a week. They are comparable to TV programs for which we are the sole audience. This experience is a tremendous creative endeavor well beyond what most of us think we are capable of when awake. Dreams most resemble TV soap operas with a prevalence of negative emotions involving many familiar characters and settings, yet the contents of others are strange and new. Our dreams tend to focus around things that are of personal importance to us, especially at an emotional level. Just as with TV soap operas, our dreams focus on key components of the story rather than include each mundane detail. Aspects may be distorted for emphasis or symbolic in order to bring more meaning. But always they are ours and important to us.

Individuals are the source of their own dreams, and their dreams are *continuous* with their waking personal concerns, experiences, and situations as well as their self-view and worldview. Overwhelmingly, people report dreaming about people and things familiar to them that come from their own memories and personal concerns. This familiarity includes the person's knowledge, experiences, life situation, and world view, plus social interactions with family, friends, and close acquaintances. Dream content is more related to the dreamer's current concerns and interests, particularly to goals that are emotionally important, than other types of themes (Nikles et al. 1998).

This idea is the most prevalent notion in the Western world today about the source of dreams and there is considerable evidence to support it.

8.1.5 A Compromise on the Source of Dreams

Dream content may be influenced by random activation of cortical areas that serve functions such as memory, emotion, senses, and movement plus occasional external stimulation, such as a noise, or internal stimulation, such as indigestion. However, that does not mean that dreaming is meaningless, because the areas stimulated contain the person's individual and meaningful memories and their customary emotional responses plus the way their brain associates the elements activated. For example, if the image of a dining room is activated, then brain networks based on experience such as forks and knives and pleasurable emotions such as eating are more likely to be activated, while others such as bicycles and fear of falling are more likely to be inhibited. However, a person that experienced a different culture might associate dining room to chopsticks rather than forks. Then, just as when awake, the brain does its best to integrate these activations and associations in a sensible way in its own more or less unique way again based on a lifetime of experience. The result is dreaming that is unique and meaningful to the individual.

However, the rules that the brain uses to integrate these elements are a bit different when in REMS than they are when awake or in NREMS. This is shown by experiments testing word association tests (Stickgold et al. 1999) and anagram puzzle solving (Walker et al. 2002) very soon after awakening from either REMS or N2. During this time the brain has not completely functionally reorganized from sleep mode to awake mode and thus still contains remnants of REMS or NREMS associative structure. The major finding was that upon awakening from REMS subjects responded differently with less common or weak word associations and anagram solutions than they did when awake or coming out of N2. Such associative structure changes during REMS suggest why dreaming results in both bizarre but creative dreams.

8.2 The Dominant View of Dreaming in the Western World

The prevailing view of dreaming in the Western World contains several elements—cultural, personal, emotional, and current events.

8.2.1 Cultural Influences on Dreaming

One way that shows that dreams are a product of our waking lives is that dreams contain elements of the culture in which we live. Some things appear to be typical of recalled dreams in all cultures, such as falling, flying, or being unable to move. However, anthropological studies show that what people report dreaming about, the amount of dream recall, and thus possibly the amount of dreaming itself are influenced by the dreamer's language, religious beliefs, social structures, and customs. Yet, there are also common elements in what neighbors, friends, and relatives report dreaming about, showing that our culture also influences dream content. People in the United States mostly dream about houses and cars, and their dreams are populated with people dressed like their neighbors. The dreams of people in small primitive societies contain huts or tents, yaks or oxen, and people dressed far differently than people in the United States.

Sociological cultural differences also influence what people dream about. This is shown in the dreams of the Japanese and people in three East African societies versus those of people in the Western industrialized world (Domhoff 1996). While Japanese men report two times as many men as women in their dreams, just as do men in the in the Western world, women's reports in Japan differ greatly. While women in the Western world report 1:1 ratio of male and female characters in their dreams, Japanese women recall a 2:1 ratio of women to male characters. This difference is thought to correspond to the intense gender segregation in Japanese society. Both Japanese men and women report much less aggression in their dreams than do their counterparts in the West. The reduction was much larger for the men than the women. Again, the dream differences are thought to relate to differences in Japanese society regarding everyday aggression.

In three male dominated societies of East Africa—the Gusii, the Kipsigis, and the Logoli—the males revealed a greater percent of male compared to female characters in their dreams, whereas the females showed ratios much closer to equal. This finding closely parallels what is found in Western industrialized societies but differs greatly from that found in Japan. Aggression in dreams showed a different pattern. The East Africa women reported much more physical aggression in their dreams than did Western women or Japanese women. They also reported more non-physical aggression than their male counterparts did. This finding, too, differed from reports from Western and Japanese women. These aggression results are most likely related to a great concern by East African women about being victimized.

Other factors, such as socioeconomic class, can have an effect on dream content. For example, people of lower socioeconomic status have more misfortune in their dreams; people in upper class have less death anxiety in their dreams (Anch et al. 1988).

8.2.2 *Influences from Waking Life on Dreaming*

We seem to prefer to dream about recent and personal waking events, thoughts, concerns, and emotions. Yet dreams are not exact reflections of the waking world but rather are more like dramas that portray things in such a way to be useful and meaningful to the dreamer. The elements of the dream are put together according to dreamers' typical ways of organizing their perceptions, knowledge, and emotional overlay. These elements and their organization may differ considerably from one individual to another.

While not very popular until the twentieth century, the following view of the source of dreams has ancient roots. Aristotle saw dreams as perceptions similar but not identical to waking perceptions. He went on to say that many of our waking perceptions are based on sensing physical stimuli, but we can still perceive these things by imagining them in our minds when the stimuli are not present. In the same way, we can imagine things in our minds when asleep. Yet, when asleep, the perceptions may be distorted since the "intellect" is not working as it does when we are awake. This phenomenon is like "eddies in a great river... (that are often) broken into other forms by collisions with other objects" (Aristotle as quoted in Borbély 1986). Additionally, to Aristotle dream content is distorted and exaggerated by our emotions left over from waking experiences.

The great popularity today of this notion about the source of dreams can be attributed to Freud. In his classic book, *The Interpretation of Dreams* published in 1900, he stressed that dreams are the creation of the dreamer's mind originating in "wish-fulfillment." Although Freud maintained that these wishes present in dreams are disguised from our awareness, they nevertheless emanate from our own minds and waking lives. And they are of great benefit for the dreamer, for they relieve the pressure coming from unfulfilled unconscious desires of waking life (see more of Freud's theory of dreaming in Sect. 9.1.1). While many of those who followed in Freud's footsteps later rejected the concept that we are not aware and cannot easily be aware of the real meaning of our dreams, they nevertheless accepted the basic idea that our dreams are a product of our mind formed out of our waking experiences, needs, and concerns.

Experimental evidence confirms that the content of our dreams is influenced by our waking world but are not usually an exact replica of it. For example (Fosse et al. 2003), subjects kept a diary of both waking events for two weeks and recalled dreams. Sixty-five percent of the dreams were found to contain some element from their diary, but less than 2 % were exact replicas of their waking experiences. Thus fragments, but only fragments, of our waking experiences are often a part of our dreams. Other research has found that recent experiences rather than older ones more frequently become a part of our dreams.

8.2.3 Emotional Influences on Dreaming

When something, especially an emotion, is experienced during the day, it is more likely to form the core of dream content during the next night or perhaps a few nights later, because various brain cell processes favor reactivating recently activated connections between cells. These core components link to other components, especially the main people in the dreamer's waking life and the kinds of social interactions they have. But they also link to features like events and settings from the dreamer's past as well as the dreamer's main interests and activities to form much of the content of the dream. However, dreams are not simply replays of what happened during the day or the past, but they draw upon these things and use them in ways for, seemingly, their own purposes. Lengthy dream journals studied by people unacquainted with the dreamer confirm this hypothesis.

8.2.4 The Influence of Current News Events on Dreaming

Mid-twentieth century psychologist and dream researcher, Calvin Hall, stated in his 1966 book *The Meaning of Dreams* that dreams seldom focus on current events such as elections, war, athletic events, or happenings recorded in newspapers. These things may be common topics of conversation, but seldom topics of our dreams. Kelley Bulkeley, Visiting Scholar at the Graduate Theological Union in Berkeley, California, has a Ph.D. in religious studies and a strong professional interest in dreams. He has investigated the implications of Hall's statement (Bulkeley 1996). He agrees that political themes are relatively rare in recalled dreams, but when they are present, they add to the understanding of the source of dreams. They show how dreams can help dreamers with their personal internal world by relating them to events that are important to them or that may have personal consequences.

Bulkeley began by studying detailed dream diaries of 12 people during the two weeks straddling the presidential election in the United States in 1992. This election contest, mainly between sitting Republican president George Bush senior, Democratic challenger Bill Clinton, and independent candidate Ross Perot, was exciting and passionately waged and dominated the print as well as electronic media for weeks. Six of the 12 subjects recorded at least one dream with some content about the election and of the total of 113 dream reports, 10 contained such content. As Bulkeley concludes, since many people during this election "felt that the political state of the United States was confusing, strange, and frightening" (Bulkeley 1996, p. 188), it should not be surprising that some people occasionally dreamed about it.

In additional data from that presidential election and the next one four years later, Bulkeley (personal communication, 2001) found three kinds of dreams related to politics: political cartoons of the mind, new political perspectives, and personal symbols.

8.2.4.1 Political Cartoons of the Mind

Dreams express in succinct and sometimes humorous ways the dreamer's waking political perspective. Here's an example from a 36-year-old man from Florida:

> I'm playing golf with Bill Clinton. I've heard people say he cheats, and I understand what they mean, because he frequently improves the lie of his ball. But he encourages the people he's playing with to do the same. He says, "It's just a game, and just for fun!"

This dreamer voted enthusiastically for Clinton in 1992, but in 1996, when he had this dream, he was not sure if he would vote for Clinton in the upcoming election. The dreamer saw the golf imagery of his dream as an expression of his concern that President Clinton is a "cheater" who frequently "improves his lies" and then tries to smooth-talk other people into letting him get away with it.

8.2.4.2 New Political Perspectives

Dreams call into question the dreamer's waking life political attitudes, leading the dreamer to think anew about his or her accustomed beliefs about a politician or a political issue. This example comes from a 44-year-old man from New York:

> I'm on a camping trip with the President and his party in a heavily wooded area. Suddenly, Clinton darts up a hill into the woods. He sees a bear approaching the camping area. None of us moves, as the President confronts the bear; Clinton is very expert and competent as he does this, not wild or frightened. He manages to drive the huge bear, the size of a Grizzly, into a snare set for him. The FBI in the entourage are angry at the close call, but the President seems unperturbed.

This dreamer said that from the start he had been skeptical of Bill Clinton's leadership qualities, but he awoke from this dream surprised by Clinton's swift, assertive, and fearless response to the threat of the huge bear. As a result of his dream, this man reconsidered his generally dim view of Clinton's executive abilities, wondering if he had been overlooking the President's skills as a fighter.

8.2.4.3 Personal Symbols

Dreams use the figures of politicians as "personal symbols" to express strong emotions that the dreamer is feeling toward some matter in his or her waking life. Here's an example from a 55-year-old woman from New Mexico:

> I'm back in college, in one of the classrooms, and Bill Clinton is one of the students. Then he's the teacher, and he asks me how alcohol manufacturers get us to drink so much. I say I haven't given the question much thought.

This dreamer had long struggled with alcoholism, and in her dream, she sees the President as the voice of "executive authority" within her, a voice that is prompting her to think more carefully about why she drinks.

8.3 Dreams Are Products of the Dreamer's Brain/Mind

The contemporary of approach toward the source of dreams in the Western World draws on the understanding of how the brain/mind works. Within the brain/mind of each of us are networks of memories from acquired knowledge and experiences, many in the form of images. There are also networks of stored information about how we conceive of ourselves and others as well our dominant modes of perceiving, thinking, and reacting. Also included are our individual world views, our hopes and fears, our life situation, our social interactions with family, friends, and close acquaintances, and our current, as well as enduring, concerns. Various components of these networks are linked with one another so that when one component is accessed it is easier to access the other linked components. Thus, a particular emotion may be linked to specific experiences, both recent and remote, that evoked that emotion during past wakefulness—or in past dreams for that matter. Some of the components form the core of the linkages while others have varying degrees of remoteness. When a core component is accessed, it is more likely that the components linked to it will be also be accessed. This linkage can also happen, but is less likely, when a more remotely linked component is the first to be accessed. On the other hand, research by Robert Stickgold and associates at Harvard (Stickgold et al. 1999) suggests that linkages to more remote components are more favored during REMS (see Sect. 11.3.2). Others maintain that even some previously non-associated or at least not obviously associated elements can also be brought into the dream.

David Foulkes (e.g., 1999), based on his studies of dream recall development in children (see Sect. 9.2.4), adds that the ability to dream gradually develops during childhood beginning at about 5 years of age, becomes well formed by age 9, but continues developing through age 12, 13. Foulkes sees this development in the ability to dream as depending on the development of visual-spatial abilities in the brain as measured by various tests during waking. Yet others interpret Foulkes's data differently (e.g., Hobson et al. 2000). For example, the low quality and quantity of dream recall at early ages could just as well be due to the fact that language ability is not sufficient to describe the dream experiences that children may actually be having.

8.3.1 The Influence of Presleep Experiences on Dreaming

Attempts to manipulate dream content by exposing people to specific experiences prior to sleep have had only mixed success. There are two types of exposure—a specific stimulus or a more complex experience.

The best success with a specific stimulus was obtained by Roffwarg and colleagues (reported in Arkin et al. 1978). Nine people wore red tinted goggles for 5 days when awake. During this time, their dreams went from containing a normal spectrum of colors to primarily only reds. Overall, there was a three-fold increase in the color red in the dreams even among those told to expect more green, the complementary color to red. Furthermore, the amount of red reported in dreams increased from the first through the third days of the experiment.

Attempts to incorporate complex experiences include using events such as social isolation, vigorous exercise, difficult or stressful mental tasks, and subliminal stimulation. Likewise, films with graphic, emotion-arousing scenes such as a difficult birth, amputation, ritual circumcision, and hard core pornography have been employed. However, these experiences only occasionally influence dream content. It has been suggested that when such attempts were successful, it was because the stimulus was related to the subject's interests, especially at an emotional level. Also, some studies suggest the influence of such experiences on dream content may not be immediate, which is what most studies look for, but occur several nights later (Powell et al. 1995).

The experience most likely to influence dream content is the sleep lab itself. It is not unusual for someone sleeping in a sleep lab, whether a part of this type of experiment or not, to report dreaming of people in lab coats, a room full of strange electrical machinery, things glued to the head, and long wires. This experience occurs about one-third of the time. This is an example of an intense interpersonal encounter that the person is living rather than something just passively viewing and therefore may be more engaging and thus more able to influence dream content.

8.3.2 Dream Incubation

Dream incubation occurs when a person is successful at determining what they will dream about before they dream. Typically this is done by concentrating their attention on the desired topic when going to sleep. For example, a person might repeat to themselves that they will dream about a particular person or an experience they once had. While little published research has been done on the validity of dream incubation, Delaney (1998) reports that several studies show high success rates. The results are better when dreamers are given help interpreting the meaning of the metaphorical content of the recalled dream showing how it related to their incubation efforts. Additionally, Nikles and colleagues (1998) found that people are more likely to incubate dreams when directed to dream about things related to their personal current concerns than if directed to dream about other things or given no directive. They also found that suggested topics related to personal concerns frequently became the central topic of a reported dream.

Dream incubation is only sometimes successful. All in all, dreams it seems are semi-autonomous. They appear to have their own agenda of what to focus on, but sometimes this focus can be influenced.

Box 8.3 Dream Incubation: Delaney's Method

Gayle Delaney, Ph.D., is a psychologist who has devoted her career to working with dreams. In her books *Living Your Dreams* (1996) and *All about Dreams* (1998) she describes in detail her method for incubating dreams. The crucial step in her method is to write down and then repeat what you want to dream about over and over again as you are falling asleep. This request could be to dream about something in particular or to answer a question. This task is the only thing accomplished dream incubators need to do. However, neophytes need to do more in order to improve on the ability to incubate dreams.

Neophytes need to begin by choosing a night when you are not overly tired and have some time both before bed and upon awakening to work on this technique. In a journal, begin by writing a few lines about what you did and felt during the day. Next, focus on an issue you would like to dream about and write out a thorough discussion of the issue. Be sure to include your feelings on the issue. Now, and this is an important but not always an easy step, compose and write a one-line request or question. As you are ready to fall asleep, repeat the request or question over and over. As soon as you awaken from a dream, or at the end of your sleep period, write down your recall of your dream(s) with as much detail as possible. Perhaps the dream obviously fulfills your request or answers your question, but it is more likely that it is metaphorical. In either case, Delaney recommends that you work with the dream to fully understand its meanings (see Box 9.1 for Delaney's dream interpretation technique.)

8.3.3 The Influence of Physiological Events on Dreaming

A common idea expressed in some ancient through contemporary writings is that dreams are generated by internal sensations such as from illness or from indigestion after eating an anchovy, onion, and green pepper pizza right before bedtime. Some Greek as well as other writers even maintained that dream content could be used to help diagnose illnesses. Although many studies have tried to relate physiological changes in the body to dream content, the results have been disappointing.

Dramatic thirst caused by 24 h without fluid intake prior to sleep failed to produce any dream content related to drinking or thirst. However, in another experiment, the subjects not only went without fluid for 24 h prior to going to sleep, but also ate salty food just before bedtime. Their dream reports contained various references to water, including snow and lakes and more specific thirst-related objects such as soda pop. Thus, strong internal physiological stimuli may sometimes contribute to what is dreamed about, but only some of the time (Empson 1993).

Overall, however, extensive studies of the relationship between physiological events including heart rate, facial muscle activity, penile erections, or a full bladder do not regularly influence dream content or amount of recall. For example, heart rate does not seem to be related to the emotionality in the dream even though it changes during strong emotions when awake. One exception is some relationship between breathing rate at the time of the dream and recalled dream content.

It is reasonable to hypothesize that those phasic events of REMS such as rapid eye movements or surges in heart rate would affect dream content. Specifically, it was hypothesized that dreams would be more intense with more perceptions rather than just thoughts and would be more bizarre during such phasic events. However, laboratory tests largely failed to confirm this hypothesis. Likewise, occurrences like K-complexes during NREMS were shown to have little effect on reported mentation. Yet, reported dream content when phasic events are more frequent, such as a high "density" of rems, have been reported to be more emotional, be more vivid, contain more activity, and be better recalled.

8.3.4 Effects of External Sensations on Dreaming

Although you, like many people, may recall having slept through a buzzing alarm clock, because you *incorporated*[1] the sound into your dream, laboratory studies show that this type of incorporation is infrequent. Various kinds of stimuli have been used in the sleep laboratory in the attempt to produce incorporation during sleep including light, sound, and touch. Of all things tried, spraying water onto the face of sleepers during REMS most frequently produces incorporation during sleep but only at 42 % in one study (Dement and Wolpert 1958). It is incorporated directly as water squirts or indirectly as a sudden shower or a leak in the roof. Even

---

[1] Incorporation occurs when a sound or some other stimulus sensed by a sleeper when dreaming is woven into the dream rather than being ignored or causing awakening.

electric shocks applied to the wrist during sleep result in reported incorporation into a dreamonly one out of five times.

Even when incorporation of a stimulus that occurs during sleep happens, it is extremely rare for the stimulus to become a dominant element in the dream. Most often it becomes some minor element in an ongoing dream. Also, higher rates of incorporation of a stimulus applied during sleep are reported when less literal representations of the stimulus are counted. For example, when the stimulus was jet sounds, dream recall containing sounds of a gas stove that spits was counted as incorporation. In another example, the stimulus of weeping sounds led to the report of squeaking footsteps in a dream being counted (Strauch and Meier 1996).

An example of this kind of research was done by Ralph Berger (1963). While his subjects were awake, he determined which names of each one's friends evoked the greatest emotional responses on recordings of their galvanic skin responses—a component frequently used in lie detection. He then spoke one of the high response names to each subject while asleep. He found evidence of incorporation in about half of the trials, but the named individual appeared in the dream in only 3 of the 48 instances of incorporation. Most of the rest were based on assonance such as "Chilean" for "Gillian" and "like" for "Mike."

8.3.5 Dreams Have Their Own Agendas

One interpretation of these data about only occasional incorporation of stimuli applied during sleep or pre-sleep experiences is that the agenda for a dream is based on a general theme such as an emotional need. Also the specific contents of the dream are there only if they, in some way, contribute to this overriding theme. Likewise, dream incubation is not always successful because the preexisting agenda for the dream may often take precedence. Another interpretation is that the dream agenda and the specific contents of the dream are randomly selected from all that is available and that presleep experiences, including incubation, and sensations during sleep are simply included in this large pool.

8.3.6 Long-Term Consistency and Change in the Dreams of Individuals

There is a consistency in a persons recalled dreams over their adult lifetime, but significant emotional events can cause changes (Domhoff 1996). Examination of the dream journals of a number of people, each with several hundred dreams, shows just how consistent our dreams are. Consistency is first noted late in adolescence and lasts for the rest of life. There are three kinds of consistency: absolute consistency—elements continue to appear at the same frequency, relative consistency—even when the appearance on elements increase or decrease their relative ratios remain constant, and developmental consistency—the change in frequency remains consistent over successive time periods.

There is only uneven evidence that aspects of the content of a person's dreams, especially social interactions and dream emotions, are influenced by their personality. However, one study showed that over a 6 to 10 year duration dream content was well correlated with psychological wellbeing. Also, successful psychotherapy can cause changes in recalled dream content (Hunt 1989).

Other studies have shown that people who have experienced a negative emotional event, such as sexual abuse, have more frequent and intense nightmares (Penn et al. 1991). Other similar observations include changes in the dreams of patients prior to surgery and in patients hospitalized for burns, and when the Dow Jones Industrial Average experienced one of its worse weekly declines, those stockbrokers who showed higher stress had dreams that were more negative such as being chased or falling. However, the best research comes from the study of the change in dreams during the course of pregnancy, divorce, and psychological trauma.

8.3.6.1 Dream Changes During Pregnancy

Pregnancy, especially the first one, is a major change in a woman's life (Maybruck 1986; Stukane 1985). During the first few months of the pregnancy, sometimes beginning even before she knows she is pregnant, the content of a woman's recalled dreams changes. Some of the dreams are obviously related to pregnancy, such as themes related to fertility and reproductive ability, miscarriage, and dangerous or intrusive fetuses. Other themes are thought to be more symbolically related, such as an increase of small animals, representing the fetus, in recalled dreams. More generally, a pregnant woman may recall dreaming more about herself than she had before.

By the middle of the pregnancy, the content of recalled dreams again changes. Now there is more critical judgment of herself and her significant other. There are concerns about being an adequate mother that emerge, as well as many of the kinds of things that can go wrong with being a mother. She may typically dream about her relationship with the prospective father as well as that of her own mother and of her comparisons with her mother. Babies rather than small animals are more likely to populate her recalled dreams. It is not uncommon for these babies to be abnormal in some way. Continuing from the earlier phase of the pregnancy are dreams of the baby as some kind of trespasser. By late middle pregnancy, the fetus in her dream recalls often are more appealing, but there are dreams of various general disasters involving not only labor and delivery but also topics such as finances, careers, and marriage.

During the last couple months of pregnancy most women report recalling many more dreams than they had previously. This increased recall seems to happen not because of having more dreams but because of waking up more often during this stage of the pregnancy (see Sect. 4.8) and thus being able to recall more of the dreams. Women recall continuing to dream of the things they did during the middle of their pregnancy, such as comparing themselves to their mother and unusual or abnormal babies, but also about changes in their body and how they are the focus of special attention by others. As the pregnancy draws to a close, they begin to recall dreaming of the birthing process itself and of their doctor.

Subsequent pregnancies also affect the dreams of the woman but with some differences. For example, recalled dreams about her ability to be a mother and comparisons with her own mother tend to be replaced by concerns about the relationship of the new child with the existing family members.

It is not entirely clear if these changes in the dreams of pregnant women are due to the psychological or the physiological changes that accompany pregnancy. However, the situation is clearer when looking at the changes that also occur in the recalled dreams of the prospective father (Siegel 1983; Stukane 1985). Since he is much less physiologically involved in the ongoing pregnancy, changes in his dream recall must be psychologically based.

After he becomes aware that he initiated a pregnancy in a woman, the prospective father recalls dreaming more about his sexual masculinity and identity. He may recall dreams with more sexual activity in them. A conflict between his machismo and his nurturance may also emerge. During the middle of the pregnancy, the themes of nurturance continue, but dreams about his general identity replace those of overt sex. He may compare himself to his father and to his family when he was a child in his dreams. At the same time he may dream of being left out of the pregnancy process, or he may even dream about being pregnant himself. He often will dream about his relationship with his pregnant partner. Later in the pregnancy, his recalled dreams about his childhood family diminish, replaced by content about his current family. He also may recall dreaming about his changes in his partner's body, what their child will be like (more often as a son than a daughter), and, toward the end of the pregnancy, the birthing process.

Note the similarities between the dreams of pregnant women and their partners responsible for the pregnancy. Early on, both focus on themselves and the changes that the pregnancy may bring for them. As the pregnancy progresses, they both begin to recall dreaming more about the pregnancy itself, the baby, and their relationship to one another.

8.3.6.2 Dreams of Depressed People

Rosalind Cartwright has done an extensive series of research studies on the dreams of people undergoing a major and usually emotionally difficult change in their lives, namely divorce (Cartwright 1989; Cartwright et al. 1998). She hypothesized that if we dream about things that are important to us, and especially if these things arouse strong emotions, then the dreams of divorcing people, many of whom are very depressed during the process, should show obvious differences from the dreams of non-divorcing, non-depressed cohorts.

Cartwright found that people who are divorcing and are depressed have their first REMS period earlier, and their REMS periods are more evenly distributed through the night. Additionally, they have noticeably more rems during their REMS. All these symptoms are considered signs of emotional overload. Further, they report recalling dreams that are shorter, more oriented to the past, more masochistic, more repetitive, and blander. Also, the themes of their recalled dreams are often that things are "all my fault." They seem impotent in their recalled dreams in the sense that as a character they are unable to do even simple things such as moving their arms. Likewise, things do not seem to work, such as drawers not opening. Also, important things like keys to the car are lost. By the end of the night, the negativity in their dreams is increased rather than reduced, and there is no progression from dream to dream through the night. Cartwright also finds that as the depression abates, these characteristics of their dreams lessen.

8.3.6.3 Effect of Psychological Trauma on Dreaming

Hartmann (1998) points to recalled dreams following traumatic events as the clearest case of showing the source of dreams. These dreams may occur for some months following the trauma but often eventually go away. (For dreams that do not fade with time following trauma, see the discussion about PTSD in Sect. 12.4.2.2). People will dream of the incident but with changes in details. The changes continue as the person dreams again and again of the incident. In spite of these changes, people will say years later that they remember the dreams as being an "exact replay" of the incident. Others will recall dreams about the incident that are more metaphorical, such as dreaming of a tidal wave or great whirlwind about to overtake them. They report feeling terrified and vulnerable during the dream. These descriptions best illustrate how emotions can be the instigating focus of dream content, because it is obvious that the emotion of the traumatic situation is on the person's mind when awake. Incidentally, Hartmann finds that such dreams can be somewhat equivalent to our own internal psychotherapist, because they enable the dreamer to work through the trauma in a "safe place," just as happens when talking to a trained therapist in the safety of the office following a trauma.

8.4 The Process of Dreaming

There was a time when it was believed that dreams occurred instantaneously, often at the time of awakening. Much of this belief can be attributed to a dream report by Alfred Maury, a nineteenth century dream researcher. He had a dream that he was in Paris at the time of the French revolution. He recalled being led to the guillotine and his head placed in it. He awakened just as the blade struck his neck only to find that the headboard on his bed had fallen on this exact location! He reasoned that the entire dream must have been instantly fabricated from the sensation on his neck caused by the fallen headboard.

The notion that dream formation is instantaneous has been contradicted by twentieth century research that found a correlation of the apparent time that had elapsed in the dream recall story with the amount of time the person had been in REMS before being awakened. However, this research used a small sample size and has not been replicated (Domhoff and Schnelder 1999). Other research using incorporation was more conclusive. For example, spraying a mist of water on a sleeper's face when in REMS then awakening them 1, 3, or 7 min later generally resulted in reported events that would have taken an equivalent amount of time after the "cloudburst," "being splashed," "feeling a bird dump on my nose." Also, Maury did not write about his famous dream until 10 years after he had it, which raises questions about the veracity of the recall. Conclusion: we probably dream in real time, although it is possible that we may at times speed the process up.

8.4.1 The Number of Dreams During a REMS Period

There may be multiple dreams per REMS period, especially for the longer bouts of REMS, somewhat like watching a single channel on TV during a sequence of different half hour shows. However, since the boundaries between dreams are not always clearly defined, it is not possible to say for certain just how many different dreams are typical per night.

8.4.2 Brain Organization During Dreaming

Evolving technologies for studying brain function such as PET scans and recordings the activity of individual or small groups of brain cells are being used to provide understandings of the process of dreaming. The primary finding is that functional organization of the brain is different during sleep than during waking, especially during REMS (see Sect. 5.4). That is, the areas of the brain continue for the most part to have the same functions that they have during wakefulness; however, the relative strength of activity in various parts of the brain differs, the organization of the connections between them is altered during sleep, and the balance of the neurochemicals is different.

The situation in the brain during NREMS is simple. During NREMS the forebrain is relatively inactive, operating at a low level. Whatever activation occurs is less frequent and less sustained. This relative inactivity is what causes the characteristics of NREMS mentation.

According to Hobson and colleagues at Harvard (e.g., Hobson et al. 2000), during REMS the situation is very much different and more complex. Overall, there is relatively more activity in the intermediate and higher levels of the brain that is more sustained because of the action of the arousal systems located in the brainstem using acetylcholine. The intermediate areas activated are parts of the limbic system involved with basic emotions, especially fear, anger, and emotions related to sexual behavior; motivations, particularly those that are related to survival; and aspects of our memories of the past. Higher areas are also selectively activated including those for our sensory processing especially the so called secondary areas that process sensory information; areas that contain our depictions about the nature of things and how they work; partial elements of our episodic memories; and the parts of the cortex that associate the these available bits of information in meaningful ways.

At the same time, there is relatively less activation of the primary sensory areas and the areas of the cortex, especially the prefrontal cortex, that provide reality checks, inhibitions, and general executive functioning (see Box 5.4). Additionally, areas important for the formation of new memories are deactivated.

One way to conceptualize this is to think of the brain as almost completely isolated from external stimulation from the rest of the body but with the brain internally stimulating some areas but not others. Figure 8.1 summarizes the functional organization of the brain during REMS and how this produces dreaming.

Overall, many brain areas important for cognitive processes are active during REMS, but some key components are not. The result is dreaming that includes elements of memories from our waking lives and experiences, emotions, and motivations but lacking in logic and reality testing. We experience this with total attention in a mainly visual mode that seems real at the time and out of our control. The result is dreams that our waking mind perceives as often bizarre and illogical but with many recognizable elements.

Mark Solms presents a somewhat different view of how the brain produces dreams based on his review of dreaming in brain damaged patients (Solms 1997, 2000). Some aspects are similar to the Activation–Synthesis Hypothesis but differ in certain key ways. Similarities included areas of the brain that are functionally altered such as (1) the lack of motor output, (2) internal rather than external activation of the forebrain, and (3) the inability to distinguish hallucinations from reality. The key differences between the Activation–Synthesis Hypothesis and Solms' view are (1) the source of activation for the initiation of dreaming is via dopamine from the midbrain, not acetylcholine from the lower in the brainstem; (2) the areas first activated are certain reward networks located in the limbic and prefrontal areas rather than simultaneous activation of multiple forebrain areas; and (3) the inhibitory influences from the frontal cortex that function to prevent awakening the sleeper are activated. In its simplest terms, according to Solms, it is arousal from the emotional areas of the midbrain that instigates dreaming, not random activation from the brainstem.

Fig. 8.1 The functional organization of the brain during REMS showing how it produces dreaming. Based on information from neurophysiological, neuropsychological and neuroimaging studies. Redrawn from (Hobson et al. 2000). Locations of areas in figure are approximate

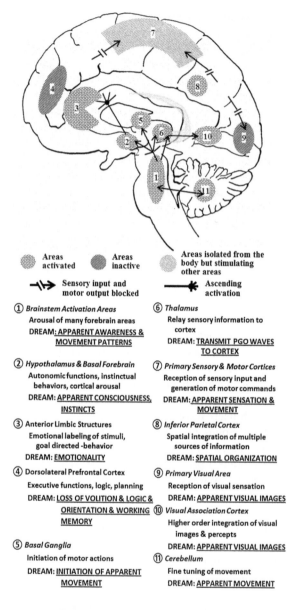

Areas activated   Areas inactive   Areas isolated from the body but stimulating other areas

Sensory input and motor output blocked   Ascending activation

① *Brainstem Activation Areas*
Arousal of many forebrain areas
DREAM: APPARENT AWARENESS & MOVEMENT PATTERNS

② *Hypothalamus & Basal Forebrain*
Autonomic functions, instinctual behaviors, cortical arousal
DREAM: APPARENT CONSCIOUSNESS, INSTINCTS

③ *Anterior Limbic Structures*
Emotional labeling of stimuli, goal directed -behavior
DREAM: EMOTIONALITY

④ *Dorsolateral Prefrontal Cortex*
Executive functions, logic, planning
DREAM: LOSS OF VOLITION & LOGIC & ORIENTATION & WORKING MEMORY

⑤ *Basal Ganglia*
Initiation of motor actions
DREAM: INITIATION OF APPARENT MOVEMENT

⑥ *Thalamus*
Relay sensory information to cortex
DREAM: TRANSMIT PGO WAVES TO CORTEX

⑦ *Primary Sensory & Motor Cortices*
Reception of sensory input and generation of motor commands
DREAM: APPARENT SENSATION & MOVEMENT

⑧ *Inferior Parietal Cortex*
Spatial integration of multiple sources of information
DREAM: SPATIAL ORGANIZATION

⑨ *Primary Visual Area*
Reception of visual sensation
DREAM: APPARENT VISUAL IMAGES

⑩ *Visual Association Cortex*
Higher order integration of visual images & percepts
DREAM: APPARENT VISUAL IMAGES

⑪ *Cerebellum*
Fine tuning of movement
DREAM: APPARENT MOVEMENT

8.4.3 Rhythmic Influences on Dreaming

Tore Nielsen (2011), Ph.D., a Professor in the Department of Psychiatry, University of Montreal where he is the Director of the Dream and Nightmare Laboratory, has reviewed research that suggests REMS dreaming and NREMS mentation are shaped by rhythmic influences that emanate from the brain (see Sect.

3.2.2). These include the 90 min REMS-NREMS ultradian cycle, the sleep-wake circadian rhythm, and the increase in REMS propensity as a night of sleep progresses. While the research done to date is far from conclusive, different aspects of dreaming seem to be affected, such as the likelihood of a dream or mentation recall, the length of recall reports, and the intensity of the visual perception.

Nielsen concludes that both the quality and quantity of REMS dreams and NREMS mentation are varied by one or several "imagery generators" with a 90 min ultradian rhythm. For example, during REMS, dream reports are longest when obtained during the middle of a REMS period but shorter before or after this; for NREMS mentation recalls the pattern is just the opposite. That is, the peak of the ultradian influence is in the middle of the REMS period and lowest during the middle of the NREMS period. In addition, qualitative aspects such as how vivid, intense, and dreamlike the recalls are seem also to vary with a 90 min frequency.

Research on REMS dreams and NREMS mentations through the night indicate circadian and sleep-dependent influences. Changes in the length of dreams as well as their organization, substance, and how well they are remembered imply circadian-like variations. Additionally, the reports obtained from the first third of the sleep period are markedly different in quality from those obtained during the remainder of the sleep period. For example, REMS dream reports get longer as the night goes on even if all the reports are gathered after about 5 min into the REMS period have elapsed. Likewise, the number of events per story, but not the number of statements in the episode gradually increase during the sleep period. Also dreams tend to become more realistic and engrossing later in sleep. However, it is also possible that these qualitative differences may be due to changes in the length of the reports that also get longer as the night goes on, so these conclusions have to be considered tentative.

Sleep-dependent influences have also been reported. Compared to shorter episodes (less than a minute), dreams during longer REMS episodes (over 9 min) are livelier, more theatrical, and more vibrant, but with more distortion, emotionality, anxiousness, disagreeableness, antagonism, and violence. In addition there are a greater variety of scenes and more scenes where the imagining is more clear. Yet elements like believability and reasonableness of the dream remain constant.

8.5   Conclusion

Dreams, like sleep, occur between two periods of wakefulness. They are influenced by prior waking and can influence subsequent waking. Cartwright captures this with the title of her book *The Twenty-four Hour Mind* (2010). Earlier in history and in other cultures people had other views of the sources of dreams such as that during a dream the dreamer is existing in a different world or that dreams have psychic properties. Today, most dream researchers agree that dreams are constructed by the same mental processes that we use when awake, but the source of material differs between individuals (Bulkeley 1997). They also seem to concur that dreaming plays a role in processing both external and internal information from waking that helps adaptation to the environment by organizing perceptions, keeping cognitive mechanisms exercised, and integrating new with existing memories. Dream researcher Bill Domhoff (personal communication, July, 2001) sees the contents of dreams as being mostly continuous with our waking lives, generally expressing our conceptions and concerns. Further, studies of a series of dreams show that there is a lot of repetition in what an individual dreams about (Domhoff 1996). Dreams contain the "conceptions, concerns, and interests" of the dreamer (Domhoff 1996, p. 153), but do not necessarily reflect how they behave during their waking lives. Domhoff does not believe that dreams are compensatory, that is bringing some kind of balance or healing to our waking lives, but other dream researchers believe that dreams can sometimes be compensatory. However, this issue is difficult to scientifically assess (Van de Castle 1994).

References

Anch, A. M., Browman, C. P., Mitler, M. M., & Walsh, J. K. (1988). *Sleep: a scientific perspective*. Englewood Cliffs: Prentice Hall.

Berger, R. (1963). Experimental modification of dream content by meaningful verbal stimuli. *Brittish Journal of Psychiatry*, *109*, 722–740.

Borbély, A. (1986). *The secrets of sleep*. New York: Basic Books.

Bulkeley, K. (1996). *Among all these dreamers*. Albany: State University of New York Press.

Bulkeley, K. (1997). *An introduction to the psychology of dreaming*. Westport, Connecticut: Praeger.

Cartwright, R. D. (1989). Dreams and their meaning. In M. Kryger, T. Roth, & W. Dement (Eds.), *Principles and practice of sleep medicine* (pp. 184–190). Philadelphia: Saunders.

Cartwright, R. D. (2010). *The twenty-four hour mind*. New York: Oxford University Press.

Crick, F., & Mitchison, G. (1983). The function of dream sleep. *Nature*, *30*, 111–114.

Dement, W., & Wolpert, E. (1958). The relation of eye movements, body motility, and external stimuli to dream content. *Journal of Expimental Psychology*, *55*, 543–554.

Domhoff, G. W. (1985). *The mystique of dreams*. Los Angeles: University of California Press.

Domhoff, G. W. (1996). *Finding meaning in dreams: a quantitative approach*. New York: Plenum.

Domhoff, G. W., & Schnelder, A. (1999). Much ado about very little: the small effect sizes when home and laboratory collected dreams are compared. *Dreaming*, *9*, 139–151.

Empson, J. (1993). *Sleep and dreaming* (2nd ed.). Hertfordshire: Harvester Wheatsheaf.

Fosse, M. J., Fosse, R., Hobson, J. A., & Stickgold, R. J. (2003). Dreaming and episodic memory: a functional dissociation? *Journal of Cognitive Neuroscience*, *15*, 1–9.

Hartmann, E. (1998). *Dreams and Nightmares: the new theory on the origin and meaning of dreams*. New York: Plenum Trade.

Hobson, J., Pace-Schott, E., & Stickgold, R. (2000). Dreaming and the brain: toward a cognitive neuroscience of conscious states. *Behavioral and Brain Sciences*, *23*, 793–842, 904–112.

Hunt, H. (1989). *The Multiplicity of Dreams: Memory, Imagination, and Consciousness*. New Haven: Yale University Press.

Maybruck, P. (1986). Contents of dreams of pregnant women. *Association for the Study of Dreams Newsletter*, *3*, 8–9.

Moorcroft, W. H. (1993). *Sleep, dreaming, and sleep disorders: an introduction* (2nd ed.). Lanham: University Press of America.

Murray, H., & Wheeler, D. (1937). A note on the possible clairvoyance of dreams. *Journal of Psychology, 3*, 309–313.

Nikles, C. D., Brecht, D. L., Klinger, E., & Bursell, A. L. (1998). The effects of current-concern- and nonconcern-related waking suggestions on nocturnal dream content. *Journal of Personality and Social Psychology, 75*, 242–255.

Nielsen, T. (2011). Ultradian, Circadian, and Sleep-Dependent Features of Dreaming. In M. Kryger, T. Roth, W. Dement, M. Kryger, T. Roth, & W. Dement (Eds.), *Principles and Practice of Sleep Medicine* (5th ed., pp. 576–584). St. Louis: Elsiver.

Penn, P., Bootzin, R., & Wood, J. (1991). Nightmare frequency in sexual abuse survivors. *Sleep Research, 20*, 313.

Powell, R. A., Nielsen, T. A., Cheung, J. S., & Cervenka, T. M. (1995). Temporal delays in incorporation of events into dreams. *Perceptual and Motor Skills, 81*, 95–104.

Siegel, A. (1983). Expectant father's dreams. *Dream Craft, 2*, 5–7.

Solms, M. (1997). *The neuropsychology of dreams: a clinico-anatomical study*. Laurence: Erlbaum.

Solms, M. (2000). Dreaming and REM sleep are controlled by different brain mechanisms. *Behavioral and Brain Sciences, 23*, 843–850.

Stewart, K. R. (1951). Dream theory in Malaya. *Complex, 6*, 21–33.

Stickgold, R., Scott, L., Rittenhouse, C., & Hobson, J. A. (1999). Sleep induced changes in associative memory. *Journal of Cognitive Neuroscience, 11*, 182–193.

Strauch, I., & Meier, B. (1996). *In search of dreams. Results of experimental dream research*. Albany: State University of New York Press.

Stukane, E. (1985). *The dream worlds of pregnancy*. New York: Quill.

Ullman, M., Krippner, S., & Vaughan, A. (1989). *Dream telepathy: experiments in nocturnal ESP*. Jefferson: McFarland.

Walker, M. P., Liston, C., Hobson, J. A., & Stickgold, R. (2002). Cognitive flexibility across the sleep-wake cycle: REM-sleep enhancement of anagram problem solving. *Cognitive Brain Research, 14*, 317–324.

Webb, W. B. (1992). *Sleep: the gentle Tyrant* (2nd ed.). Boston: Anker.

Van de Castle, R. (1994). *Our Dreaming Mind*. New York: Ballantine Books.

Chapter 9
Modern Theories of Dreams and Dreaming

Contents

Although there have been theories about dreams and dreaming throughout history, the currently influential ones emerged in the twentieth century. First were the psychoanalytic-based theories and later were the theories based more on the science of sleep and scientific methods for studying dreams and dreaming. We will now turn our attention to both groups of theories.

Portions of this chapter have been adapted from Moorcroft (1993) with permission of the publisher. Specific references to statements in this chapter that can be found there and in multiple, widely available sources are not included in the text. A selection of these sources is listed below and can also be consulted for verification or more detail. (Cartwright 2010; Kryger et al. 2011; Ameen et al. 2002). Related ideas about dreams and dreaming can be found in Chap. 11.

W. H. Moorcroft, *Understanding Sleep and Dreaming*,
DOI: 10.1007/978-1-4614-6467-9_9,
© Springer Science+Business Media New York 2013

9.1 Psychoanalytic Theories of Dreams and Dreaming

The primary psychoanalytic theories of dreams and dreaming are those of Freud and Jung.

9.1.1 Freud[1]

> One of the most common types of dream-formation may be described as follows: a train of thoughts has been aroused by the working of the mind in the daytime. During the night this train of thoughts succeeds in finding connections with one of the unconscious tendencies present ever since his childhood in the mind of the dreamer, but ordinarily repressed and excluded from his conscious life. By the borrowed force of this unconscious help, the thoughts, the residue of the day's work, now become active again, and emerge into consciousness in the shape of a dream.
>
> -Freud 1958, p. 265

Sigmund Freud's ideas are widely recognized in the Western world. Many of the concepts he introduced are now an accepted part of our culture, including the existence of the unconscious. Yet many of his radical ideas, when isolated from the historical context in which Freud wrote, may seem to be bizarre and overly emphasize issues of sexual conflict. Thus, in order to understand Freud's perspective of dreams and dreaming better, we shall begin by taking a brief look at what influenced Freud's theories.

Born in 1856 to Jewish parents, Freud lived and practiced medicine in Vienna during the time of the decline of the Hapsburg Empire and the reemergence of anti-Semitism, with its atmosphere of strict Victorian moral codes. Living in this Victorian society influenced Freud and his thinking, and it is not surprising to find that it also influenced his theories.

Freud developed his psychological theories, including those of dreams, from his experience with his troubled patients and his own life events. In 1900, he published what many regard as his most important work, *The Interpretation of Dreams*. In his writings, Freud emphasizes three basic aspects (Hunt 1989): (1) why dreaming occurs, (2) how dreams are formed, and (3) from these, a method of dream interpretation.

Because his approach was new and unique, Freud's ideas were the basis for the theories of many others who followed him, and these other theories also adopted much of his new terminology. Therefore, as we discuss his theories, we will also emphasize the more important terms of this theory.

---

[1] This summary of Freud's theories on dreaming is from his groundbreaking book *The Interpretation of Dreams* published in 1900. It is interesting and relatively easy to read.

According to Freud, dreams have two related functions: (1) to release psychic tension from unconscious wishes and (2) to keep sleep from being interrupted. Dreams then compromised between these two.

Freud believed that all behaviors, including dreaming, are motivated by powerful, inner, unconscious forces. These unconscious forces are so strong that they may be too disturbing to think about openly when awake. Yet, the pressure of these unconscious forces needs to be released to keep the individual from going crazy. But there exists a *censor* that simply will not allow conscious awareness of these forces.[2] However, during sleep, the mind transforms the unconscious forces into a *disguised* version as a dream in order to get past the censor and allowing *wish fulfillment*. The undisguised, underlying content of the dream Freud called the *latent* (or hidden) *content*. Its disguised version, what is remembered upon awakening, he called the *manifest content*.

Freud considered the transformation from latent to manifest content an important psychological process called *dream work* that has several components. *Secondary revision*[3] occurs when thoughts and impulses are logically transformed into a visual format, and a storyline is added through the process of *dramatization*. Freud believed that we may use aspects of our recent experiences, which he called *day residue*, to precipitate some of the images of our dreams. These images are combined with memories, including those of childhood, to become the dream during the process of secondary revision.

Two or more unconscious thoughts often merge together into a single image or event in our dreams. When this merging occurs, our sleeping brain has gone through the type of dream work called *condensation*. In turn, many single images or events in our manifest dream may be *overdetermined*, that is determined by the condensation of numerous latent dream thoughts. This process can be done because much of the manifest content of dreams is *symbolic*, and a symbol is capable of conveying multiple meanings.

Another term Freud used to describe dream work was *displacement*. This process is a part of censorship. If an unconscious desire, emotion, or thought is too threatening to the dreamer, it is transformed into an insignificant component of the dream. Freud saw many neutral objects and events in his own and his patients' dreams as displaced sexual thoughts or desires. Hence to Freud, a dream of a box and a knife was actually about a vagina and a penis in a disguised form.

---

[2] The censor, for the same reason, also causes poor retention of dreams.

[3] Over his 49-year professional career, Freud used secondary revision in different ways including: (1) putting finishing touches on the dream to make it more story-like and (2) revising the manifest content of the dream when retelling it to make it smoother and more logical. To illustrate this second type of secondary revision, recall your own experiences of waking up and reviewing your own dreams. Perhaps, you dreamed of a casual acquaintance being in your class. But you believe the person was your friend, and your mind changes the memory of the dream to be consistent with your belief. Now when you recall the dream, it was your friend who was in class.

Because dreams are protective disguises of unacceptable unconscious/latent thoughts, dreamers themselves cannot understand them fully without the help of an analyst. Freud developed and used the dream interpretation technique of *free association* on the manifest content to uncover the true meaning of dreams, the latent content. He famously said that dreams are "...the royal road to knowledge of the unconscious activities of the mind." In order to accomplish this, his patients were instructed to talk freely about whatever came to mind when thinking about their dream. They were to talk without judgment, evaluation, or criticism. Freud then used the associations to trace from the manifest content back to the dream's latent content. His method also relied heavily on *symbol substitution*—replacing the symbols in a manifest dream with their fixed latent equivalents. Symbol substitution needs to be done by the therapist. After weeks, months, or years of analysis, the conflicts that generate dreams, which also cause waking psychological problems, would be "worked through" and Freud would close the case.

Freudian analysis of dreams is still practiced today but is not as popular as it once was because of its heavy emphasis on sex[4] and childhood experience and also because of the enormous amount of time it takes. Also it relies heavily on the skill and training of the psychoanalyst. Different psychoanalysts often come to different interpretations of the same dream. Yet, we owe a big debt of gratitude to Freud for introducing the notion of a dynamic unconscious to the Western world and for linking dreams to the psychology of waking life and starting us on the road to our current understanding of dreams.

Freud has been much criticized for a variety of reasons. His methods are said to be too "arm chair" with little true empirical data. His theories have been called too narrow. He has been labeled as sexist. His ideas are based too much on abnormal patients and himself rather than a good cross section of people. His notions have been called anti-religious. There are too many criticisms to detail here, but some of them become apparent in the ideas and theories of those who departed from his footsteps to whom we now turn our attention.

9.1.2 Jung[5]

Dreams, I maintain, are compensatory to the conscious situation of the moment.
-Carl Jung 1974, p. 38.

---

[4] Psychoanalysts, including Freud, have denied the popular conception of an overemphasis on sex in psychoanalytic theory and practice. To some extent they are correct in that there is more to the theory and practice than just sexual motives, yet sex is a heavy emphasis.

[5] The synopsis of Jung's theories is derived from his books Dreams, (1974) and Man and His Symbols, (1964). Also used were Mahoney's (1966) review of Jung's work, The Meaning in Dreams and Dreaming: The Jungian Viewpoint, and portions of Bulkeley 1997 and Delaney 1998.

Carl Jung was a Swiss psychologist and close colleague of Freud for several years. He broke from Freud in 1913 when he realized his views of dreams were taking a much different direction than those of his mentor. While Freud was an excellent and very systematic writer, Jung was not. He is not always easy to read and he was more scattered in the topics he wrote about. As a result, it is more difficult to comprehend and describe Jung's theories and methods. Nevertheless, several key points are obvious and commonly mentioned.

Jung built upon Freud's theories of dreams, expanding and adding to them. Although Jung believed that wish-fulfilling dreams did exist, he did not agree with Freud that wish-fulfillment should be the sole criterion for interpreting a dream. Dreams provide a *compensatory* function by bringing forth unconscious perspectives to *complement* the waking points of view, a process he called *individuation*. Dreams aim at psychological self-healing designed to enhance a "balance" of emotional well-being. Dreams reveal, not conceal. In this way, dreams are more positive in Jung's view than they are to Freud. Dreams serve as our partners, not our opposers.

Here is a specific example: A man who is not psychologically whole walks by a ladder on the side of his house. He does not consciously note that this ladder has a broken rung. But this information is taken in and enters his unconscious without his realizing it. That night, he dreams that he falls off a ladder and breaks his leg, objectively telling him about the ladder. But, it simultaneously contains a subjective truth. It also means that a "rung" of his personality is in need of attention before it causes him to fall. This information was brought to this dream by his unconscious because his conscious had not taken note of these very important bits of information. In this way, dreams can aid the dreamer in maintaining health, be it physical or emotional.

To Jung, the unconscious is more comprehensive than it is to Freud. In addition to containing repressed feelings, instincts, and personal memories, it also contains aspects that are a part of every human's unconscious, what Jung calls the *collective unconscious*. The collective unconscious is composed of *archetypes*, which are predispositions, instincts, or elements that all people have inherited from primitive humans—a kind of natural wisdom. They resemble blue prints into which the individual fills in details. They are seen in the similarities of the motives and images in the dreams, fantasies, and myths from the past and present. Archetypes form a link between the ways in which we consciously express our thoughts and a more primitive, more colorful, and a more imaginative form of expression. In a sense, archetypes are *universal symbols* available to everyone. Several of the important archetypes include the persona, the shadow, and animus and anima.

- The *persona* is like a mask of personality, the image of ourselves that we endeavor to project to others and to ourselves. We "put our best face forward" as it were.
- The *shadow* is the dark, repressed aspects of personality that press for recognition. These are our traits and attitudes that we hide from ourselves and try to hide from the world. They are poorly integrated into our personalities. For

example, a respectable but overly puritanical young woman might have a sexually uninhibited, wild female motorcycle gang member who often appears in her dreams, chasing her and causing her problems. These aspects of the shadow need to be appropriately integrated into the rest of the person, and it is up to the unconscious to insure that they are.

- The *animus* is the male element in the female unconscious and the *anima* is the female element in the male unconscious. A very masculine man may appear to have nothing feminine about him. But underneath, there are very feminine aspects that are carefully guarded and hidden in order to prevent being described as "feminine." It is because of this attempt to repress as much of this femininity as possible that the anima accumulates in the unconscious and must be brought out through dreams.

Dreams may seem strange to us, not because of a censor that causes obfuscation, but because of the special symbolic language of the unconscious—images, symbols, and metaphors. But Jung also believed that dreams could provide prospective visions of the future in the sense that they may show potentials for what might be. Nevertheless, they are not absolute predictions.

In contrast to Freud, Jung's methods of dream interpretation centered on helping a "normal" person find its meaning. He sees dream interpretation as a joint process between the dreamer and the therapist. The most important steps are first to find the *context* of the dream, then *amplify* the dream.

9.1.2.1 Context

The first step is for the dreamer to describe their waking life in relation to the dream. Without this knowledge, it is impossible for the therapist to interpret a dream correctly.

9.1.2.2 Amplification

Amplification is the main technique developed by Jung for use in dream interpretation. This technique refers to the process of elaboration on or expansion of the images and ideas present in dreams in order to reveal the messages of the dream while not drifting too far from the dream's manifest content. There are two kinds of amplification, personal and objective.

Personal amplification involves asking the dreamer to explore and describe any and all possibilities of their own associations, such as thoughts, feelings, and recollections, but being careful to not stray too far from the dream. Each image is discussed to make possible associations to the dreamer's life. For example, perhaps there was a flowering plant in the dream. The dreamer might talk about how the plant looked, what its shape was, the color, size, and smell of the flowers. The dreamer might then talk about their view of flowers in general, how to grow them, problems with them, and what use they might have. The dreamer should also relate feelings about flowers. These associations are also discussed to determine possible explanations for dream images.

The second step is *objective amplification*. Elements of the dream that are a part of the dreamer's culture and the more universal collective unconscious are described by the dream analyst. To do this properly, a great deal of knowledge regarding the nature of the collective unconscious is required of the therapist.

Jung also advised people to meditate on or have *interior dialogue* with the characters in the dream, a kind of active imagination. For it is the dreamer who knows his or her dream better than anyone else and therefore can interpret it most accurately. Some consider this process Jung's third technique for interpreting dreams.

Jung also believed that interpretation requires working with more than just one dream. An analyst and dreamer working together with a *series of dreams* can provide the best interpretation. Dreams in a series can throw light on one another and possibly show progression of ideas or events.

Jung suggested that dream analysis is not really a technique that can be learned and applied according to a certain set of rules. If specific rules are used, the individual personality gets lost too easily. The intuition, imagination, and intelligence of both the analyst and the dreamer are very important and must be freely shared. Dream interpretation should come from the dreamer with the help of the analyst. It should come from what exists in the dreamer's psyche so that it can serve the dreamer in the best way possible.

The main criticism of Jung is that he is close to being mystical in his views and theories. Also, like Freud, his method has been called too "arm chair" and subjective.

9.1.3 Other Psychoanalytic Dream Theories

Certainly Freud and Jung can be considered the most important and influential of the psychoanalytic dream theorists. Others are also noteworthy, not because they have shown us a new path by which to understand and work with dreams, but they have modified the path of Freud and Jung in some significant way that deserves our attention.

9.1.3.1 Adler[6]

Alfred Adler was an Austrian psychiatrist who was a member of Freud's inner circle until he broke away with his own ideas. The key for Adler was that people

---

[6] Sources for the section on Adler include Bulkeley 1997; Carskadon 1993; and Weiss 1986.

strive to achieve superiority and avoid inferiority. Also, he believed that the conscious and unconscious do not oppose one another. His ideas about dreams are consistent with these basic notions, although he did not focus on dreams as much as Freud did, and his ideas are not as well developed and even contain some internal inconsistencies.

To Adler, dreams focus on the dreamer's lifestyle and relate to the dreamer's everyday existence. Therefore, therapists can use persons' dreams to learn of their typical beliefs, behaviors, and attitudes. Dreams attempt to solve the problems of dreamers, yet are often ineffectual because they are "self protective fantasies" created to defend the dreamers' impression of superiority and self-worth. In a sense, dreams are failed adaptations to waking reality and give no real help, but interpretation of them can be helpful to see these failures that are in need of waking work. Dreams anticipate or prepare for the future, yet seldom are specific solutions for interpersonal problems carried from a dream to waking life, so in a sense, dreams fail. Rather, a mood is carried from the dream to waking life.

According to Adler, dream interpretation requires a trained therapist, but the interpretation is more of an art lacking rules other than to stay within the dreamer's unique logic and language. Free association should be used as well as looking at the emotional context of the dream. Contrary to Jung, Adler believes there are no universal symbols in dreams.

9.1.3.2 French and Fromm[7]

Thomas French and Erika Fromm, both classically trained psychoanalysts, focused on Freud's notion of the ego; hence, they are known as ego psychologists. The goal of ego psychology is to strengthen the ego against anxiety and better adapt to the demands of social reality. This is a waking life orientation and thus a more practical approach than that of Freud's.

To French and Fromm, every dream has a "focal conflict" involving a current life problem. This focal conflict is personal or interpersonal with emotional overtones. The recalled dream reveals what this conflict is and how the dreamer is trying to solve it. In longer dreams, the same conflict in the dreamer's past is also presented to see what did and did not work. Every element in the dream is connected to the conflict in some way.

Dream interpretation, according to French and Fromm, needs to be done by a trained therapist who uses "empathetic imaginations" from a psychoanalytic viewpoint to guide the session. However, the therapist does not simply dictate conclusions to the dreamer but also carefully checks for evidence that this empathetic imagination is correct. In the process, the therapist moves between the parts of the dream to the whole and back again. Success with the process is

---

[7] Sources for the section on French and Fromm include Bulkeley 1997; Weiss 1986.

determined when there are no inconsistencies with parts of the interpretation and the dreamer is enthusiastic about feeling that the interpretation is insightful.

9.1.3.3 Boss[8]

Medard Boss was a Swiss psychiatrist who trained and worked with Jung. However, he came to reject the notion of the unconscious and the notion that there are special messages delivered through dreams. Rather, he aligned with a philosophy called existential phenomenalism that asserts that we exist solely in relationship to people and things. This "being-in-the-world" occurs in the world of our dreams as well as our waking world, so we must treat our dreams as an experience rather than as containing symbols and metaphors. As such, dreams mirror our present and open future potentials and possibilities. Dream experiences are more restricted and dimmer than waking existence, but they characterize how the dreamer relates to the waking world.

The key to working with dreams, for Boss, is to focus on the experience. We should strive to get the obvious meaning from the dream. His method, called *explication*, was not as clearly outlined as was that of Freud and Jung, but contains the following elements.

Start by looking at what is in the dream, but also notice what is not in the dream. Then note the relationship of the dreamer to the elements of the dream and how the dreamer responds to them. Make special note of how the dreamer relates emotionally to these elements. As much as possible, one should try to relive the dream. Stay as close to the recalled dream as much as possible while exploring its details and one's reactions to them. Try to get an "increasingly refined account" of it.

It is necessary for the dreamer to have the guidance of a trained and knowledgeable therapist to find the "significances" of the dream to the dreamer's waking life. The therapist does not need to know the client's life history or even the predream life situation. The therapist does not offer interpretations but does comment on the dream as an existential experience and offers "helpful comments and hints" such as, "Is there anything similar to waking life?" The dream means nothing more than what the dreamer can see revealed in it and how it points to the dreamer's individual traits. The dream experience is the focus.

For Boss, dreams can be useful in psychotherapy because they can point to constrictions in the dreamer's personality, but they can also disclose potentials for growth. They can be transforming experiences. He also emphasizes that we should pay special attention to very unusual dream phenomena.

---

[8] The information for this section on Boss was taken from Bulkeley 1997; Delaney 1998; and Domhoff 1985.

9.1.3.4 Hall[9]

> In short, the images of our dreams are pictures of our conceptions. We study dreams in order to find out what people think during sleep—Calvin Hall 1966, p. 10.

Calvin Hall was a university professor of psychology prior to becoming the Director of the Dream Research Institute in Santa Cruz, California. His dream theory derives from Freud's basic concepts but differs in its details. Hall found many of the details of Freud's and Jung's theories to be turgid, unscientific, and impractical. He derived his notions by applying the scientific method to the study of dreams in order to determine precisely *what* people dream about (see Sect. 7.4.2). The following discussion is from his book, *The Meaning of Dreams* (1966).

Unlike Freud and Jung, who used patients' or clients' dreams as the basis of their theories, Hall derived his ideas from the study of thousands of dreams collected from hundreds of "normal" people. Yet, it is interesting to note that in the end, he concluded that Freud was essentially correct about the nature of dreams, for Hall's normal subjects dreamed in the same way as Freud's disturbed patients. For example, Hall's male subjects often revealed the Oedipal complex[10] in their dreams, just like Freud's male patients. The details of the content and focus may differ between patients and a non-clinical population, but the basic underlying processes are the same.

To Hall, a dream is "a succession of images, predominantly visual in quality, which are experienced during sleep" (Hall 1966, pp. 2–3). These images represent the ideas or conceptions of the dreamer that are typically found below the level of consciousness. He did recognize that external, sensory stimuli sometimes generate dream content, but he said that they are neither responsible for the generation of the dream nor are they typically accurately portrayed. For example, a ringing telephone may become a fire alarm in a dream. Also people, things, or events of our recent waking experience may also show up later in our dreams. For Hall, dreams are *continuous* with the person's waking personality and thoughts.

Hall believed that people dream only of things that are of personal importance to them but not current events, even catastrophic ones. For example, none of the hundreds of dreams he collected from many U.S. citizens shortly after the first atomic bomb was dropped on Japan contained any reference to that event. Neither do people dream about other impersonal things such as politics, economics, sports, business, or work. Rather, dreams are very personal—a *letter to oneself* about things that are important to the dreamer.

Dreams particularly reveal what dreamers really think of themselves by getting behind their waking self-facades. In this regard, Hall pointed out that each aspect of the dreamer's personality is often symbolized by a different character in a dream, that is, the personal subjective portrayal of others as found deep in the

---

[9] In 1953, Hall wrote a short and easy-to-read book about his dream theory called *The Meaning of Dreams*. It was republished in 1966.

[10] A boy's desire to sexually possess his mother and kill his father.

minds of dreamers. Yet dreamers may have more than one conception of themselves and others. Some of these conceptions may even be contradictory, since logic is not important in dreaming. These various conceptions may all manifest themselves within one dream or some in one dream and others in another dream.

Additionally, dreams are not generated by our impulses, rather they show our attitudes toward our impulses. When asleep, our mind is free of external controls and free to indulge in impulse gratification.

The contents of dreams also reflect a person's worldview such as whether other people are generally kind and generous versus generally nasty and aggressive. Dreams also show how dreamers view the space that they live in or how it affects them. This subjective world is never an exact replica of the "real" world, and two different people will certainly have two different views of the same "real" world.

Finally, and most importantly, dreams show the dreamer's conflicts and problems. Most of the information gained from dreams comes from this source. Hall defined conflicts as opposing conceptions that are constantly struggling and fighting with one another within a person. The real authentic problems, rather than the delusions and pretensions of waking life, surface in dreams.

Since the dreamers create their own dreams, they determine who is in them and what things become a part of them. Furthermore, everything in a dream is there for a purpose and is important. How these things are included and combined is usually very clever. The dream is a very creative product, but it comes out of our unawareness. We do not consciously create our dreams.

Symbols are an important aspect of dreams. Hall believed that they serve the same function in dreams that they do in waking life. He called symbols pictorial metaphors, and he emphasized that they are intended not to obscure, but to clarify. They express the dreamer's thoughts better, and they convey meaning more precisely and economically. Symbols are an efficient and concise way of presenting complex and hard to understand ideas and they can often make visible things that are otherwise invisible, such as feelings.

But the presence of symbols in dreams does make it more difficult to assess the meaning in dreams. Thus, there is the need for dream analysis or interpretation. Interpretation of a dream means to turn the symbols back into ideas. Since dreamers are the ones who created the dreams and chose what symbols to use, the dreamers themselves should be an important part of the interpretation process. Most interpretation should be easy, because dreams are relatively transparent. If a dream does not make sense on the face of it then the dreamer must work with its parts and symbols to get at its meanings. If that approach is not successful, then the dreamer should try free associating to each symbol.

Hall believed that the dreamer is the best person to interpret their own dream since the dream is a product of the dreamer's mind. Anyone who is clear thinking and is willing to let go without suppressing or controlling or trying to edit can free associate. Hall also advised against reading some theory *into* a dream; rather, he advocated reading the meaning *out of* the dream. The goal of dream interpretation is to convert images into verbal ideas.

Hall believed that you should not work with only a portion of a dream. A dream is "an organic whole" and should be analyzed that way. Moreover, he recommended looking at a series of dreams rather than each dream separately. Each dream is like a chapter in a book, while each chapter may contain a lot of information. Only by reading the whole book can you understand what the author is saying. Similarly, Hall believed you should consider the interpretation of one dream only as a hunch until verified by the interpretation of other dreams.

Hall also recognized the occasional occurrence of what he called spotlight or bareface dreams whose meanings are obvious, and thus need little interpretation. If such a dream is available, use this one first, then work with other, more complex dreams in the series.

In sum, Hall, like Jung, broadened the scope of Freudian dream interpretation by emphasizing the importance of working with a series of dreams and the personal, contemporary nature of dream content. He also eliminated the need for a trained analyst to interpret dreams, believing instead that each of us is best capable of interpreting our own dreams.

9.1.4 Comment

The theories reviewed to this point are based on psychoanalytic concepts. They can be considered to be "arm chair" theories based on insights and intuitions gained from working with patients as opposed to being based on objective data. Furthermore, they are in most cases very difficult or impossible to test. While this does not necessarily mean they are wrong, the likelihood of their being wrong is greater than a data-based theory, no matter how intuitively correct they seem to be. Unlike what is in much of the rest of the book, they are included not because they are correct and have stood up to objective testing over time, but because they are of historical and intellectual importance. Calvin Hall was the exception. He was not a clinician, and he based his ideas on scientific analysis of everyday dreams he collected from non-patient populations. His theories are included in this section because they emanate from the psychoanalytic theories.

We now turn to the dream theories of the latter half of the twentieth century and beginning of the twenty first. These theories were developed in the era of intense scientific study of sleeping and dreaming that resulted from the discovery of REMS and as a result are very much different from the psychoanalytic-based theories. We begin with an influential theory that uses knowledge of brain functioning as its starting point.

Box 9.1 Dream Interpretation (From Delaney 1996 and 1998)
All methods of dream interpretation are based on the interpreter's theory of dreams. Sometimes the theory is described in great detail, but in other cases, it is just loosely mentioned or implied. Some methods are strongly

intertwined with one theory of dreaming, especially the psychoanalytic, others are eclectic combining aspects of several theories, and still others have a few basic assumptions about dreaming but are essentially pragmatic. Taking a look from the other direction, it should also be noted that some proponents of theories of dreaming are indifferent about dream interpretation, believe it is a waste of time, or even believe it is counterproductive. Yet, there is evidence that working with dreams can be useful in psychotherapy (Pesant and Zadra 2004; Siegel 2010).

It is a good idea when considering a dream interpretation method to begin by asking the following questions:

1. How do the theoretical assumptions behind the method influence the interpretations?
2. What are the roles of the dreamer and the interpreter? Can both roles be played by anyone, or does the interpreter need to be highly trained?

The answers can tell a lot about how narrow or broad the method is and whether you want to invest a lot of time in it.

The following are six of types of methods most frequently used by experts and amateurs alike. They can be used individually but often can and are used in combination.

1. *Cultural-Formula*

   In the Cultural-Formula method, the dreamer is told what the components of the dream mean. It is among the oldest approaches to dream interpretation and, to varying degrees, some or most of the meanings of the components may be tied to a particular culture. This method is a part of Jungian and New Age dream interpretation. The assumption is that the culture implicitly agrees on the meaning of certain objects and actions, but it takes someone who has carefully studied these meanings or been schooled in them to recognize them in the dreamer's dream or record them in a book often organized like a dictionary.

2. *Psychotheoretical-Formula*

   With the Psychotheoretical-Formula, a trained analyst interprets the themes and images of the dream for the dreamer. The analyst uses a specific psychological theory to match particular components with interpretations. Freudian and Jungian analysis is example of this method. The ordinary person cannot do the interpretation, because it requires working knowledge of the theory and considerable experience.

3. *Associative*

   In the Associative method, the dreamer gives associations, semantic and also emotional, to components in the dream. It was Freud who first espoused using the associations of the dreamer to help with the interpretation. Later, others believed that Freud allowed dreamers to follow a train of associations too far from the dream itself, and they encouraged dreamers to stay closer to the dream with their associations, such as Jung's personal amplification technique (Sect. 9.1.2.2). In another example, the Dream Interview Method of Gayle Delaney (1991, 1996) asks the dreamer to describe components of the dream as if talking to someone from another planet who knows little of the planet earth. The dreamer is to give literal definitions as well as emotional feeling about the component. Since we create our dreams based on our personal meanings and feelings to understand the meaning of the dream, it is helpful to garner these individual meanings and feelings.

4. *Emotion-Focusing*

The emphasis of the Emotion-Focusing method is for the dreamer to assume the role of an image in the dream, be it people, animals, plants, or even inanimate objects, and act it out. The dreamer may alternate between two images as they carry on a dialog. Or in a group setting, others in the group may be asked to assume the role of some of the other images and interact with the image that the dreamer assumes. The idea here is to have the dreamer get to the often intense feelings associated with the images of the dream, and the best way to get to these feelings is to experience them. The Gestalt approach of Fritz Perls (1969) champions this method.

5. *Personal-Projection*

Personal-Projection involves someone other than the dreamer projecting a mixture of cultural associations, psychotheoretical associations, personal associations, and emotional responses onto the dreamers' dream. This method has been around for eons. The method of Ullman and Zimmerman (1979) is a modern version. A small group of people discuss the dream of one other group member as if it is their own, projecting their feelings and associations onto its components. At this point, the dreamer is only to listen. Then, the dreamer tells if any of the projections help to interpret the meaning of the dream. The idea is that sometimes other people can see the meanings in our dreams that we are unable to see until they are pointed out by others.

6. *Phenomenological*

The object of the Phenomenological approach is to get the dreamer to fully re-experience the images and feelings of the dream from an individual perspective. The dreamer is to describe in as much detail as possible precisely what happened in the dream as the dream is being re-experienced. There is no presumptuous or restrictive dream theory allowed to get in the way of experiencing the dream just as it was dreamed. Re-experiencing the dream can enlighten the dreamer about new attitudes and feelings and even new ways of being. Medard Boss is credited with championing this method. Delaney's Dream Interview Method (1991, 1996) also loosely fits in this category; after the dreamer defines the components of the dream, the dreamer is asked if the components remind him or her of anything from waking life.

Other ways of working with dreams have been suggested (Siegel 2003; Savary et al. 1984) including

- working with a partner or group
- automatic writing—writing all feelings, thoughts, and associations that come to mind about the contents of the dream
- assessing what message could be brought to the person's waking life
- write how two characters or other components of a dream would converse with one another
- start by telling the dream in the present tense a couple of times while focusing on your feelings, body sensations, and associations
- tell the dream again from different perspectives such as that of different character
- try drawing the dream or make a series of drawings like a cartoon strip
- make as list questions you have about the dream and its parts then choose one or two of the most central questions and answer them
- select an image from the dream then let the dream come alive and focus on the symbol then describe/define as if to someone from another planet including how you feel about it
- what the image is doing in this dream, and what it reminds you of
- finish by reflecting on things like what new insights, possibilities, healing, or peace you have gained.

Note: This description of the various approaches to dream interpretation is intended only for a basic understanding of what has been and can be done. It is virtually impossible to do actual dream interpretation from such brief descriptions. The reader who would like to try dream interpretation is directed to consult books that detail one or more of these theories.

From my experience, I find Delaney's Dream Interviewing technique (1991, 1996) method the most useful with Faraday's (1972, 1974) and Ullman's (Ulman and Zimmerman 1979) methods as close seconds. Most people who have seriously tried these methods of dream interpretation are impressed with how well they seem to work. Insights about themselves as well as people and events in their lives are commonly gained. Yet, the question remains whether the interpretation uncovers the actual reason the dream was put together or whether it is a projective, yet meaningful, response to the dream (Crick and Mitchison 1983; Hunt 1989).

As Hartmann (2010) points out it is unreasonable to think that any dream can be completely and fully interpreted. Dreams are a unique creation that cannot be put into words or even pictures without losing some of their content. Nevertheless, there are insights that can be gained from incomplete interpretation of a dream especially if the dream as a whole is always kept in the forefront.

I add a caution, however, that dream interpretation takes a lot of time and effort to do even a single dream of average length and complexity. If you were to do this for several dreams each week, it would be very costly in time and effort. For most of us, that time and effort may probably be better used in other ways. And yet for some people, regular dream analysis may be useful; for others, occasional dream analysis may be a good idea especially in the context of psychotherapy (Pesant and Zadra 2004; Siegel 2010), for troubling recurrent dreams or nightmares, or for recreational and intellectual stimulation.

9.2 Scientific-Based Theories of Dreams and Dreaming

Scientific-based theories of dreams and dreaming differ considerably from the psychoanalytic theories.

9.2.1 Activation-Synthesis

In the late 1970s, Alan Hobson and Robert McCarley of the Department of Psychiatry at Harvard Medical School first described their influential activation-synthesis model of dreaming (Hobson and McCarley 1977) as an extension of their reciprocal interaction model for the control of NREM/REMS cycling (see Sect. 5.3.6) and how the brain causes dreaming (see Sect. 8.4.2). The theory has undergone revisions since then to incorporate new data and the neural network model of brain functioning, and the synthesis part of the theory has been more defined. The following is from the latest version of the theory (Hobson et al. 2000).

According to the activation-synthesis model, dreaming during REMS is result of the REM-ON area configuring the functioning of the brain differently by *activating* several forebrain systems while a few others are deactivated (see Sect. 8.4.2). The activated areas include those for awareness, eye movements, instincts, vestibular sensations (sense of body position and acceleration), memory consolidation, and emotions. Areas involved in the production of various motor movements and the secondary procession of sensory information are also activated, but the motor output to the muscles for body movement are blocked. Simultaneously, the areas involved in the primary reception of most sensory information are not activated, causing most of the information from the senses to be ignored. That is, there is isolation from reality. Importantly, the site of executive control, the dorsal lateral prefrontal cortex located approximately just inside the front of your temples, is deactivated. The result of this area of the brain not being online is the unquestioned acceptance while dreaming that we are having waking experiences without any realization of their frequently illogical and unfeasible nature.

Meanwhile, the activating and activated structures are interacting and the resulting information is then *synthesized* into a unified, perceptual whole.[11] The result is the experience of a dream isolated from reality but that seems real at the time with heavy emphasis on emotional and sensory content. It includes much that is familiar because the areas of the forebrain that are activated are also responsible for the storage of *your* preexisting memories, *your* typical emotional responses, and *your* typical way of synthesizing this information. In this way, the aspects of your life and personality become part of your dreams and, thus, the contents of your dreams are very meaningful to you. This important aspect of the activation-synthesis model has frequently been ignored or missed by its critics.

Seligman and Yellen (1987) describe a classroom demonstration that illustrates synthesis. The instructor crumples a string of sequentially blinking, miniature, Christmas tree lights into a loose ball. The lights now appear to blink randomly. The instructor then turns on a tape of Beatles' music. Soon most students report that the lights appear to blink in synchrony with the song. When the instructor turns the music off, the randomness of the blinking again becomes apparent to the students. This demonstration shows how a pattern is imposed on something un-patterned. It is irresistible. We cannot help but do it, because our brain does it automatically when awake and when dreaming.

When awake, our sensory information is usually very much related to our motor information and seems "normal." For example, when we stroke a furry cat, we see and feel our hand moving across the fur at the same time that we sense the muscles of our arm producing the stroking movements. Also, sensory events are usually sequentially continuous when we are awake. For example, when we watch a baseball game, we see the pitcher wind up and throw, then the batter swings, next the ball is rocketing toward the left field bleachers, the batter is running the bases, and the scoreboard changes the score. In contrast, discontinuities are more common in dreams. The pitcher winds up, the batter swings, and starts to run, but is now running up an escalator at an airport in a frustrating effort to get to class. The reason for discontinuities is that when asleep, the activation of the various components is random and varies in strength. Thus, at any time, the activated components may not be so well related; yet the brain synthesizes them as best it can into a single entity. The result is often the bizarreness we perceive in our dreams. For instance, the sensory part of our brain may be activated to produce the image of a wall, while the muscle command area of the brain is sending out signals to produce walking, so we dream of walking through a wall. For similar reasons, we may experience abrupt, bizarre scene shifts. We are in a boat at one instant and in class the next. The difference between dreaming and being awake, then, is not the process of activation

---

[11] The process of synthesis during dreaming is no different from what occurs when you are awake. All of us constantly synthesize the currently available sensory and motor information with our present emotional state and then draw upon our memory banks of similar experiences and meanings in order to try to make it coherent. Also see Box 8.2.

and synthesis, but the source of the activation—more external, and sequential, when awake, almost entirely internal and random when in REM.

Originally, the activation-synthesis theory was developed to explain REMS dreaming. Later, the same mechanisms were extended to explain stage 2 dream-like mentation that is frequent toward the end of the sleep period (Hobson et al. 2000). This process is thought to result from an "admixture" of REMS and N2 sleep. The length, strength, and closeness of the REMS periods to N2 sleep without intervening N3 sleep cause some components of REMS to occur during N2 sleep in a weaker intensity insufficient to trigger REMS but sufficient to cause mentation. Nielsen (2000) describes a similar, more elaborate, and data-based theory.

A colleague of Hobson at Harvard, Robert Stickgold, has updated and elaborated upon aspects of the activation-synthesis theory of dreaming (Stickgold, unpublished manuscript). Since the original formulation of the activation-synthesis hypothesis, data from neurophysiology, cognitive neuroscience, dream recall content, and postmodern literary theory have added to the specification of the synthesis component. According to Stickgold, the bizarreness in dreams has been found to be not entirely random. Rather, there are rules that restrain the transformation of objects into other objects and determine the degree of plot continuity. Analysis of dream content shows that people tend to morph into other living things but not inanimate objects and vice versa. Furthermore, people are more likely to morph into other people than into animals, rocks into chairs than into flowers, and so forth. Also, the memories that are sequentially activated during dreaming tend to be associated, resulting in immediate plot coherence, but the memories that are non-sequentially activated during dreaming are not so associated, resulting in strange twists and turns in the plot when the dream is viewed in its entirety. The result is like a meandering social conversation that twists and turns as the most recent topic leads to the next association, and soon people are talking about things far different from what they were discussing just a few minutes ago. This experience is in distinction to a good lecture where remote, as well as recent, topics are very tightly related, even after an hour or more. A good lecture, unlike a social conversation or dream, has a specific goal in mind from the very start.

Box 9.2 Implications of the Activation-Synthesis Theory for Dream Interpretation

Dream construction, dream experience, and dream interpretation are all worthy topics of study but are independent of each other (Stickgold, unpublished manuscript). The construction of the dream is done from randomly stimulated elements without any intent of specific meaning or plot. While experiencing the dream, the dreamer's mind links its parts together as best it can to form a coherent plot. During interpretation, meaning for the dreamer that can be very useful is sought from the elements and the plot. This linkage can be done because the components of the dream, and the way they are joined to form a plot, come out of the dreamers own mind and are thus meaningful to them. For example, if you have exaggerated concerns about your personal safety, then your descriptions of your waking and dreaming life will be filled with threats to your physical well-being. Thus, your dreams may contain information that is relevant to you and revealing about you. Such information can be useful in psychotherapy. However, the results of the interpretation cannot be used to infer an intended plot or any intention for the elements whether symbolic or otherwise. Thus, according to Stickgold, there is no need for dreams to have intent in order to have meaning. Experiential meaning and interpreted meaning cannot legitimately be projected backwards to infer intent.

Criticisms of the activation-synthesis theory have been many and varied as follows:

- It is too neurological or too narrowly scientific to describe what dreaming is really about
- It is based on animal brain research that may not apply to a mental function in humans
- Evidence suggests the instigation for dreaming occurs in the cerebral cortex, not the brainstem
- There are people who have REMS and do not dream, and there are people who dream but do not have REMS
- Lucid dreaming is said to disavow the notion that higher mental functions of the forebrain play only a secondary role in dreaming, for many lucid dreamers can control the dream
- Objective analysis of dreams shows that only a small portion of their content is bizarre, but the activation-synthesis hypothesis only describes how bizarreness occurs; and, as mentioned earlier
- Random stimulation of the forebrain that results in dreaming cannot explain the meaningfulness, focus on current concerns, and their pattern of sequencing through the night.

Others have dismissed these criticisms in various ways, such as they show a misunderstanding of the theory.

As an update and extension of the activation-synthesis model, Hobson has developed a general model of the brain-mind called AIM (e.g., Hobson et al. 2000). It purports to model the nature of mental processes in sleep, waking, and some abnormal states. AIM stands for the three factors in the model. A is activation level of activation in the brain. I is relative source of input, internal versus external, to the activated areas. M is the information processing mode that is related to the relative levels of various neurotransmitters at the moment. The interaction of the current level of these three factors determines the instantaneous state of the mental processes in the brain/mind whether awake, asleep, dreaming, or in an abnormal mode. Dreaming occurs when A is high, I is internal, and the M component is dominated by acetylcholine.

9.2.2 Solms[12]

A somewhat different view by Mark Solms of how the brain causes dreaming based on studies of his and other's brain damaged patients was presented in Sect. 8.4.2. Like Hobson and colleagues, Solms maintains that dreams occur because of a functional reorganization of the higher portions of the brain, but the specific details of that reorganization differ. The key for Solms is the direction of information flow that results in dreaming. When awake, sensory stimuli coming primarily from external sources activate the sensory areas of the cortex that in turn activate nearby perceptual and stored memory areas of the cerebral cortex. These, in their turn, activate the limbic areas that are considered important for goal-seeking, appetitive, and volitional activities, and that influence the motor output system. However, during sleep, there is a different flow of information. The functioning of the primary sensory areas in the cortex that are responsive to external stimuli is attenuated. This attenuation allows internally generated stimuli, together with the small amount of external stimuli that still gets through, to first arouse the goal-seeking, appetitive, volitional, and emotional areas of the limbic system before any sensory or memory areas become involved. Motives instigate dreams because the only thing that eliminates dreaming is damage to the area of the brain involved with motivation. The generation of abstract (symbolic) thoughts derived from past experiences follows. The result is symbolic and primarily movie-like visual-spatial hallucinations. Meanwhile, the reflective mechanisms of the dorsal lateral prefrontal cortex are not operative during sleep and thus do not distinguish these resulting hallucinations from reality and awakening. In summary, dreams are the result of "abstract thinking… converted into concrete perception" (Solms 1997, p. 241).

Solms tentatively expresses some support for Freud's ideas about the source of dreams; that is, dreaming is motivated by our wishes yet is the guardian of sleep. These potentially arousing wishes are channeled away from waking into the sleep perpetuating hallucinations of dreaming, since neurological patients reporting the cessation of dreaming also describe their sleep as disturbed, which Solms admits needs to be objectively verified in a sleep laboratory. Furthermore, patients who exhibit loss of inhibition and regulation following damage to, or disconnection of, deep prefrontal regions, possibly Freud's censor, report an absence of dreaming.

Solms's theories have been criticized from a number of fronts on a number of grounds. Yet, his data and some of their implications have had a major effect on how dreaming is viewed by theorists from a number of perspectives. In particular, Hobson's group has recognized much of Solms's data as being important and informative but disagrees with some of the interpretations. For example, Solms describes damage to the motivational system that eliminates dreaming but, according to Hobson's group, this is damage to much more than the motivational

---

[12] (1997, 2000).

system. Others criticize Solms for being too neurological and not psychological enough in his theory.

Dr. Solms reviews parts of these ideas at http://www.youtube.com/watch? v=9nmVzXxdUeU&NR=1&feature=endscreen from 20:19 to 24:43.

9.2.3 Cognitive Dream Theories

Cognitive dream theory approaches dreams not as brain processing of perceptual experiences, but as a type of cognition or information processing (Carskadon 1993). These theories assume that dreams reprocess memories and knowledge using the same basic methods that the waking mind does. The focus is more on the process of dreaming than on the particulars of dreams' contents, sources, or significances. Unlike neuroscience approaches, they do not reduce dreams to the activity of the brain. Unlike clinical approaches, they do not see unconscious motivation for dreaming nor hidden meanings in dreams. The interest is on how dreaming is similar to and how it differs from waking cognition. Within this framework, there are different cognitive dream theories. We will examine two of the more prominent ones.

9.2.4 Foulkes

David Foulkes (1999), as a cognitive dream theorist, maintains that dreams are not simple perceptual phenomena but are a way of thinking. The main difference between waking cognition and dreaming is that the dreaming mind is not regulated by sensory stimulation or even self-control. It processes information that is broader in scope and less associated than when awake. Yet, as in waking, the brain attempts to provide a coherent synthesis in a narrative format of the information currently available. The result is recombinations of waking experiences, knowledge, and memory that simulate waking reality.

Dreaming thus depends on the ability to access and cognitively process recent experiences, knowledge, and other memories. It is also related to language production and high-level cognitive constructive processes of the human mind. For this reason, Foulkes maintains, animals do not dream because they are not capable of such cognitive processes.

Foulkes comes to his understanding from rigorous series of studies of sleep laboratory dream recall from children of various ages (see Sect. 7.5.1). He sees the ability to dream gradually developing during childhood beginning at about 5 years of age as language abilities and cognitive processes continue to develop. Although a few recalls could be obtained from children beginning at age 3, they were so short and not dream-like that Foulkes dismisses them as dreaming. He sees the ability to dream becoming well formed by age 9 but continuing to develop through age 12–13.

Although dreams are the result of the "natural powers of the mind" that are the same as when awake and the content of dreams is systematic, coherent, and has a specific structure, there is no intention behind dream content. However, dreams do extend the dreamer's range of experiences and contribute to self-consciousness. They constitute a model of the waking world that is not a simple replay of the past but as something that could have happened.

9.2.5 Hunt[13]

Harry Hunt, a psychologist at Brock University in Canada, takes a broader approach than Foulkes. He says the study of dreaming needs to take information from a variety of sources, not just from subjects in the sleep laboratory or patients in the therapist's office. For Hunt, dream data also comes from anthropological studies, dream journals, and those special dreams that people tend to notice and remember. In fact, he maintains, home dreams, not the ones from the lab, really tell what dreaming is all about. Such data show that there are a variety of types of dreams:

- Personal-mnemic dreams: containing everyday matters from the dreamer's waking life;
- Medical-somatic dreams: reflecting the physiology of the dreamer's body, especially illness;
- Prophetic dreams: Omens or other images of the future;
- Archetypal-spiritual dreams: encounters with ethereal or supernatural forces that are especially vivid and powerful often accompanied by very strong sensations;
- Nightmares: terrifying and upsetting;
- Lucid dreams: being conscious that one is dreaming while dreaming.

Some of these types of dreams occur frequently, such as the personal-mnemic dreams, while other types, such as the archetypal-spiritual dreams, are rare but typically intense and not likely to occur in the sleep laboratory. Each type has its own combination of cognitive processes and perhaps different functions.

Hunt also maintains that dreams are not limited to being either stories or imagery. They are both. One or the other can instigate the dream. Personal-mnemic dreams come from more grammar-oriented processes while the rarer, intense dreams are more image oriented.

Hunt believes that Foulkes and Freud focus only on the personal-mnemic dreams; thus, their theories are incomplete. Furthermore, some dreams are verbal propositions that are transformed into images—the theories of Freud, Foulkes, and Hobson focus on these—while other dreams start as visual-spatial images that are transformed into linguistic forms—the theory of Jung focuses on these types of dreams. This disparity leads to disagreements and disputes between the various theorists. But

---

[13] Derived from Bulkeley 1994, 1997 and Hunt 1989.

in reality, most of the various theorists have an accurate view of some dreaming, but none is comprehensive enough to account for all kinds of dreaming. In the end, a true theory of dreams and dreaming has to encompass all types of dreaming.

9.3 Other Contemporary Theories

9.3.1 Hartmann[14]

The theory of dreaming by Ernest Hartmann, a Boston psychiatrist and long-time dream researcher, has three major aspects: the functional structure of the brain when dreaming, the emotional focus of dreams, and an aspect of personality related to dreaming. This theory is based in part on (1) recent brain research and theories, (2) his clinical impressions working with people and their dreams, and (3) his and others' empirical research on dreams and dreamers.

For Hartmann, what is most important for understanding dreams and dreaming is what happens in the cortex, for it is there that conscious experience occurs. The functional structure of the cortex is made up of neural nets. These nets are the synaptic connections between several or several hundred neurons active at any given time. Actually, it is a network of nets. That is, there are nets scattered about the cortex, sometimes widely scattered, that are networked together at specific times for specific functions. A mental event, be it a thought, memory, or an image, is the activation of a certain configuration of the net. There are different activation patterns for different contents of the mind.

Parts of the net are more tightly woven than other parts. A tight weave serves specific functions such as grammar, image recognition, or detailed memory recall. They may have networked connections that are rather tightly defined with specified pathways. However, when dreaming, the network is more loosely and more broadly connected. When dreaming, neural activation tends to wander around networks and explore different connections (see Fig. 9.1). As a result, dreaming cognition is less linguistic, logical, and goal directed than waking cognition. Additionally, there are fewer direct paths from input to output. Deduction and making lists are not as possible. When dreaming, cognition is more metaphoric, bizarre, and novel.

There are always disturbances in the network of nets. These disturbances can be caused by emotions resulting from behavioral stress, trauma, and conflicts. The greater the emotion, the greater the disturbance. The disturbance (emotion) focuses the content of the dream, and the nature of the network causes the disturbance to be metaphorically pictured rather than literally pictured. This process is most clearly seen in the dreams of adults following a trauma. They may dream of being overwhelmed by a tornado, an earthquake, or some similar catastrophe. As the

---

[14] From Hartmann's 1998 book, *Dreams and Nightmares: The New Theory on the Origin and Meaning of Dreams.*

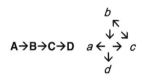

Fig. 9.1 On the *left side* is a representation of the organization of the functional neural networks during waking, and on the *right side* a representation during dreaming (modified from Hartmann 1998). Additionally, the nets represented by the letters are tighter during waking than during dreaming

emotion changes with the passing of weeks and months, the metaphor also changes. For example, guilt may be represented as hurt small animal or not supervising children who then get run over by a car. This same process also occurs, albeit not as obviously, in all dreams.

Hartmann also has found that some people apparently have looser, broader networks as their typical mode of functional brain organization. Behaviorally, he describes their personalities as having "thin boundaries." They have a rich fantasy life and have trouble telling reality from fantasy. They are daydreamers and are more open to experience. They have difficulty focusing on one thing. Their thoughts and feelings merge. Artists of various types tend to fall into this category.

In contrast, there are people who usually have apparently tightly woven, closely networked nets. They focus on one thing at a time. They clearly differentiate thoughts from feelings, reality from fantasy, self from others. They have a clear and well-compartmentalized sense of self that is well defended. They think of themselves as thought people. Many businessmen fall into this category.

These are the extremes. Most people are somewhere between these extremes, with thicker boundaries for some things and thinner boundaries for others.

The nature of individuals' boundaries relates to their dreams. People with thin boundaries have more dream recall, and their dreams have more vividness, more interaction between characters and are more emotional than those of people with thick boundaries. People with thin boundaries are more likely to have nightmares.

One friendly critic (Domhoff 1999) of Hartmann's theory says that parts of the theory are not well grounded in objective research. The idea that emotions direct the focus of dreaming needs to be tested rather than form the starting place for the theory. Further, Domhoff maintains that Hartmann does not have a reliable methodology to use in studying the place of emotions in dreams. Finally, Domhoff contends that Hartmann presents no data that systematically show that dreams change over time in adults. In fact, much data (see Sect. 7.5) suggest otherwise.

9.3.2 Domhoff

Psychologist G. William Domhoff (2001) of the University of California, Santa Cruz, has developed what he calls "A New Neurocognitive Theory of Dreaming."

It is based on the data of Solms, brain imaging during sleep, Foulkes data and theory, and the Hall and Van de Castle method of studying dream content.

Domhoff sees dreaming as a developmental, cognitive process resulting from the maturation and maintenance of a network of certain forebrain structures. Dreams are produced in accordance with a continuity principle using the present concerns of relevance to the dreamer and a repetition principle based on emotional concerns from the dreamer's past. The brain structures involved are those described by Solms and the images of the brain during sleep. The cognitive development aspect is from Foulkes's research showing that dreaming develops gradually during the first decade of life. Domhoff points out that this cognitive development may be the result of the maturation of the brain structures necessary for dreaming. The continuity and repetition aspects come from his findings and others using the Hall and Van de Castle scales, showing that most recalled dream content is continuous with the dreamer's waking life yet with considerable repetition of characters, social interactions, misfortunes, negative emotions, and themes unique to the individual dreamer. The repetitive content may emanate from the activity in the portions of the brain responsible for emotionality.

The parallels between waking cognition and recalled dream content suggest that figurative thinking, using symbols and metaphors, may also be an important element of dreaming. The emphasis in dreams are concerns about self and others (see Sect. 7.4.2.1). Yet, recalled dreams having psychological meaning does not imply that dreaming is purposeful. Rather, he agrees with Flanagan (see Sect. 11.3.5) and Foulkes that dreams are the spin-off of the evolutionary development of sleep and consciousness.

9.4 Dream Theories Based on Function

In a sense, all theories of dreams are intertwined with notions of the functions of dreaming. However, some notions of the functions of dreaming are not as elaborated as the theories presented in this chapter and are therefore presented in Chap. 11.

9.5 Conclusion

In this chapter, we have reviewed several important and representative theories of dreams. Some of these theories are basically psychological in their nature, while other theories are based more on the physiology of the brain. Some see dreams as "improvisationist" in that the dreamer combines whatever elements of mental activity that happen to occur. Others see dreams as a "stage play" in that the dreamer starts with a story and brings in the elements necessary to portray that story. Hobson and colleagues would be an example of improvisationists, while Freud and Jung are examples of stage play. Other views are that dreams are either a compromise between primitive and disruptive tendencies and more advanced mental processes, or as non-linguistic, emotional expressions on the same level as waking mental processes. Examples of the first type are Freud and Hobson and colleagues, while an example of the second is Jung. There are those who insist that we reject subjectivity and study dreams only in the laboratory, believing that method is of prime importance. In contrast are those who say we should start with the dream itself and allow the methods to follow from their nature.

Not everyone agrees that dreams are meaningful or even that a chapter such as this one should be included in this book. Many of my colleagues in the Sleep Research Society conclude that since the activation-synthesis theory has shown that dreams are a result of random activation by the pons of the cortex, dreams are a meaningless epiphenomenon. Others reach the same conclusion from a psychological perspective that dreams are the result of the lawful integration of more or less, randomly activated, recent and long-term memories. Although this process results in a structured storyline, there is no communicative intent. Hence, dreams do not mean anything, and interpretation of them is meaningless.

Each of these dream theories has been criticized. The proponents of one theory have easily found and often vocally proclaimed the weaknesses of the others. It is not necessary to detail the individual criticisms of these theories since, in the end, we would be left with a welter of confusion or with nothing. We included the theories in this chapter—however imperfect—for two reasons. First, they are all we have at the moment. While not perfect, some, if not all, may contain aspects of the truth about what dreams really are. In the future, more accurate theories will probably adapt the best parts of them, or at least use them as a springboard to even better theories. Second, current approaches to dreams in the scientific laboratory, in the therapists' offices, in the popular press, and in the minds of modern humans are heavily influenced by these theories. Until something better comes along, they cannot be ignored.

Meanwhile, we recognize that such theories can even be useful. Such theories help organize the available knowledge and suggest further research. They also offer opponents of one or another of the theories, a clear and focused target for criticism. Both the research and criticisms generated help further our knowledge and perhaps will be the basis from which a future "Sleep-Einstein" will develop an equation that more truly shows the nature of dreams.

References

Ameen, S., Ranjan, S., & Nizamie, S. (2002). *The reinterpretation of dreams*. Retrieved from Mental Health Reviews: http://www.psyplexus.com/excl/dicp.html.
Bulkeley, K. (1994). *The wilderness of dreams*. Albany: State University of New York Press.
Bulkeley, K. (1997). *An introduction to the psychology of dreaming*. Westport: Praeger.
Carskadon, M. A. (Ed.). (1993). *Encyclopedia of sleep and dreaming*. New York: Macmillian.
Cartwright, R. C. (2010). *The twenty-four hour mind*. New York: Oxford University Press.
Crick, F., & Mitchison, G. (1983). The function of dream sleep. *Nature, 30*, 111–114.
Delaney, G. (1991). *Breakthrough dreaming*. New York: Bantam.

Delaney, G. (1996). *Living your dreams.* San Francisco: HarperSanFrancisco.
Delaney, G. (1998). *All about dreams.* New York: HarperCollins.
Domhoff, G. W. (1985). *The mystique of dreams.* Los Angeles: University of California Press.
Domhoff, G. W. (1999). Using Hall/Van de Castle dream content analysis to test new theories: an example using a theory proposed by Ernest Hartmann. Annual meeting of the Association for the Study of Dreams. Santa Cruz.
Domhoff, G. W. (2001). A new neurocognitive theory of dreams. *Dreaming, 11,* 13–33.
Faraday, A. (1972). *Dream power.* New York: Berkley Books.
Faraday, A. (1974). *The dream game.* New York: Harper & Row.
Foulkes, D. (1999). *Children's dreams and the development of consciousness.* Cambridge: Harvard University Press.
Freud, S. (1900). *Interpretations of dreams.* New York: Modern Library.
Freud, S. (1958). *The standard edition of the complete psychological works of Sigmund Freud,* vol. 12. London: Hogarth
Hall, C. (1966). *The meaning of dreams.* New York: McGraw-Hill.
Hartmann, E. (1998). *Dreams and nightmares: The new theory on the origin and meaning of dreams.* New York: Plenum Trade.
Hartmann, E. (2010). The dream always makes new connections: The dream is a creation, not a replay. *Sleep Medicine Clinics, 5,* 241–248.
Hobson, A., & McCarley, R. (1977). The brain as a dream state generator: an activation-synthesis hypothesis of the dream process. *American Journal of Psychiatry, 134,* 1335–1348.
Hobson, J., Pace-Schott, E., & Stickgold, R. (2000). Dreaming and the brain: Toward a cognitive neuroscience of conscious states. *Behavioral and Brain Sciences 23,* 793–842 and 904–1121.
Hunt, H. (1989). *The multiplicity of dreams: Memory, imagination, and consciousness.* New Haven: Yale University Press.
Jung, C. G. (1964). *Man and his symbols.* New York: Dell.
Jung, C. G. (1974). *Dreams.* Princeton, NJ: Princeton University Press.
Kryger, M. H., Roth, T. R., & Dement, W. C. (Eds.). (2011). *Principles and practice of sleep medicine* (5th ed.). St. Louis: Elsevier.
Mahoney, M. F. (1966). *The meaning in dreams and dreaming: The jungian viewpoint.* Seacaucus: The Citadel Press.
Moorcroft, W. H. (1993). *Sleep, dreaming, and sleep disorders: An introduction* (2nd ed.). Lanham: University Press of America.
Nielsen, T. A. (2000). A review of mentation in REM and NREM sleep: "Covert" REM sleep as a possible reconciliation of two opposing models. *Behaviora Brain Science, 23,* 851–866.
Perls, F. (1969). *Gestalt therapy verbatim.* Moab: Real People Press.
Pesant, N., & Zadra, A. (2004). Working with dreams in therapy: What do we know and what should we do? *Clinical Psychology Review, 24,* 489–512.
Savary, L. M., Berne, P. H., & Williams, S. K. (1984). *Dreams and spiritual growth: A Christian approach to dreamwork.* Ramsey: Paulist Press.
Seligman, M. E., & Yellen, A. (1987). What is a dream? *Behavior Research and Therapy, 25,* 1–24.
Siegel, A. (2003). *A mini-course for clinicians and trauma workers on posttraumatic nightmares.* Retrieved from http://www.asdreams.org/magazine/articles/seigel_nightmares.htm.
Siegel, A. B. (2010). Dreaming and Nightmares. In J. F. Pagel (Ed.), *Sleep medicine clinics: Dream interpretation in clinical practice: A century after Freud* (pp. 299–313).
Solms, M. (1997). *The neuropsychology of dreams: A clinico-anatomical Study.* Laurence: Erlbaum.
Solms, M. (2000). Dreaming and REM sleep are controlled by different brain mechanisms. *Behavioral and Brain Sciences, 23,* 843–850.
Ullman, M., & Zimmerman, N. (1979). *Working with dreams.* New York: Dell.
Weiss, L. (1986). *Dreams analysis in psychotherapy.* New York: Pergamon Press.

Part IV
Why We Sleep and Dream

Sleep has persisted in evolution even though it is apparently maladaptive with respect to other functions. While we sleep, we do not procreate, protect or nurture the young, gather food, earn money, write papers, etc. It is against the logic of natural selection to sacrifice such important activities unless sleep serves equally or more important functions.

-Alan Rechtschaffen (1998)

Why do we and other animals sleep? One answer to this enduring question about how this is accomplished was already covered in Part II of this book: physiological, especially brain, mechanisms that produce sleep. But this still leaves the why question, namely what functions do sleep serve?

Since sleep is so pervasive, at least among mammals and birds, there must be some compelling reason or reasons for sleep. Yet, there is no comprehensive understanding of, much less complete agreement about, the functions of sleep. It persists as one of the most enduring and puzzling mysteries in science (Frank 2006).

Some promising explanations have emerged. It seems as if we are just on the threshold of understanding why we sleep. It is like being in a room with several doors that are just a bit open allowing us a peak of what is inside. With a bit of effort, we may be able, in the future, to open one or more of those doors and get a clearer view. Meanwhile, in the next two chapters we will peek into many doors in order to review many of the current theories of sleep, especially those that remain active and viable or that are new and exciting.

First, let us be clear about what is meant by function (Carskadon 1993). Function means purpose. Function equals instrumental value, that is, it makes a difference. Function means the effect or effects that are accomplished. But there are different levels of purposes, instrumental values and effects, ranging from essential to enhancing to convenient to trivial to detrimental. Consider the functions of your nose. It is a vital component of the respiratory system, a convenient place upon which to rest glasses, an enhancer or detractor of facial beauty, and a most annoying place of irritation when you have a cold.

A function may be a component of a larger system or sequence. Again, your nose is a part of the respiratory system and a component of your face. Some of its functions are in relation to the greater whole.

Some functions are absolutely necessary; the system would fail without them. Other functions may not be necessary, but the system works better or faster with them. These could be considered accessory theories. You can breathe through your mouth, but it is generally better to do so through your nose. Still other functions may be enhancing or convenient but could be easily replaced or done without. There are ways that glasses could be kept on your face rather than to rest them on your nose. Finally, other functions may be superfluous or even detrimental. A stuffy nose is a good example. At this point in time we do not know if there is a single unifying theory of sleep, several accessory theories, or a combination of both. Or for that matter we do not know if sleep serves the same functions in all animals, which is unlikely.

Often the question is put too simply: "What is the function of sleep?" Turn the question around and ask, "What is the function of wakefulness?" There is no one, simple answer to either question. Thus, perhaps we must ask, "What are the functions of sleep?" and seek answers on many levels, from cellular, such as maintenance and energy balance, to behavioral, such as memory consolidation and emotional balance (Hauri 1979). Furthermore, we need to remember that "sleep and wake are mutually interacting and cyclic phenomena" (Hauri 1979, p. 252), and thus a theory of sleep necessarily also involves implications for wakefulness.

In an interesting twist, Nicolau and colleagues (2000) posit that it is not so much that sleep has evolved, but that it is waking that has evolved. Specifically, with the development of the forebrain during evolution, homeotherms developed a new wake that is different from their endotherm reptilian forebearers. The old wake of reptiles became N3.

Then too, a theory or explanation of the functions of sleep must be consistent with the other myriads of details that are known about it, many of which have been presented earlier in this book. Most importantly to Kreuger and Obal (2002), the loss of consciousness that occurs during sleep must be explained in an adequate theory of sleep.

There are essentially four scientific strategies used in the search for the functions of sleep: description, correlation, stimulation, and deprivation (Rechtschaffen 1998). Each has its strengths and weaknesses.

- Description: points to possible functions, but there may easily be other explanations for the observations. For example, it is easily observed that sleeping animals typically close their eyes, but that does not mean that the function of sleep is to protect the eyes. It is more likely that closing the eyes facilitates sleep.
- Correlation: sleep correlated with something suggests possible function, but other explanations are possible. For example, if sleep is correlated with some aspect of personality, we do not know if sleep causes that aspect, or that aspect causes sleep, or a third factor causes both.

- Stimulation (experimentation): suggests internal changes to which sleep responds, but stimulation can increase or decrease sleep independent of need. For example, a sleeping pill is shown to stimulate sleep. Research can show the brain mechanisms by which the pill stimulates sleep, but it may have nothing to do with natural mechanisms, hence function.
- Deprivation: reveals what happens without sleep, but the results could be responses to sleep- preventing stimuli themselves rather than affecting sleep directly. For example, rats kept awake by forced running show consequences, but it is not clear if the consequences are from the lack of sleep or the continuous running or stress.

The best clues to the functions of sleep come when there is research using several different methodologies from more than one type of strategy that consistently lead to the same conclusion.

You may ask, "Why is it important to seek out and understand the functions of sleep and dreaming?" The answer is, we can never really know what sleep is until we understand its functions. This in turn influences our (Meddis 1979):

- attitudes toward our own sleep;
- research endeavors—a good example is the dramatic change in sleep research that occurred when it was realized that sleep is active and not passive;
- treatments for sleep/wake disorders;
- and contributions to our basic understanding of human beings and the world in which we live.

We will begin our review by examining the overall functions of sleep and NREMS in Chap. 10, then look at the functions of REMS and dreaming in Chap. 11.

References

Carskadon, M. A. (Ed.). (1993). *Encyclopedia of sleep and dreaming*. New York: Macmillian.

Frank, M. G. (2006). The mystery of sleep function: Current perspectives and future directions. *Review of Neuroscience, 17*, 375–392.

Hauri, P. (1979). What can insomniacs teach us about the functions of sleep? In R. Drucker-Colin, M. Shkurovich, & M. Sterman (Eds.), *The functions of sleep* (pp. 251–271). New York: Academic Press.

Kreuger, J. M., & Obal, F. (2002). Functions of sleep. In T. Lee-Chiong, M. Sateia, & M. Carskadon (Eds.), *Sleep medicine* (pp. 23–30). Philadelphia: Hanley & Belfus, Inc.

Meddis, R. (1979). The evolution and function of sleep. In D. Oakley, & P. HC (Eds.), *Brain, behavior, & evolution* (pp. 99–125). London: Methuen.

Nicolau, M. C., Akaarir, M., Gamundi, A., Gonzalez, J., & Rial, R. V. (2000). Why we sleep: The evolutionary pathway to the mammalian sleep. *Progress in Neurobiology, 62*, 379–406.

Rechtschaffen, A. (1998). Current perspectives on the function of sleep. *Perspectives in Biology and Medicine, 41*, 359–390.

Chapter 10
Functions of Sleep and NREMS

Contents

10.1 Aspects of Sleep that a Theory of Sleep Needs to Consider

As a beginning to our exploration of the possible functions of sleep, let us briefly review the many unique characteristics of sleep (after Rechtschaffen 1998).

Portions of this chapter have been adapted from Moorcroft (1993) with permission of the publisher. Specific references to statements in this chapter that can be found there and in multiple, widely available sources are not included in the text. A selection of these sources is listed below and can also be consulted for verification or more detail (Cartwright 2010; Cirelli and Tononi 2008; Frank 2006; Horne 2006; Kryger et al. 2011; Siegel 2005; Vassalli and Dijk 2009).

W. H. Moorcroft, *Understanding Sleep and Dreaming*,
DOI: 10.1007/978-1-4614-6467-9_10,
© Springer Science+Business Media New York 2013

- Sleep is found in all mammals, birds, and apparently reptiles; it may also occur in some or all amphibians, fish, and invertebrates.
- In mammals, the nature and amount of sleep are influenced by size of their body, their age, what they eat, how safe their sleeping site is, and the environment they inhabit.
- Sleep cannot be replaced by waking rest.
- Sleep is rhythmic in that it tends to occur at regular times each nychthemeron.
- Sleep results in physiological and psychological changes that do not easily occur otherwise.
- Sleep is a time of quiescence with a loss of consciousness and reduced interaction with the external environment.
- Sleep is actively produced by the brain.
- NREMS and REMS alternate in mammals.
- Sleep has similar development in all young mammals.
- There are unique brain waves in sleep such as the slow waves, K-complexes, and spindles of NREMS and the brain waves of REMS that are similar to wakefulness.
- Different types of sleep have different levels of brain metabolism; during NREMS it is low, but high in REMS.
- Sleep types differ in thermoregulation, which occurs during NREMS but not in REMS.

Generally, sleep is somewhat responsive to what happens in the daytime. Some waking activities have been found to affect sleep, such as increasing body temperature with exercise, sitting in a hot tub of water, or gaining or losing weight. Equally important are factors during waking that do not affect sleep, or do so to a very limited extent. Among them are increased metabolic rate, prolonged bed rest, and sensory deprivation (Rechtschaffen 1998). The most consistent result of sleep deprivation is an increase the need for sleep and the need for what happens during sleep.

Box 10.1 Historical Overview of Sleep Theories[1]

Throughout recorded history, speculations about the causes and functions of sleep usually reflected the prevailing understanding of physiology subsequently modified to be consistent with new discoveries. Along the way, prevailing psychological and religious ideas have also had an influence.

The ancient Greeks often viewed sleep as caused by and causing distributions of heat in the body. A slight cooling of the temperature of the blood was thought by Aristotle to cause sleep because of a resulting redistribution of warm blood into the center of the body. He also stated that heat causes fumes from eaten food to leave the veins and go to the head. There the fumes cool and sink to lower parts of the body, which draws heat away from the body making one sleepy.

---

[1] From Borbély 1986 and Horne 1988.

A rather curious explanation came out of the twelfth century by Hildegard von Bingen, who often wrote about medicine and nature in a mystical way. She made a connection between sleep and food and the biblical Fall of Adam. She described how food and rest nourished the body. Prior to the Fall, the sleep of Adam was a kind of deep contemplation, and food was partaken visually—simply delighting and edifying the soul and spirit. The Fall weakened and enfeebled the body and thus made eating and sleeping necessary to rejuvenate it once again.

The sixteenth century physician Paracelsus endeavored to relate medicine and nature. His advice was to rise with the sun and retire at sunset. This habit would eliminate tiredness caused by working and thus refresh the body.

During the seventeenth and eighteenth centuries, physiology and metaphysics were combined to explain sleep. Sleep resulted when the "animal spirits" were drained off from the body by work and activity, resulting in exhaustion. Or, sleep occured because the brain separated nervous spirits out of the blood during wakefulness. Or, sleep happened when the liquor in the brain got used up or thickened while being awake and thus could not fill the small vessels and nerves that serve the sense organs and muscles. Interestingly, these notions led to opposing views on how to improve sleep: some espoused no pillows, so that blood flowed to the head while others suggested many pillows to encourage blood to flow from the head.

The discovery of oxygen led to a new theory of sleep around the turn of the nineteenth century. Oxygen in the air we breathe yields "ether of life" that the blood transports to the brain for storage. From the brain, it is distributed into nerves and muscles to produce motion, but it is apparently used up during wakefulness and needs to be replenished by sleep. Later in the nineteenth century, other oxygen-based theories emerged. Sleep was seen as a result of a lack of oxygen, especially in the brain. This phenomenon occurred, according to one theory, because certain substances, such as lactic acid and creatine, were higher in the tired body and these substances absorb oxygen.

Passive theories of sleep were also common during the nineteenth century, especially the notion that sleep is due to a lack of stimulation. Dr. Edward Elapariede of France developed one such popular theory of the time. He saw sleep as an active instinct like a process that serves to avoid fatigue. In short, we cease sleeping when we have had enough sleep!

Early in the twentieth century, many "bottle" theories were proposed. These theories liken the body to a bottle that gradually fills up with one substance or another, called "humors," that induce sleep. Sleep rids the bottle (body) of this poison. The putative humors included known substances such as lactic acid, carbon dioxide, and cholesterol, as well as poorly defined substances given names like leucomaines and urotoxins. There was a flurry of research on these substances early in the twentieth century, especially with the "hypnotoxin" of Legendre and Pieron but with poor success. Later, in the 1960s, research again flourished, this time with success, leading to a current knowledge of several sleep substances (see Sect. 5.1).

During the twentieth century, as the understanding of brain functioning advanced, there have been many neurophysiological theories of sleep. Prominent among these theories was Pavlov's notion of "cortical inhibition," that is sleep resulting from inhibitory influences located in the cerebral cortex. Subsequent theories and research have shifted the location of such inhibitory areas to lower parts of the brain and have included active excitatory areas as also being important.

10.1.1 If Sleep were not Essential...

- Some animals would not sleep; however, there is no convincing evidence of this in any species.
- There would be no recovery of lost sleep; however, sleep deprivation leads to sleep rebound.
- There would be no serious consequences of losing sleep; however, harmful consequences of sleep deprivation have been described in many studies including the intrusion of microsleeps and lapses into wakefulness and deterioration of performance.

Other than animals with no brain or a very simple one, there are no animals that fulfill any of these assertions.

10.1.2 Sleep is Like Hunger and Eating

It can be useful to compare sleep to another important activity, namely eating (Division of Sleep Medicine at Harvard Medical School 2007). Not eating for a while results in the uncomfortable feeling of hunger. Hunger is a means to ensure that we eat the nutrients required to live. Likewise, that we get uncomfortably sleepy when awake for a long duration and are refreshed after sleeping may not indicate a function of sleep but rather be a means to see that we obtain sleep. Just like the effects of hunger can be separated from the benefits of food consumption, so too might the effects of sleepiness be separated from the functions of sleep. That is, sleepiness is a powerful internal drive that encourages us to get the benefits that sleep provides.

Box 10.2 Rechtschaffen's Sleep Deprivation Experiments in Rats
Starting in the mid-1980s, Al Rechtschaffen and colleagues at the University of Chicago did a series of experiments involving depriving rats of sleep in an attempt to learn more about the functions of sleep (e.g., Rechtschaffen et al.

1989; Rechtschaffen and Begrmann 2002). Their basic procedure was to have an experimental rat and a control rat share a floor that was a disk mounted over a shallow pool of water. The rats are separated from each other by a wall and each had constant access to its own food and water. When a computer monitoring the experimental rat detected sleep-onset, it caused the disk to rotate slowly which quickly awakened the experimental animal and disturbed its mate whether awake or asleep. As a result, the experimental rat gets only brief snatches of sleep before it is awakened, only 10 % of its normal total sleep, but the control rat gets almost 75 % of its normal amount, because it can sleep whenever the experimental rat is awake and the disk is not moving. Nevertheless, when deprived of sleep in this way, the experimental rats died after 2–3 weeks while their mates continued to live.

For some of the experiments, the rats were selectively deprived of either REMS or SWS, the equivalent of N3 in humans, rather than all sleep. Unless otherwise noted, the results were the same except that they survived about twice as long with the selective sleep stage deprivation. In some of the experiments, the rats were allowed uninterrupted sleep when it looked like they were approaching death, typically after 12–20 days of sleep deprivation. They recovered completely within a couple of weeks.

During individual experiments in this series, the rats were variously monitored for numerous physiological parameters and examined postmortem for many more. Originally, few noteworthy abnormalities were found other than they gradually did become disheveled looking, lost weight, and preferred a much warmer room temperature. Notably, the researchers could find no major changes in the gross anatomy of the body, microanatomy, synaptic activity, chemistry, or functioning of the brains of these animals. But later review of these studies (Evenson 2009) revealed three kinds of malfunctions: (1) metabolic problems shown by a loss of weight in spite of increasingly greater eating that was most likely due to the increased need for energy because of malfunctions in the immune system, oxidative stress, and injury to cells; (2) indications of decreased resistance to infections; and (3) disruption of the system of anabolic hormones including thyroxin, growth hormone, and prolactin. The first two of these types of abnormalities are consistent with antioxidant decline. Therefore, maintaining oxidative balance may be an important function of sleep. In the end this research, coupled with observations of the effects of less severe sleep deprivation in humans, leads to the conclusion that the effects of sleep deprivation are insidious, affecting the functioning of many systems in the body and the brain.

There are three major criticisms of this rodent research. First, Michael Bonnet (personal communication) maintains that it is not sleep deprivation that is occurring in the experimental rats but sleep fragmentation since they get brief snatches of sleep before being quickly awakened. The results pertain not to lack of sleep but to sleep disruption. Second, Horne (2000, 2006) states that the effects may have been directly caused by stress of the procedure. The experimental rats occasionally got wet from falling into the water if asleep as the disk began rotating so they had to continually be alert to the rotation of the disk. This stress was coupled with sleep deprivation in the experimental rats, and since REMS may be an anodyne for stress, they may have shown more symptoms than the less stressed controls. However, it has been pointed out that (1) stress causes effects, such as diarrhea, increased plasma corticosteroids, and reduced food consumption not seen in these rats, and (2) the experimental rats showed effects not seen in other stressed rats, such as eating more and sleeping when the opportunity occurs. Horne also cautions about generalizing these results to humans, since rats do not spend much time in relaxed wakefulness, but humans do. Thus, sleep may have a different role to play in humans. One of the scientists involved in this research counters that "normal humans and laboratory rats exhibit comparable physical signs in response to sleep deprivation where the scientific evidence is sufficient for comparisons to be made" (Evenson 2009).

10.2 Sleep is for the Body

Commonly proposed theories about the functions of sleep can be split into two categories: **restoration** theories and **adaptation** theories. That is, some functions seem to reinstate resources used or damaged by being awake while other functions help the organism function better in its environment. Restorative theories focus on one of the key characteristics of sleep: it is a period of inactivity. This leads to the possibility that such inactivity is an important function of sleep. The two major possibilities are that the inactivity of sleep allows (1) restoration of bodily processes that are depleted during wakefulness and (2) conservation of energy resources.

10.2.1 Sleep Provides Rest and Restoration

Today, most people when asked would probably say that the function of sleep is for some kind of rest and restoration of the body. We go to bed tired, worn out, and exhausted, but usually awaken refreshed and revived following a night of sleep.
  Support for this theory comes from several areas.

1. Sleep appears to have evolved out of periods of rest that alternates with periods of activity in most animals. It is possible that this pattern we call sleep occurred to enable greater rest and even restoration of tissues and organs worn down by waking activity.
2. Wound healing can be hindered by sleep deprivation (Gumustekin et al. 2004).
3. The levels of anabolic hormones such as growth hormones, prolactin, luteinizing hormone, and testosterone are highest during sleep while catabolic

hormones such as the corticosteroids are low during normally phased sleep periods (see Sect. 6.1.7). Men with greater N3 have higher growth hormone secretion than men with less N3 (Van cauter et al. 2000).

4. Smaller animals have higher metabolic rates and generally sleep more than larger animals with lower metabolic rates.
5. Two different research projects out of the University of Chicago—Rechtschaffen's rat deprivation studies (see Box 10.2) and more recently Van Cauter's human studies (see #3 above, Sect. 3.1.3, and Box 6.3)—have shown that sleep is necessary for certain body functions to stay within normal limits.

Other notions of the rejuvenating value of sleep focus on the brain and cognitive functions discussed later in this chapter.

Yet, simple rest and restoration ideas of the function of sleep are too simple to be the only answer. Left unanswered are questions such as what is restored and why is sleeping the only, or best, means of doing so? Restoration thus may be a part of the explanation, but not a major part. However, there is evidence contrary to the hypothesis of a rest and restoration function for sleep (Rechtschaffen 1998 among others).

1. In spite of an increase of growth hormone during sleep, there is a mean decrease in protein synthesis due mainly to fasting that occurs then.
2. The level of muscle activity, hence wear and tear, during waking has a very low correlation with sleep length.
3. Short periods of sleep deprivation of 1–3 days does not result in obvious dramatic and permanent breakdowns of the body.
4. Also it is not clear why unconsciousness, a key component of sleep, is necessary for rest and restoration, when simple inactivity while awake would seem to accomplish the same ends.
5. Some mammals sleep half a brain at a time, because they need to keep their bodies moving (see Sect. 2.4) suggesting that the benefit of sleep is not primarily for the body.
6. Sleep duration does not influence somatic growth in children (Jenni et al. 2007).

10.2.2 Sleep Conserves Energy

Arguments for: Sleep is a time of reduced levels of body temperature and energy consumption. During sleep a decrease of 1–2° can reduce energy use by up to 10 % in humans and even more in some other endotherms.[2] Such a reduction is cost-effective (Walker and Berger 1980). This temperature reduction during sleep leads to the hypothesis that sleep serves the function of conserving energy, especially when little is to be gained from being awake and active (Obál 1984; Webb 1979). The energy savings during sleep comes from two sources: (1) a lack

---

[2] Animals that regulate their body temperature by producing heat through internal means.

of body and brain activity and (2) a lowering of body temperature regulation set point. It is the lowering of the set point during sleep that conserves considerable energy (Berger and Phillips 1995).

Evidence to support this theory comes from several sources. As endothermy evolved in birds and mammals, so did NREMS with its lowered set point. Likewise as baby mammals mature there is a parallel development of endothermy and NREMS. Animals with less energy reserve have more to gain from lowered temperature during sleep and they generally do have a greater requirement for sleep. And those animals that sleep more typically have higher core body temperatures and metabolic rates.

A second version of this purported function for sleep focuses on energy use. Sleep is a time of enforced rest that sets limits on activity and thus energy expenditure in order to help balance an animal's species-specific energy budget to keep it at a level that is affordable. Energy cost of activity varies inversely with body size. Indeed, longer sleeping species tend to be those that are small with higher metabolic rates. Additionally, there is greater sleep in immature animals when more energy must be directed toward growth. On a different note, the significant reduction of activity in the brain, a high energy consumer during waking, that accompanies NREMS contributes greatly to the reduction of energy usage.

Arguments against: The correlation between body size and sleep is not perfect since animals that have a safe place in which to sleep tend to sleep more than those that do not, regardless of body size. Likewise, those that consume food with a high caloric density also sleep more, because they do not have to spend as much time to obtaining food. Little energy is replenished during sleep. Glycogen restoration is increased only during early sleep with little change during the rest of sleep.

Many higher mammals spend considerable time awake but relaxed, which can result in conservation of energy. Also an inactive but alert animal is more likely to be safer from predators, yet saving energy. However, "… rather than sleep for 8 h overnight, if we sat relaxed and read a book instead (assuming that we could stay awake), then the small further increase in energy saved by sleeping rather than resting like this is equivalent to only the calories provided by a slice of bread or a handful of peanuts—a meagre reason for sleeping!" (Horne 2006).

Finally, hibernating animals are conserving considerable energy from both inactivity and much lower body temperatures, but when they come out of hibernation they show signs of sleep deprivation. This suggests that energy conservation cannot be the primary reason for their sleep.

10.3 Sleep is for Behavioral Adaptation

Arguments for: One of the behavioral theories of sleep can be summed up by the phrase, "It's safer to be asleep." There are times in the 24 h day when an animal may be less safe. The danger might be from other animals attacking it when it is more vulnerable. The immobility of sleep attracts less predator attention and reduced responsiveness to the environment. Webb (1983) has termed this **"adaptive non-responding"** during times of potential danger. Adaptive non-responding is under circadian control and resembles an evolutionarily developed instinct. It may be more important in more advanced animals (Horne 1983).

Another threat might be from an accident when the animal is less able to perceive danger in its environment. For many animals, including human beings, nighttime is more dangerous. Our main sensory receptor, our eyes, is built to respond best during daylight. We can see at night, but not well. This fact makes us and other animals like us more susceptible to stumbling over a cliff or other natural dangers. For some other animals, daytime is the dangerous time. Their sensory receptors are adapted to perceive things in the dimness of nighttime while they are less easily perceived by others. However, during daylight they are more easily seen and thus more vulnerable. During such dangerous times, it is safer for them to be asleep (Meddis 1983).

Paralleling the safety function of sleep may be a function related to food availability (see Sect. 2.4). It is not effective for an animal to be active during those parts of the day when its food is not as available, such as when its food is sleeping! From a cost/benefit basis, it is better to be asleep when there is little likelihood of securing much food (Meddis 1975).

Arguments against: The adaptive non-responding hypothesis, intuitive as it is, is almost impossible to test scientifically, because it is difficult to determine the degree of predatory susceptibility. Also, it has been argued that sleeping animals may be less aware of potential predators, thus at greater, not less, risk of danger. In fact, there is less NREMS and REMS in some animals when they are in the presence of predators. Additionally species that are more likely to be preyed upon have less REMS while some carnivores, who have little to fear such as lions, sleep the most. Some researchers counter that the nature of the typical sleeping habitat also needs to be considered. Animals who have a safe sleeping habitat tend to sleep more than those animals that do not have a safe place to sleep. Being asleep in a safe place is clearly an advantage. Yet, for all versions of this hypothesis, it is not clear why sleep with unconsciousness is necessary when waking behavioral inactivity or dozing (see Sect. 2.4) would do the same thing. Finally, some aquatic mammals move while asleep which increases their vulnerability and animals show sleep rebound following sleep deprivation, which would not be necessary if sleep were for adaptive non-responding.

10.4 Sleep is for the Brain/Mind

Benefits of sleep for the brain/mind can be divided into two types, cognitive and biological. The biological benefits are like upkeep. During sleep the brain can rid itself of substances that accumulate during wakefulness and restore what has been depleted. Also repairs to the physical structure of the brain can be made. The cognitive benefits involve sleep serving higher order needs such as brain development (see Sect. 11.1.1.1) or memory. Yet, the cognitive and biological functions are related because cognitive changes require changes in the biological structure and/or functioning of the brain—changes that are called plastic. Such plastic changes can occur in the chemical, anatomical, and local cell realms.

10.4.1 Cognitive Benefits of Sleep

The brain/mind clearly suffers more than the body from insufficient sleep of good quality. The result is cognitive impairment. While inactive rest may be beneficial for the remainder of the body, such as muscles, rest provides no such benefit for the brain. Only sleep will suffice. Even during quiet restfulness, meditation, or "zoning out," the brain is still very active. This is like a computer whenever it is turned on. It consumes about the same amount of power whether it is running a program or simply waiting for instructions. It may be that brain cells get tired from constant activity during waking and are unable to persist in working at a high level. PET scans during prolonged wakefulness reveal greater functional reductions in prefrontal and parietal association areas compared to the primary sensory and motor areas. This suggests that a small grouping of cells, referred to as local cells rather than the whole brain, are "tired."

Biological benefits are more easily achieved when brain activity is reduced. Only during N3, which is SWS in animals, is this condition met. This activity reduction applies to the cerebrum but not to the brainstem. The functions of the brainstem are rigidly determined, with little possibility for adaptability or change. In contrast, the cerebrum is plastic, allowing greater flexibility in behavior and learning but requiring more upkeep and maintenance. Thus, if sleep has an essential function, it would most likely be to provide the higher parts of brain with the benefits of reduced activity.

10.4.1.1 Sleep Aids Memory

There has been a great deal of research and theoretical focus on the benefits of sleep for memory. In order to create a memory, something must change in the brain such as a functional reorganization of the structures that are responsible for storage of the memory (Wamsley and Stickgold 2011). This is not a singular event. Rather new memories undergo a series of changes over hours, days, weeks, and even months. During this time meaning is extracted and insights are realized. They are integrated with other memories and made more permanent or weakened or eliminated if they are less essential. This entire process is known as memory consolidation. Much evidence has been accumulating that sleep plays an important role in various types of memory consolidation. Thus, we may both sleep to remember and sleep to forget (van der Helm and Walker 2011).

There are four lines of research used to study the importance of sleep for memory consolidation in both animals and humans: (1) demonstrating that memory consolidation is diminished by sleep deprivation, (2) finding changes in brain functioning that occur during sleep following learning (3) showing that stimulating the brain during sleep improves memory, and (4) revealing that there are replays of recently learned information in the brain during sleep. We will explore each of these lines of research in turn.

1. **Deprive Sleep Following a Learning Session** Either total sleep deprivation or selective deprivation of one of the stages of sleep is done. For comparison, other subjects are allowed to a normal night of sleep. Memory for the task is measured in the next day or days later. The classical study of this type was done by Jenkins and Dalenbach (1924) who found newly learned verbal matter was retained better after sleep. Subsequent studies have confirmed this finding and suggested that N3 is more important than REMS for this kind of task. More recently, the detrimental effect of a lack of sleep prior to the formation of new autobiographical memories has been demonstrated (van der Helm and Walker 2011), especially for more emotionally positive events but less for negative emotional events.

   Biopsychologist Carlyle Smith of Trent University in Canada developed the concept of REM windows (e.g., Smith 1996) with this type of research. A REM window is a period of time following complex cognitive learning when the occurrence of REMS is crucial for consolidation. Other REMS periods are either not as important or of no importance. For example (Smith and Rose 1996), rats had to learn to find a platform that was not visible, because it was submerged just below the surface of a large tank of cloudy water. The animals deprived of 4 h of REMS after a 4 h delay following the end of the training session showed memory deficits for the task the next day. The memory deficit did not occur if the 4 h of REMS sleep deprivation occurred either immediately following the end of training or begun after an 8 h delay. Other experiments have shown REM windows for other tasks in both animals and humans, but the timing of the window varies with the task and other influences. Also when protein synthesis is suppressed during a critical REM window then memory is compromised.

   Critics have pointed out that memory impairment resulting from acute sleep deprivation may simply be the result of an increased drive for sleep, in other words sleepiness. Lapses caused by microsleeps (see Sect. 3.1.2) could be due to the activation of sleep-promoting processes, rather than the brain being "tired." Situations such as jet lag, the sleepiness after a heavy meal, or falling asleep in a boring environment point to reasons for sleep other than for benefiting the brain/mind. They also note that the dysfunctions from a lack of sleep may be due as much to the disruption of the circadian rhythms that accompany sleep deprivation as from the lack of sleep itself. It has also been pointed out that there are no clinical signs of memory problems in people who have taken drugs for years with the side effect of severely reducing if not eliminating REMS. Rechtschaffen (1998) adds that while sleep deprivation worsens performance and higher order cognitive and creative mental processes in humans (see Sects. 3.1.2–3.1.4 and 12.1.2), these results would seem to have little parallel in animals, leaving no reason for animal sleep. Also, the amount of sleep, either REMS or NREMS, is not related to the size of the cerebral cortex. For example, elephants have a very large brain but need a relatively small amount of sleep, while rats with much smaller and less developed brains need a considerable amount of sleep.

Finally, in many of the REM window experiments, the REM window is defined by looking at the data after the experiment is done and the location of the window changes with changes in the task or even the strain of the rat used. Thus, any effect observed on memory of the task cannot simply be attributed to the disruption of consolidation by REMS deprivation.

2. **Changes Occur in Sleep and in the Brain Following Learning** Examples include: post-learning changes such as the duration or proportion of sleep stages, rapid eye movement density, and changes in the NREM/REM cycles in both animals and humans. For example, changes in delta waves and sleep spindles have been related to memory consolidation and REMS has been found to increase after learning. More recent research focuses on changes in cells and synapses. In general, there have been positive results in animal studies for sufficiently learned complex tasks, but not for simple tasks.

   A difficulty with these kinds of studies is the assumption that the only thing the subject is learning the imposed new task. Actually, the mind of the subject is not otherwise blank and idle while waiting for the learning task.

3. **Stimulation of the Brain During Sleep** Brain stimulation during sleep following something newly learned can improve memory for it. One example is improved memory of a complex task because of replaying background sounds during REMS that were present when the learning was occurring. Another example is improved by memory of learned facts when cortical excitability is reduced during N3.

4. **The Pattern of Activity in Neurons During Sleep After Learning** The brain repeats the pattern of activity involved in recent learning during subsequent sleep. Bruce L. McNaughton's group at the University of Arizona saw this in the activity of hippocampal cells during sleep in rats that had experienced new things during the prior waking period. For example (Poe et al. 2000), brain activity of rats was recorded while they ran a rectangular track for food. Each part of the track was associated with activity in different cells in the hippocampus. Some days the animal kept running the same familiar track, but on other days, novel portions were added that caused additional cells in the hippocampus to be activated. During subsequent REMS the patterns of activity in the hippocampus that were present when the animal was running the track occurred again. Also, the replay was timed in such a way to strengthen synaptic connections.

   http://www.Teachersdomain.Org/Resource/Oer08.Sci.Life.Reg.Sleep/   shows similar research from a different researcher.

   Other research has found evidence of replays during sleep of something newly learned in the cat cortex (Amzica et al. 1997) and in the human cortex (Laureys et al. 2001). For example, brain areas that were active while learning a task were uniquely reactivated during subsequent sleep. However, as of yet, there is not much evidence that such reactivation has any subsequent consequences, and this activity could merely be a carryover of activity from waking.

Overall the evidence seems convincing that sleep is important for post-learning consolidation of various kinds of memories. Additionally, sometimes task performance that had deteriorated is restored during sleep in the absence of further practice. Every stage of sleep, except N1, has been linked to some form of memory consolidation. For example, emotionally charged memories are consolidated better after REMS rather than NREMS. Other studies show sleep involved in memory, but without such clear linking of a particular stage of sleep with a particular type of memory (Smith 2010).

Kavanau (1997) among others has a slightly different take. He maintains that the primary reason for sleep is to periodically reactivate brain circuits containing memories, for both innate behavioral patterns and learned ones, in order to maintain them. Without periodic stimulation, the synapses that are part of these circuits chemically degrade, resulting in weakened memories. In the higher animals, such reactivation of brain circuits can only be done during sleep because, while awake, the same brain cells are too preoccupied with sensory input and body movements are too disruptive.

Sleep may be necessary for learning and memory, because it helps to maintain an adequate supply of new synapses necessary for the creation of new memories. Infant mammals sleep so much, because they have a great deal to quickly learn requiring additional availability of new synapses. As maturity sets in the rate of new learning slows and older memories have become more permanent. Thus, the need for sleep reduces.

One criticism of the idea that sleep is important for memory is that stress is often a component of the learning situation. The stress may come from a negative reinforcer, such as mild but unpleasant electric shock in the animal studies or uncertainty about receiving a positive reinforcer, such as rewarding an animal only for correct responses or a person trying to not look like a fool when learning something new. Also sleep deprivation is stressful. For example, stress alone can sometimes increase REMS.

There are several sources of rebuttals to the stress argument. In most experiments, controls undergoing much the same procedure, hence much the same stress, have shown no significant increase in REMS when the task was not learned or when there was nothing new to learn. Also stress during the learning and testing situations cannot explain the existence of REM windows. In addition, memory problems can continue for up to a week following sleep deprivation—long after the stress of the deprivation has dissipated. Finally, REMS increases following some kinds of learning but decreases during others, such as learned helplessness. Stress should have the same effect on sleep regardless of the type of learning.

Other criticisms emanate from the fact that reduction of specific stages of sleep by either some medications taken for nonsleep problems or brain damage in humans does not seem to cause memory problems. However, it has been pointed out that the reduction of sleep stages caused by medications is not as complete and continuous as critics imply and research methods have not used a thorough methodology to test the claims that memory is not impaired in these people.

To some sleep experts, the evidence is not solid enough to conclude firmly that sleep plays a general role in the consolidation of memory. They point out that studies supporting a role for sleep in the consolidation of human procedural learning have made contradictory claims about similar learning tasks. Some concluded that REMS but not NREMS is important, others stated just the reverse, and yet others claimed that both sleep states are essential. Also, numerous studies have shown that depriving animals of REMS has no effect on learning or memory (Ameen et al. 2002). Others have meticulously detailed the problems with certain key studies and whole groups of certain kinds of studies (e.g., Siegel 2003). Also, the idea that sleep is needed for memory consolidation cannot account for the fact that REMS is very high in human fetuses but drops after birth when the baby has so much to learn. Yet, while such weaknesses exist, when the results of many studies using several very different methods point to the same conclusion, and the weaknesses of one method are not found in the other methods, then it is reasonable to conclude that sleep plays a role in memory consolidation. Additionally, Horne (2006) has acknowledged that the evidence is clear that some kinds of learning does benefit from NREMS. However, this has been demonstrated only with simple tasks and the benefits are not all that large.

A great discussing of the benefits of sleep for memory plus other related topics by several top people in the sleep field can be found at http://www.science friday.com/segment/02/08/2013/science-of-slumber-how-sleep-affects-your-memory.html.

10.4.1.2 The Importance of the NREMS-REMS Sequence for Memory

A related theory is that NREMS and REMS play complementary, serial roles necessary for consolidation of some kinds of learning (Walker and Stickgold 2010). The research on discrimination learning by Robert Stickgold, PhD, Director, Center for Sleep and Cognition at Harvard Medical School is an example of research supporting this theory. In one experiment (Stickgold et al. 2000), subjects were trained on a visual discrimination task that required them to identify the orientation of three short diagonal lines imbedded in a field of short horizontal lines flashed on a computer screen for a fraction of a second. Selective sleep deprivation experiments showed that memory enhancement took place in a two-stage process during the night following the training. Both early NREMS followed by late REMS during the same night of sleep are required. It has been pointed out, however, that a different group of researchers, using the same task, has gotten somewhat different results.

Guiditta and colleagues also posit the importance of the sequence of NREMS-REMS for memories (e.g., Ambrosin and Giuditta 2001). They maintain that

NREMS strengthens or selects "adaptive memories" and weakens "non-adaptive memories," and the subsequent REMS stores the results. Cartwright (2010) suggests that during NREMS new information is matched with existing related long-term memories resulting in consolidation. Then, during REMS, the actual strengthening occurs. Under these kinds of views, it may require several rounds of NREMS/REMS alternation within a night or even over several nights to effectively complete the process.

We will further explore the issue of the importance of sleep for memory in Sect. 11.3.4 on the role of dreaming in memory consolidation.

Box 10.3 Can We Learn While We Sleep?

The idea of sleep-learning has been a topic of science fiction, as well as of scientific investigation. Numerous studies have been done to determine whether or not we can learn while we are asleep (Badia 1990; Eich 1990; Kleitman 1972). In one experiment, sleeping subjects were presented 10 Chinese words and their English equivalents. Later, when awake, they were tested for their memory of these word equivalents. The data showed that learning had not occurred. In another study, 21 subjects were presented with 96 sets of questions and answers at 5 min intervals throughout the night of sleep. The EEGs of all the patients were monitored, and it was discovered that the percentage of items recalled during wakefulness decreased as alpha wave frequency, a sign of wakefulness, decreased. Other research has been unable to verify that implicit learning[3] may take place during sleep. It was concluded that sleep-learning is a very weak phenomenon at best and therefore an impractical way to acquire any new learning.

On the other hand, sleep-learning may possibly be state-dependent learning. That is, what is learned when asleep may be recalled only when again asleep. Thus, you would have to be tested during sleep to demonstrate what you have learned during previous sleep. For example, sleeping subjects were instructed to make a specific response, such as, "your nose will itch and you will scratch it," to a word, in this example ITCH. Later, these words, mixed in with other new words, were spoken to the still sleeping subjects. Sometimes the suggested response occurred, but only if the suggestion was given during REMS, and only if the cue word was later spoken during REMS. Appropriate responses to the cue words were still seen 5 months later in some of the subjects. None of the subjects were able to recall any of the words or the suggested responses when awake.

There has also been some evidence that more elementary kinds of learning, such as classical (Pavlovian) conditioning and habituation involving things like heart rate and eye blinks (Carskadon 1993), or associating tones with smells may occur during sleep (Arzi et al. 2012).

---

[3] Learning without awareness.

The data from studies on sleep-learning have been disappointing to those who expected useful, easy, and efficient learning during sleep. Most authorities in the Western world do not believe new learning of any significance occurs while sleeping that transfers to the waking state. Neither explicit nor implicit learning have been shown to occur during sleep and be manifested during wakefulness when the to-be-learned material was presented during the absence of wake-indicating alpha waves. In contrast, Russian researchers conclude that sleep-learning is a hardy, viable, and useful phenomenon. However, their conclusions are based on highly trained subjects and include no direct measurement of sleep. In fact, the information to be learned was presented early and late in the sleep period when a lot of wake or alpha waves were likely to be occurring.

Sleep-learning is appealing to many students because it seems almost effortless. But it is based on the implicit assumption that nothing of value or use occurs during sleep, thus the unoccupied brain is available for learning. As apparent throughout this book, this assumption is unfounded.

10.4.2 Biological Benefits of Sleep for the Brain

The biological benefits of sleep for the brain may be chemical and/or anatomical with an emphasis on local cells.

10.4.2.1 Chemical Benefits of Sleep for the Brain

Two chemical things happen in the brain during sleep—reducing the levels of unwanted chemicals and increasing the levels of desirable ones. While we are awake the brain is unable to clear away all the byproducts of its high level of activity. The most noteworthy of such byproducts is adenosine. During NREMS, when brain activity is much lower, the brain can clear away the excess adenosine and other accumulated substances. Also, while the activity level of the brain during sleep is substantially lowered, there remains some activity with a lower metabolic rate. This lower metabolic rate is speculated to be favorable for the replenishment of chemicals necessary for good brain function. Simply stated, sleep may give the brain a chance to replenish chemicals, such as glycogen (Bennington and Heller 1994, 1995), used by the high metabolic rate that occurs during wakefulness.

While this makes sense intuitively, there is little direct experimental support for it. Neither is there any evident brain damage in sleepdeprived animals that may have excess of undesirable chemicals in their brains but depleted stores of necessary chemicals. Furthermore, protein synthesis increases during NREMS that requires sufficient availability of chemical resources. Also, if sleep is necessary to restore something used up during waking, then infants should sleep less rather than more than adults.

10.4.2.2 Anatomical Benefits of Sleep for the Brain

Moruzzi (1966) suggested that sleep is for the slow recovery and stabilization of synapses involved in plastic activities of learning, memory, and consciousness. Sleep begins when brain cells that have been active release pent up chemicals that in turn initiate several biochemical processes that help strengthen active synapses. The result is maintenance of individual synapses, but also the integration of new synaptic patterns initiated by new experiences. These integrated patterns result in greater flexibility in behavior but within a contextual framework. Kavanau (1997) has speculated that use-dependent synapses are stabilized during sleep, free of sensory input interference. Krueger (e.g., Krueger and Obál 1993; Krueger et al. 1995; Krueger et al. 1999) also views sleep as necessary for the maintenance of synapses that have not been recently stimulated during wakefulness. This need arises because such synapses are components of important circuits for memories that can weaken from disuse.

Tononi and Cirelli (Tononi and Cirelli 2006; see also Krueger et al. 2009) have a different view. They see N3 as functioning to reduce the number of synapses in the brain. This is because when we are awake, we produce many new synapses that eventually can cause the brain to become cluttered and inefficient. When the number of synapses is reduced, savings occur in the amount of energy the brain uses, reducing the amount of space the new synapses take up, and allowing more room for new synapses for new learning. The synapses that survive, usually the recently activated synapses, are the ones that are most strongly and effectively involved in memory storage and other useful functions. The rest are eliminated. The net result is better efficiency in the brain with beneficial effects on performance. Support for this notion is gained from the biological mechanisms found in all species that have been studied—flies, mice, rats, hamsters, and sparrows. During waking, synaptic potentiation is favored, while during sleep the opposite is dominant.

Somewhat in contrast, Siegel (2005) notes that in general protein synthesis in the brain is greater during N3. Likewise there is some evidence that new neurons can develop in some parts of the brain but are hindered by a few days of sleep deprivation. This suggests that sleep may be important for the creation of new brain cells.

10.4.2.3 Benefits of Sleep for Local Cells in the Brain

Traditionally, sleep was thought to be controlled by certain areas of the brain exerting influence on the rest of the brain. More recently, all parts of the brain are thought to play an important role in the control of sleep (Vassalli and Dijk 2009).

According to James Krueger, a neuroscientist at Washington State University, whole brain sleep onset and duration are coordinated and organized by specific brain areas such as the basal forebrain area, thalamus, and pons (see Sect. 5.3.1). But numerous experiments have shown that destruction of these areas results in only temporary disruption of sleep, but the sleep may not be as well organized. Thus these areas are actually not the source of sleep but only play a role in organizing it. Rather it is the regions of the brain that have been overly active during waking that require sleep and thus determine the need for sleep (Rectol et al. 2009; Krueger et al. 2009). For example, rats make greater use of their eyes during the light of day but of their whiskers in the dark of night. If they are awake during the night, there is more SWS in the area of the brain to which the whiskers connect. In contrast, sleep following wakefulness during the day results in more SWS in the visual areas.

When brain cells are active, there are changes in their chemistry. Sleep begins when groups of cells that have been active release such chemicals that cause an alteration of firing patterns in these circuits to which these cells belong. When enough of these local circuits are in this altered state, sleepiness occurs. Local circuits are interconnected with larger circuits and chemical signals. Global sleep emerges when these multiple local sleep states collectively influence the sleep coordinating and organizing areas in other parts of the brain. Thus, sleep is neuron *use* dependent, not simply wake dependent and the *primary* reason for sleep is to benefit local groups of brain cells rather than benefit the entire brain or the entire organism or even other organs in the body.

Additional evidence that sleep occurs at a local level includes:

- Electrical activity indicative of sleep can be shown to occur in local groups of cells.
- Local cellular events that combine to produce a coordinated output have been shown to occur in the brain. For example, as mentioned in Sect. 5.3.7.1, individual cells in the SCN have their own circadian firing patterns that coordinate with one another resulting in the circadian rhythms of the entire animal.
- Adenosine tends to build up in local areas because of activity in that area. The adenosine, in turn, causes a local slowing of EEG potentials.
- There is no area of the brain that when destroyed permanently eliminates NREMS.
- Sleeping one side of the brain at a time occurs in some aquatic mammals and in many birds (see Sect. 4.2), showing sleep is not a whole brain phenomenon.
- There are anterior-posterior and right-left differences in EEG power during sleep.
- As sleep progresses through the night, there are different changes in the EEG in different regions of the cortex.
- There are regional differences in brain electrical activity during sleep that follows sleep deprivation. Such differences are not seen during waking.
- The transition from wake to sleep may not occur in all parts of the brain simultaneously.

- Research by in Russia Pigarev et al. (1997) shows that parts of the cortex may be asleep, while other parts are awake and vice versa for 20–30 mins.
- A column of cortical cells may be in a wake-like state about 10 % of the time even though the animal is asleep (Krueger et al. 2009).
- The several sleep disorders, such as narcolepsy (Sect. 13.2) and REM behavior disorder (Sect. 13.7), are consistent with the idea that parts of the brain can be asleep, while other parts are awake. Also, lucid dreaming (see Sect. 7.1) and the effects of sleep deprivation (see Sects. 3.1.2–3.1.4 and 12.1.2) suggest the same thing.

Unlike many other posited functions of sleep, this function requires loss of consciousness. The loss of consciousness is both a necessary condition for and a consequence of these local processes.

On the other hand, there is evidence that changes to local cells that occur from disproportional use during waking can dissipate if waking continues, suggesting that sleep is not always necessary for localized restoration.

10.5 The Functions of Individual Sleep Stages

Some of the functions of sleep are best explored by considering each stage of sleep rather than sleep as a whole. Some of the putative functions are derived from the nature of each of the stages, and although rarely occurring in the real world, stages of sleep have been selectively deprived in the sleep laboratory and the resulting changes in physiology or behavior used to infer functions of the deprived stage. The functions of NREMS will be covered here. The functions of REMS will be covered in Chap. 11.

10.5.1 The Function of NREMS

We will start with a review of some of the characteristics of NREMS that have implications for its functions:

- General slowing of the body and brain activity and functions;
- Decreased body temperature;
- Changes in the levels of release of some hormones;
- Certain areas of the brain actively produce NREMS;
- Decrease in the turnover of acylcholine; norepinephrine, and serotonin;
- An increase of many types of pathogens in the body cause NREMS to increase;
- Selective deprivation of NREMS causes both more attempts to initiate it and NREMS rebound when uninterrupted sleep is resumed;
- Sudden awakening from NREMS results in sleep inertia.

Overall, there have been relatively few studies of selective NREMS deprivation, so most of the hypotheses about its functions are derived from its characteristics. They are divided into hypotheses about restoration, brain maintenance, conservation, and preparation for REMS.

10.5.2 The Function of N3

N3 sleep is thought to have specific functions.

10.5.2.1 N3 is for Restoration

As indicated in the discussion about sleep in general, a very old and prevailing notion is that sleep provides some kind of rest and restoration for the body. More recently it has been thought to primarily benefit the brain. Both are most often thought to occur during NREMS, especially N3.

N3 is Primary for Restoration of the Body

Many lines of evidence are marshaled in its support of the hypothesis that NREMS, especially N3, has restoration benefits for the body, but these are not always without qualifiers or alternate explanations.

- The longer you are awake, the more intense is your subsequent N3. Conversely, N3 intensity decreases exponentially with the length of sleep. An explanation is that the longer you are awake, the greater the wearing down of the body and/or using up of vital resources that can only be built back up during N3. However, this explanation is weak, because the relationship between length of wake and subsequent SWS, the equivalent of N3 in animals, is not found in all animals.
- During NREMS, there is a decrease of catabolic hormones and an increase of anabolic hormones in the body (Sect. 10.2.1). The anabolic hormones tend to build up and restore the body, while the catabolic hormones tend to wear the body out.
- Growth hormone is present only during the first N3 period of the night in adult humans. It is even more prevalent during N3 in children. However, it has been pointed out that growth hormone may not always do what its name implies (Horne 1988), and the relationship between SWS and growth hormone has not been found in most other mammals.
- Sleep deprivation, or deprivation of N3, results in a rebound during subsequent undisturbed sleep, showing that the body has a need for N3 and will make an effort to obtain it even if the opportunity is delayed, which implies N3 has an homeostatic function.
- Likewise, if deprived of N3 early in the night, there will be more of it later in the night.

- There is a high amount of N3 in children, with slow declines during adulthood and much less or none at all in retirees (Sect. 2.3). This decline parallels that of metabolic rate in humans. In other species with no decline in SWS with advancing age, there is no decline in metabolic rate.
- However, the increase of N3 following exercise sometimes observed in the past is no longer viewed as supportive evidence, because these effects are mediated by the resulting increase in body temperature (Carskadon 1993).
- There are increases in the capability of the immune system that occur during NREMS. Further, many illnesses cause enhanced sleepiness, and the resulting extra sleep has been shown to be beneficial to recovery from illness (see Sects. 4.9 and 6.2.1).

N3 is Primary for Restoration of the Brain

Other hypotheses focus on the brain rather than the body as the beneficiary of N3. This is thought to be offline maintenance. Slowing down of brain activity that occurs during N3 allows repairs. Horne (1988) points out that in larger, more advanced animals, the body does not need a special period of rest, because it gets enough from quiet wakefulness. Smaller animals spend most of their waking time active and may need sleep to get rest. However, this does not apply to the cerebrum, which is constantly active during wakefulness. It may need sleep to rest and rejuvenate. Horne also points out that extra brain stimulation during waking increases N3 but has no effect on REMS.

Horne (1992) seems to argue that N3 in humans is most important for the functioning of the prefrontal part of the cortex, since sleep deprivation results in reversible deficits in functions typically associated with this area of the brain. Also, people with psychological disorders known to involve the frontal cortex have less N3.

As mentioned above, synapses have to be selectively weeded out to maintain the more useful ones, while eliminating the less useful ones that could clutter up the brain. There is some thought that this is mainly accomplished during NREMS. This may be especially important for memory consolidation.

10.5.2.2 N3 is for Conservation

The hypothesis that sleep has a conservation function was discussed above. Some researchers maintain that only NREMS or only SWS, N3 in humans, serves that function, not all of sleep. Specifically, they posit that NREMS functions to conserve energy by reducing metabolic rate, energy expenditure, and temperature in the body and brain.

Supporting evidence includes the fact that several studies in humans and other mammals show a high correlation between metabolic rate and amount of NREMS suggesting that as metabolism increases, so does the need to conserve. In altricial species,[4] the development of metabolic rate and SWS parallel each other. Also, some animals increase SWS during times of fasting caused by the reduced availability of food. However, critics say that these data are confounded by equally high correlations of these factors with body size and feeding habits.

A temperature regulation function of NREMS is supported by the fact that:

- NREMS is a time of regulated, controlled, and active cooling of the body (see Sect. 6.1.6) by a decrease in heat production coupled by changes in mechanisms that allow increased loss of body heat. This process is in contrast to REMS, which is a time of uncontrolled body temperature regulation (see Sect. 6.1.6).
- One theory sees the development of NREMS occurring during evolution about the time that warm-blooded animals evolved (see Box 11.2). This development is viewed as a necessity to prevent negative effects resulting from being too warm for too long.
- It has been argued that SWS is the first stage on a continuum toward hibernation (see Sect. 4.2). While hibernation conserves maximal amounts of energy by maintaining minimal metabolic levels, so does SWS, only to a lesser extent.
- Heating the body just a degree or two increases the amount of subsequent N3 (see Box 6.1). It is as if the body is using the cooling that accompanies N3 to balance off the increased heating of the body when awake in an effort to maintain a constant daily average body temperature.
- Heating the basal forebrain area, which includes portions of the nearby anterior hypothalamus, increases N3. This may be the location of the body's thermostat that regulates average daily body temperature.
- During free-running conditions (see Sect. 3.2.1), N3 occurs during the peak of the circadian body temperature rhythm.
- Extended sleep of 12 h or more often includes the return of some N3, when circadian body temperature is again on the rise.
- To be sure, some of the decrease in body temperature during NREMS is due to its typical co-occurrence with the low of the circadian body temperature rhythm and to the recumbent, reduced activity position typically assumed during sleep. However, a significant part of the decrease is due to NREMS sleep itself and occurs whenever NREMS sleep happens.

See also the discussion of how NREMS is thought to prepare for REMS in Sect. 11.2.

10.5.3 The Function of N2

Little attention has been paid to the possible function to N2 sleep called "light quiet sleep" in cats and some primates, probably because it is harder to

---

[4] Those whose infants are born relatively immature.

manipulate. However, Meddis (1975) has speculated, more than concluded from data, about the functions of this stage of sleep.

Light quiet sleep, or N2, is seen only in cats and primates; thus it is most likely of more recent evolutionary development. In cats, it is similar to N3 except for less amplitude of the slow waves, which is consistent with the greater ease to awaken an animal from light quiet sleep. In primates, K-complexes are a kind of isolated slow wave with a characteristic shape. Spindles and K-complexes have been observed to occur in response to stimuli and might serve to jam out stimuli not important enough to need or to cause arousal (see Sect. 3.2.2).

If these things are true, then it follows that N2 sleep is a more advanced way of obtaining behavioral quiescence while simultaneously sustaining a higher level of selective vigilance. Indeed, those primates who are more vulnerable while asleep have more light quiet sleep.

More recently there is evidence that N2 may be important for the subsequent performance of procedural memory tasks such as simple motor skill tasks.

Box 10.4 Core and Extended Sleep

Jim Horne, psychologist and longtime sleep researcher of Loughbrough University in England, has a novel and interesting notion of sleep (Horne 1983a, b; 1988, 2006). He contends that sleep is of two functional types that he calls *core sleep*, that he has also called obligatory sleep, and *extended sleep*, that he has also called optional sleep (see Fig. 10.1).

It is necessary to obtain core sleep first. It consists mainly of restorative, homeostatic, and other benefits, especially those involving brain mechanisms. Core sleep contains a high proportion of N3 but also some other NREMS stages and a little REMS. The need for this kind of sleep builds with wakefulness, especially waking brain effort. It is a "deeper sleep" necessary for normal alertness and cognitive functioning when awake.

Extended sleep is secondary to core sleep and more flexible. It can be extended or shortened in accordance with environmental demands. It is more for safety, energy conservation, and efficiency kinds of functions. It can also function as relief from boredom but may accommodate brain restitution if necessary. Extended sleep contains a high proportion of REMS. It is on a circadian schedule but may also be governed by behavioral needs. It may vary with the seasons to act as a time occupier when the environment is less habitable.

Fig. 10.1   The hypothetical relationship of core sleep to extended sleep with increasing duration of sleep

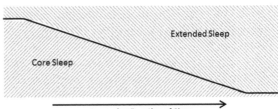

Increasing Duration of Sleep

Core sleep compared to optional sleep can be thought of like appetite. Hunger based on nutritional needs compels eating until satiated. However, more food than the body requires may be consumed especially if it is readily obtainable with little cost.

Core and extended sleep have different proportions in different animals. Core sleep is more important for animals higher up in the phylogenetic tree, with their more advanced brains. Although these higher animals can and do engage in relaxed wakefulness, relaxed wakefulness can only relax the muscles. It cannot "relax" the brain; only sleep can. Extended sleep is more important in smaller, less advanced insectivores and rodents, that is, animals that tend to have high levels of activity when awake, in order to conserve energy. For them and others, a safety function may also be an important aspect of extended sleep. Other factors that determine the relative proportions of core and extended sleep include immaturity, a safe sleeping habitat, and body size. For example, vulnerable animals have less core NREMS (Meddis 1983).

According to this theory, both core and extended sleep mechanisms are operating at sleep onset in all animals. However, core sleep starts with greater strength early in the sleep period but then declines, leaving primarily extended sleep later in the sleep period. The rate of decline of core sleep varies between animals. Figure 10.1 summarizes the proportion of extended sleep and core sleep during a long period of sleep.

Human core sleep appears to be approximately three NREM/REM sleep cycles, about 6 h, but with a lot of individual variation (Benoit 1985). It is the minimum necessary sleep in adults, but children need more. The extended component can be varied by 1–2 h per nychthemeron via napping or lengthening the main sleep period (Horne 1983b). According to this theory, human extended sleep probably originally developed to provide a time of safety, yet was flexible enough to enable humans to accommodate their daily sleep/wake schedule to the seasonal changing durations of daily light at the more extreme latitudes.

Others agree with Horne that there are these two kinds of sleep but do not agree that extended sleep is as optional as Horne implies (Benoit 1985; Stampi et al. 1990). To some, extended sleep may more properly be described as "necessary but flexible" (Benoit 1985, p. 438). That is, it can be foregone for a while, but eventually it needs to be recovered. Other extended sleep may be a way of occupying time that is unproductive and does not need to be recovered if missed, but may help us feel our absolute best. Or, perhaps, we can do without extended sleep in the short run, but not in the long run (Stampi et al. 1990).

In contrast to absolute differences between core and extended sleep, Bonnet and Arand (1995) posit a more gradual logarithmic change of the benefits of sleep with large benefits occurring in early sleep, but increasingly small benefits as the sleep period goes on.

There are several lines of criticism that have been leveled against the core sleep/extended sleep theory. The main ones are:

1. Dement and others cite MSLT and other data showing high levels of chronic sleep deprivation in the Western world and problems resulting from it. 6 h is just not enough sleep for most people. Chronic sleep deprivation leads to many negative effects (see Sects. 3.1.2–3.1.4 and 12.1.2). For example, in one experiment people were limited to 4, 6, or 8 h bedtime each night for 14 nights. Those allowed 8 h showed no cognitive performance deficits. However, significant accumulating reductions in cognitive performance occurred in those allowed 6 h that were even worse in those allowed 4 h. However, others counter by pointing to flaws in the data and logic.
2. Given the opportunity, most people can easily extend their sleep for at least a few nights. One explanation is that they are dissipating stored up sleep debt because of chronic sleep shortage, rather than temporarily engaging in optional sleep. However, more research is needed to understand how much sleep is required to recover from different amounts of sleep shortage.
3. Experiments show that people who, for a couple of nights get more hours of sleep, subsequently show increased alertness, better psychomotor performance, and improved mood during the rest of the day (Carskadon 1993).

10.6 Conclusion

This chapter has focused on the possible functions of sleep, especially NREMS. Chapter 11 continues by focusing on the functions of REMS and dreaming.

Although great progress has been made at elucidating the functions of sleep, firm conclusions seem elusive. A stumbling block may be the effort to find the one, primary, overriding function for sleep. It just may be that there is no primary function of sleep; sleep may serve a variety of functions with considerable overlap between animal species, yet differences according to the needs of the species. Many of the criticisms of each suggested function of sleep occur because that function cannot explain all of the data about sleep. If sleep does not have one overriding function but rather many different functions, then much of this type of criticism evaporates. In the end, sleep may be a convenient opportunity to accomplish several needs that vary according to the requirements of the species and that change during development within a species.

Overall, however, it appears that sleep is more beneficial for the brain than the rest of the body. Mental performance suffers most when normal sleep is deprived. Evidence is mounting that this occurs because sleep is needed for normal brain functioning, especially for maintaining neuronal structures and brain chemistry within certain limits while also allowing for plasticity sufficient for consolidating memories. The unconsciousness of sleep may be a necessary condition for such maintenance to occur without interference from sensory inputs and motor outputs. That is, the brain needs to be essentially "off line" to accomplish this maintenance. Simple relaxed wakefulness does not suffice.

Two things are striking: (1) sleep varies greatly among species yet all species need sleep, and (2) sleep changes dramatically during development within most species. These factors have to be taken into account when formulating a theory of the functions of sleep. For example, smaller mammals need to eat more relative to their body size than larger mammals. Thus, smaller mammals need to spend more time feeding with little if any extra time for relaxed wakefulness. Without relaxed wakefulness, their need to sleep may be important for energy savings. When evolution brought about today's larger animals who needed to spend less time feeding and who had progressively more complex brains, relaxed wakefulness was possible and beneficial. However, this complex brain requires sleep to maintain efficient functioning.

Similarly infants of most species need more sleep than they do as adults because of the needs of the growing and maturing brain that has a lot of new memories to create and sort out. When mature, this function becomes less time consuming and thus less sleep is needed.

References

Ambrosin, M. V., & Giuditta, A. (2001). Learning and sleep: The sequential hypothesis. *Sleep Medicine Reviews*, pp. 477–490.

Ameen, S., Ranjan, S., & Nizamie, S. H. (2002). *The Reinterpretation of Dreams.* Retrieved from Mental Health Reviews: http://www.psyplexus.com/excl/dicp.html.

Amzica, F., Neckelmann, D., & Steriade, M. (1997). Instrumental conditioning of fast (20 to 50 Hz) oscillations in corticothalamic networks. *Proceedings of the National Academy of Sciences of the United States of America, 94,* 1985–1989.

Arzi, A., Shedlesky, L., Ben-Shaul, M., Nasser, K., Oskenberg, A., Hairston, I., et al. (2012). *Humans can learn new Information during Sleep.* Retrieved from Nature Neuroscience: http://www.nature.com/neuro/journal/vaop/ncurrent/full/nn.3193.html.

Badia, P. (1990). *Memories in sleep: Old and new.* In R. R. Bootzin., J. F. Kihlstrom., D. L. Schachter (Eds.), Sleep and cognition (pp. 67–76). Washington: American Psychological Association.

Bennington, J. H., & Heller, H. C. (1994). Does the function of REM sleep concern Non-REM sleep or waking? *Progress in Neurobiology, 44,* 433–449.

Benington, J. H., & Heller, H. C. (1995). Restoration of brain energy metabolism as a function of sleep. *Progress in Neurobiology, 45,* 347.

Benoit, O. (1985). Homeostatic and adaptive roles of human sleep. *Experientia, 40,* 437–440.

Berger, R. J., & Phillips, N. H. (1995). Energy conservation and sleep. *Behavioral Brain Research, 69,* 65–73.

Bonnet, M. H., & Arand, D. L. (1995). Are we chronically sleep deprived. *Sleep, 18,* 908–911.

Borbély, A. A. (1986). *The secrets of sleep.* New York: Basic Books.

Carskadon, M. A. (Ed.). (1993). *Encyclopedia of sleep and dreaming*. New York: Macmillian.

Cartwright, R. C. (2010). *The twenty-four hour mind*. New York: Oxford University Press.

Cirelli, C., Tononi, G. (2008). Is Sleep Essential? *PLoS Biol, 6*(8), e216. doi:10.1371/journal.pbio.0060216 .

Division of Sleep Medicine at Harvard Medical School. (2007). *Why do We Sleep, Anyway?* Retrieved from http://healthysleep.med.harvard.edu/healthy/matters/benefits-of-sleep/why-do-we-sleep.

Eich, E. (1990). Learning during sleep. In R. R. Bootzin, J. F. Kihlstrom, & D. L. Schachter (Eds.), *Sleep and cognition* (pp. 88–108). Washington: American Psychological Association.

Evenson, C. (2009). Comparative research approaches to discovering the biomedical implications of sleep loss and recovery. In C. Amlaner & P. Fuller (Eds.), *Basics of sleep* (2nd ed.). Westchester: Sleep Research Society.

Frank, M. G. (2006). The function of sleep. In T. Lee-Chiong (Ed.), *Sleep: A comprehensive handbook* (pp. 45–48). Hoboken: Wiley.

Gumustekin, K., Seven, B., Karabulut, N., Aktas, O., Gursan, N., Aslan, S., et al. (2004). Effects of sleep deprivation, nicotine, and selenium on wound healing in rats. *International Journal of Neuroscience, 114*, 1433–1442.

Horne, J. A. (1983). Interacting functions of mammalian sleep. In W. P. Koella (Ed.), *Sleep 1982* (pp. 130–134). Basel: Karger.

Horne, J. A. (1983b). *Mammalian sleep function with particular reference to man*. In A. Mayes (Ed.), Sleep Mechanisms and Functions in Humans and Animals—An Evolutionary Perspective (pp. 262–312). Birkshire, England: Van Nostrand Reinhold.

Horne, J. A. (1988). *Why We sleep*. New York: Oxford University Press.

Horne, J. (1992). *"Core" and "optional" sleepiness*. In R. Broughton, & R. Ogilvie (Eds.), Sleep, Arousal, and Performance (pp. 27–44). Boston: Birkanser.

Horne, J. A. (2000). REM sleep: By default? *Neuroscience and Biobehavioral Reviews, 24*, 777–797.

Horne, J. (2006). *Sleepfaring*. New York: Oxford University Press.

Jenkins, J., & Dallenbach, K. (1924). Obliviscence during sleep and waking. *American Journal of Psychology, 35*, 605–612.

Jenni, O. G., Molinari, L., Caflisch, J. A., & Largo, R. H. (2007). Sleep duration from ages 1 to 10 years: Variability and stability in comparison with growth. *Pediatrics, 120*, e769–e776.

Kavanau, J. L. (1997). Memory, sleep and the evolution of mechanisms of synaptic efficacy maintenance. *Neuroscience, 79*, 7–44.

Kleitman, N. (1972). *Sleep and wakefulness*. Chicago: Universtiy of Chicago Press.

Krueger, J. M., & Obál, F. J, Jr. (1993). A neuronal group theory of sleep function. *Journal of Sleep Research, 2*, 63–69.

Krueger, J. M., Obál F, Jr., Kapás, L., Fang, J. (1995) Brain organization and sleep function. *Behavioural Brain Research 69*(1-2), 177–185.

Krueger, J. M., Obál, F, Jr, & Fang, J. (1999). Why we sleep: A theoretical view of sleep function. *Sleep Medicine Reviews, 3*, 119–129.

Krueger, J. M., Szentirma, E., & Kapas, L. (2009). *Biochemistry of sleep function: A paradigm for brain organization of sleep*. In C. Amlander (Ed.), Basics of Sleep Guide (pp. 69–74). Westchester, Illinois: The Sleep Research Society.

Kryger, M. H., Roth, T. R., & Dement, W. C. (Eds.). (2011). *Principles and practice of sleep medicine* (5th ed.). St. Louis: Elsevier.

Laureys, S., Peigneux, P., Phillips, C., Fuchs, S., Degueldre, C., Aerts, J., et al. (2001). Experience-dependent changes in cerebral functional connectivity during human rapid eye movement sleep. *Neuroscience, 105*, 521–525.

Meddis, R. (1975). On the function of sleep. *Animal Behavior, 23*, 676–691.

Meddis, R. (1983). The evolution of sleep. In A. Mayes (Ed.), *Sleep mechanisms and functions in humans and animals: An evolutionary prespective* (pp. 57–106). Berkshire: Van Nostrand Reinhold.

Moorcroft, W. H. (1993). *Sleep, dreaming, and sleep disorders: An introduction* (2nd ed.). Lanham: University Press of America.

Moruzzi, G. (1966). The functional significance of sleep with particular regard to the brain mechanisms underlying consciousness. In J. Eccles (Ed.), *Brain mechanisms and conscious experience*. New York: Springer.

Obál, F, Jr. (1984). Thermoregulation and sleep. In A. A. Borbely & J. L. Valat (Eds.), *Sleep mechanisms* (pp. 157–172). New York: Springer.

Pigarev, I. N., Nothdurft, H. C., & Kastner, S. (1997). Evidence for asynchronous development of sleep in cortical areas. *NeuroReport, 8*, 2557–2560.

Poe, G. R., Nitz, D. A., McNaughton, B. L., & Barnes, C. A. (2000). Experience-dependent phase-reversal of hippocampal neuron firing during REM sleep. *Brain Research, 855*, 176–180.

Rechtschaffen, A. (1998). Current perspectives on the function of sleep. *Perspectives in Biology and Medicine, 41*, 359–390.

Rechtschaffen, A., Bergmann, B. M., Everson, C. A., Kushida, C. A., & Gilliland, M. A. (1989). Sleep deprivation in the rat: X. integration and discussion of the findings. *Sleep, 12*, 68–87.

Rechtschaffen, A., Bergmann, B. M. (2002). Sleep Deprivation in the Rat: An update of the 1998 paper. *Sleep, 25*, 18–24.

Rectol, D. M., Schei, J. L., Van Dongen, H. P., Belenky, G., & Krueger, J. M. (2009). Physiological markers of local sleep. *European Journal of Neuroscience, 29*, 1771–1778.

Siegel, A. (2003). *A Mini-Course for Clinicians and Trauma Workers on Posttraumatic Nightmares.*   Retrieved   from   http://www.asdreams.org/magazine/articles/seigel_nightmares.htm.

Siegel, J. M. (2005). Clues to the functions of mammalian sleep. *Nature, 437*, 1264–1271.

Smith, C. (1996). Sleep states, memory processes and synaptic plasticity. *Behavioural Brain Research, 78*, 49–56.

Smith, C. (2010). Sleep states, memory processing, and dreams. *Sleep Medicine Clinics, 5*, 217–228.

Smith, C., & Rose, G. M. (1996). Evidence for a paradoxical sleep window for place learning in the Morris water maze. *Physiology and Behavior, 59*, 93–97.

Stampi, C., Moffitt, A., & Hoffman, R. (1990). Leonardo Da Vinci's polyphasic ultrashort sleep: A strategy for sleep reduction? *SleepResearch, 19*, 408.

Stickgold, R., James, L., & Hobson, J. A. (2000). Visual discrimination learning requires sleep after training. *Nature Neuroscience, 3*, 1237–1238.

Tononi, G., & Cirelli, C. (2006). Sleep function and synaptic homeostasis. *Sleep Medicine Reviews, 10*, 49–62.

Van Cauter, E., Leproult, R., & Plat, L. (2000). Age-related changes in slow-wave sleep and REM sleep and relationship with growth hormone and cortisol levels in healthy men. *Journal of the American Medical Association, 284*, 861–868.

van der Helm, E., & Walker, M. P. (2011). Sleep and emotional memory processing. *Sleep Medicine Clinics, 6*, 31–43.

Vassalli, A., & Dijk, D.-J. (2009). Sleep function: Current questions and new approaches. *European Journal of Neuroscience, 19*, 1830–1841.

Walker, J. M., & Berger, R. J. (1980). Sleep as an adaptation for energy conservation functionally related to hibernation and shallow torpor. *Progress in Brain Research, 53*, 255–278.

Walker M. P., & Stickgold R. (2010). Overnight alchemy: sleep-dependent memory evolution. *Nature Reviews Neuroscience 11*, 218.

Wamsley, E. J., & Stickgold, R. (2011). Memory, sleep, and dreaming: Experiencing consolidation. *Sleep Medicine Clinics*, pp. 97–108.

Webb, W. B. (1979). *Theories of sleep functions and some clinical implications.* In R Drucker-Colin, M Shkurovich, & M B Sterman (Eds.), The functions of sleep (pp. 19–35). New York: Academic Press.

Webb, W. B. (1983). *Theories in modern sleep research.* In A. Mayes (Ed.), Sleep mechanisms and functions in humans and animals - an evolutionary prespective (pp. 1–17). Berkshire, England: Van Nostrand Reinhold.

Chapter 11
The Functions of REMS and Dreaming

Contents

11.1 The Functions of REMS

We will start with a review of some of the characteristics of REMS that have implications for its functions:

- **Unique Characteristics** REMS has phasic, especially rapid eye movements, as well as tonic events. It usually follows NREMS. Neither the length nor the strength of REMS is affected by the preceding waking episode or by extra REMS obtained during the prior sleep period. However, deprivation of REMS

Portions of this chapter have been adapted from Moorcroft, 1993 with permission of the publisher. Specific references to statements in this chapter that can be found there and in multiple, widely available sources are not included in the text. A selection of these sources is listed below and can also be consulted for verification or more detail. (Cartwright 2010; Kryger et al. 2011; Horne 2006; Siegel 2005).

W. H. Moorcroft, *Understanding Sleep and Dreaming*,
DOI: 10.1007/978-1-4614-6467-9_11,
© Springer Science+Business Media New York 2013

causes some "REM pressure" and rebound. When length of sleep is shortened, the duration of REMS is sacrificed before the duration of NREMS is reduced. The duration of REMS is decreased by anxiety in humans and increased by stress in the rat.

- **Brain** There are REM-on and REM-off areas of the brain. Theta waves are prevalent in the hippocampus during REMS. Some parts of the brain are more active during REMS than during any other state, but a few parts are less active. Much of the cortex is aroused. Increased brain temperature occurs during REMS. There is high use of acetylcholine but low use of norepinephrine and serotonin in the brain during REMS.
- **Body** Muscles for movement are inhibited during REMS. There is an absence of body temperature regulation during REMS. Irregular heart rate, blood pressure, and respiration are common during REMS, as are penile erections and vaginal engorgement. REMS consumes considerable amounts of metabolic energy.
- **Cognitive/Behavioral** Rich and copious dreaming occurs during REMS. There is a lack of reflective thought during REMS. Animals with a safe sleeping site typically have more REMS as do smaller animals. Unlike NREMS, REMS appears to be dispensable; vulnerable animals have less, and some animals, such as dolphins, and people on certain medications seem to get along quite well without it. Percent of REMS varies greatly among species, yet there are generally higher amounts of REMS in altricial[1] species, in early development, and in adulthood.

Box 11.1 REMS is a Syndrome, Not a State

We treat REMS as if it is a single, unified entity. However, in reality, REMS may be not so much a unified state as a convenient assemblage of components (McCarley and Massaquoi 1992) that need to be recruited in a specific order (Hobson et al. 1986). Not only is this concept shown by the fact that various and separable brain systems are involved, but also because various components of REMS occur before the onset of full-blown REMS. For example, the neck muscle potential may decrease several seconds or more before the onset of other polysomnographic signs of REMS, and there is a decrease of sweating indicating turning off this thermoregulatory mechanism 2–3 min prior to polysomnographic onset of REMS. Several of the components of REMS can be dissociated using experimental techniques in the lab (Morrison and Reiner 1985; Siegel 1989). For example, REM without muscle paralysis can be produced by brain damage in the brainstem near the locus coeruleus, and muscle paralysis without REM can be produced by extra acetylcholine in these same brain areas. Additionally, the drug

---

[1] Altricial refers to being born relatively immature and unable to care for itself as opposed to precocial meaning being born relatively mature and able to care for itself.

reserpine can cause PGO waves to occur during waking. In reality, REMS is the coordinated concurrence of several phenomena rather than a unified state.

There has been more research and speculative focus on REMS than on the other sleep state, probably because of its paradoxical nature (see Sect. 2.1.1). An early idea was that REMS was needed to prevent hallucinations and mental illness. However, this notion was soon refuted. In fact, REMS deprivation can even temporarily help some people with severe depression. Unlike NREMS, which is proportional to the amount prior wakefulness, REMS seems related to the circadian temperature rhythm. The propensity for REMS increases when body temperature is at its lowest, but shows the least likelihood when body temperature is at its peak and for a few hours thereafter (Borbély 1986). Yet, this explanation cannot entirely account for REMS. Some rebound of this stage occurs following deprivation, suggesting that it is too important to be missed. Something is both necessary and uniquely, or at least most easily, obtained by this stage of sleep, yet there is no severe psychological deterioration if it is missed.

Cohen (1980) has emphasized that some of the functions of REMS seem to be preparatory, while others are adaptive. That is, some functions anticipate future needs and insure that the organism is ready for what may come, while others respond to what the organism has experienced and attempt better or more efficiently to utilize that experience. The preparatory functions he includes are the stimulation of the brain for proper growth, the repair and maintenance of the brain, and the exercising of brain circuits for genetically based behaviors. These functions help insure that the brain is ready to respond appropriately in the future when called upon. The adaptive functions include memory work on new learning, modulation of emotions, and the psychological benefits of dreams.

11.1.1   REMS as Preparatory

REMS may help prepare for the future.

11.1.1.1   REMS as Beneficial for Growth

Because REMS occurs for lengthened periods during fetal and infant development, it is natural to think that this sleep state may be necessary for the proper development of brain synapses and related brain maturation (e.g., Turek and Zee 1999; Shaffery et al. 2002). It is widely recognized from studies of sensory systems, especially vision, that stimulation of the growing brain is necessary for normal synaptic connections to be made between cells. In fact, the immature brain has too many neurons and synapses. Only those that are shown to be functionally beneficial through use are maintained.

But, external stimulation may not be sufficient. Or, it may be too random and irregular. And prior to birth there is little stimulation in the uterus. An internal source of stimulation that is more controlled and more predictable is necessary to stimulate the growing nerve tissue appropriately and speed its structural growth and physiological maturation, while allowing less useful connections to be thinned out. It is proposed that REMS provides this autostimulation. In this way, REMS is additive and complimentary to sensory input during waking.

Experimental verification comes from studies showing that deprivation of REMS during maturation can result in less brain development and later behavioral and sleep problems (Corner et al. 1980; Mirmiram 1986). REMS deprivation in kittens worsens adult visual deficits produced by abnormal early sensory input (Oskenberg 1987). Also, if PGO spikes are suppressed in kittens by surgically removing the parts of the brain necessary for their genesis, functioning of the visual areas of the nervous system develops abnormally (Davenne and Adrien 1987).

However, it is possible that the high amount of REMS in immature animals occurs simply because the brainstem, where REMS sleep is controlled, matures before the forebrain, where NREMS is controlled (Nicolau et al. 2000). Also the fact that some aquatic mammal infants lack REMS during infancy suggests that REMS may not be all that necessary for development. Also the role of REMS for brain development and maintenance may not be uniform throughout the brain and some but not all aspects of brain plasticity seem to depend on sleep (Vassalli and Dijk 2009).

11.1.1.2 REMS as Beneficial for Maintenance

The autostimulation during REMS later in life is thought necessary to maintain synaptic connections. Typically, REMS decreases in the adult from what it had been earlier, but it does not disappear (see Sect. 2.3). It is a predictable source of internal stimulation that maintains and self-corrects the functional pathways of interaction between brain cells. Supportive observations (Oswald 1980) include the decrease in REMS during senility, less REMS in mentally retarded individuals, an increase in REMS following brain poisoning—presumably while the brain is trying to repair the damage—and a decline in REMS in people with organic brain dysfunction (Kryger et al. 1989). Other researchers have shown that the decrease in the amount of REMS sleep is correlated with the decline in the level of cognitive ability in the elderly but not in young people (Prinz 1980).

REMS has been hypothesized to contribute to the maintenance of not only sensory and motor systems but also brain circuits for inherited innate behaviors (Jouvet 1998). Higher animals that rely on learning only irregularly use their inherited but nevertheless necessary behaviors. Without regular use, the inherited neural networks may weaken and eventually not be ready when needed. During

REMS these neurons are regularly being stimulated in a stereotyped and highly organized manner, thus ensuring their daily activation (Hobson 1988). That is, REMS may function as a reliable, patterned circuit check that additionally may improve the functioning of the nervous system rather than just maintain it.

Evidence for this idea comes from cats with lesions in a specific part of the brainstem that removes the inhibition of muscles of movement during REMS. These animals do not show random behaviors but seem to be acting out certain kinds of genetically programmed behaviors that occur during emotional states. It is as if they are tuning up their fight/flight response (Horne 2000).

Similarly, REMS has also been hypothesized to activate periodically the brain's internal reward system to keep it active (Jouvet 1998; Ellman and Weinstein 1991). The high amount of REMS in immature mammals is thought to keep this system in a state of readiness in the face of insufficient external stimulation.

On a related note, REMS erections and may be an outward manifestation of brain circuit checks for innate behaviors. The only other functional speculation for these phenomena appeared in a paper about the memory effects of REMS, by (Crick and Mitchinson 1986) that mentioned erections in a section entitled "Side Effects of REMS." They first point out that erections are not a result of the erotic content of dreams and then continue with (p.245).

> There seems no obvious reason why erection should not also be inhibited in sleep. One may wonder whether this phenomenon might have selective advantage in evolution. It would not, after all, be too surprising if this particular state of male readiness for sexual intercourse contributed to the number of offspring fathered. However, this assumes that the female of the species will be in easy proximity to the male during or shortly after sleep. One wonders, therefore, if REMS penile erection has been observed in animals such as tigers, which are solitary except for brief periods of sexual intercourse, as opposed to lions, which constantly sleep in close proximity to each other.

11.1.1.3 REMS as Beneficial for Brain Restoration

Throughout life, levels of some neurotransmitters, especially catecholamines and hypocretin, that are heavy utilized when awake may need to be replenished, their receptors restored, or other related mechanisms reinvigorated during REMS when cells using them are much less active (Turek and Zee 1999). For example, activity in the locus coerulus is much curtailed during REMS, giving it a chance to increase its catecholamine receptors. There may be a similar effect in other parts of the brain involving other norephinephrine, dopamine, and serotonin receptors. REMS deprivation causes a large reduction of the amplitude of inhibition in the brainstem caused by noradrenalin. This may explain the rebound of REMS following its deprivation. There is some but not universal research support for this notion. However, while deprivation of REMS for 1–3 days lowers the levels of norepinephrine in the brain, chronic sleep deprivation does not have much effect on these receptors (Turek and Zee 1999).

11.1.1.4 REMS and the Orienting Response

Adrian Morrison, Professor in the Laboratory for Study of the Brain in Sleep in the Department of Animal Biology School of Veterinary Medicine at the University of Pennsylvania, and colleagues (Morrison and Reiner 1985; Morrison et al. 1990; see also Horne 1988) likens the features of REMS to the components of the orienting response found in awake animals. The orienting response is the name for behavioral and physiological responses made by an animal when confronted by unexpected or novel stimuli. During the orienting response, the animal freezes for a few moments in a state of heightened alertness. The muscle inhibition of REMS may be similar to freezing of muscle activity during orientation, and the low voltage fast brain activity with PGO spikes and hippocampal theta rhythm of REMS may correspond to the heightened brain alertness of the orienting response. Additionally, the low activity in the sympathetic nervous systems and the suppression of homeostatic responses, such as the restriction of body temperature regulation, that occur during REMS are also consistent with the orienting response. Additionally, awakening out of REMS, compared to awakening from NREMS, results in higher levels of arousal for 30 or more minutes (Lavie 1989). The major difference between REMS and the orienting response is the sustained duration of the former compared to the transient nature of the latter. Another way of looking at this is that REMS is a substitute for wake by maintaining brain activation while also maintaining sleep.

11.1.1.5 REMS and the Sentinel Function

As you just read, REMS has been hypothesized to prepare the brain for awakening. Others have labeled this the Sentinel Function of REMS (Snyder 1966). There is greater sensory awareness of the external environment during REMS than during NREMS, and the brain can decide if external stimuli are familiar or unfamiliar, safe or threatening. Brain electrical responses to sensory stimuli during REMS but not NREMS are more like those of waking. Animals arouse more quickly and more completely from REMS than from NREMS and are more ready to cope with danger (Horne 2000). REMS increases toward the end of the night as waking approaches, which could prepare the brain for awakening but could also be an effort of the brain to counteract the propensity to wake (Horne 2000).

Countering sentinel function of REMS is the fact that in animals the greater the exposure to danger, the less the amount of REMS (Horne 2000). For example, rats sleeping near cats have less REMS, not more. Additionally, the sentinel hypothesis does not address why there is the muscle paralysis in REMS.

11.1.2 REMS as Adaptive

REMS may help adaptation to the present and past.

11.1.2.1 REMS and Brain Temperature

REMS functions to keep the brain, especially the brainstem, warm during sleep, while much of the rest of the body cools (Wehr 1992). Suggestive evidence for this comes from the fact that the marine mammals that sleep one side of the brain at a time (see Sect. 2.4) show very little if any REMS. This is possible because their constant motion keeps their metabolic activity high, which in turn keeps the temperature of the brainstem up, making REMS unnecessary. Also, the temperature of sea water shows little 24 h variation which may help sustain brain temperature in these animals. Direct evidence includes more the fact that brain temperature does increase during REMS, there is some increase in REMS in cool conditions, and greater REMS at the low point of the circadian brain and body temperature cycle. Also REMS occurs in all endothermic[2] mammals, but it is not clear that it is present in reptiles and lower animals that are ectothermic.

However, there are data that are inconsistent with this idea, such as cats having less REMS at lower room temperatures (Horne 2000). Also, this notion does not explain the muscle paralysis seen during REMS (Horne 2000).

11.1.2.2 REMS and Drives

REMS has been postulated to modulate the expression of drives. This modulation allows the animal more flexibility and adaptability in its waking drive gratification. Casual observation of human behavior suggests REMS deprivation disinhibits aggressive, sexual, or eating behaviors. Direct evidence comes from studies that show REMS deprived rats exhibit more excited drive behaviors. But these experiments involved stimulated or extreme responses and therefore the results may be limited to extremes.

11.1.2.3 REMS and Memory

REMS is thought to play an important role in memory because during REMS conditions may be right for the consolidation. During REMS the brain is free from competitive uses (Kavanau 2001); there is a high rate of protein synthesis

---

[2] Endothermic animals are those that sufficiently produce their own body heat as opposed to exothermic animals that rely on their environment for most of their body heat. They are sometimes called "cold blooded".

consistent with maintenance of neural components needed for memories, and the flow of information reverses during REMS now going from the neocortex to the hippocampus. Additional details of the reputed role of sleep in memory are presented in Sects. 10.4.1.1 and 10.4.1.2.

Other evidence in humans shows that emotional material is recalled better after REMS, but NREMS is without effect. For example, Cartwright (1974) gave subjects crossword puzzles, word-associations, and story completions to do. They ranged from neutral to emotional. Half of the subjects then stayed awake, and the other half had REMS between the time they started working on the problems and when they finished them. The more emotional the problem, the more REMS influenced performance. REMS changed the way the subjects saw the emotional problems. The intervening waking period had no effect.

11.1.2.4 REMS and Emotion

In most people, sleep deprivation increases negative mood and decreases positive mood (Walker 2009 and Sect. 11.1), strongly suggesting that a function of sleep is mood regulation. A number of studies show that morning mood in nondepressed people is affected by the amount and quality of their recent sleep (Cartwright et al. 1998). Sleep of sufficient length and quality improves morning mood. When deprived of sleep for one night, morning mood scores in these people are significantly lower. Sleep generally elevates mood. For example, Zohar et al. (2005) showed that sleep deprivation increased negative emotional outcomes of disrupting waking events, while reducing the positive gain that comes with gratifying or goal-directed events in medical residents.

It is REMS that has been postulated to play an important role in the regulation of mood and emotions. REMS is thought to result in "enhanced effective adjustment" and "greater interpersonal skill and inventiveness" (Cohen 1980, p. 315), leaving most people more flexible and adaptive when awake (Horne 1988). REMS is said to tame or modulate drives by reducing drive-motivated behaviors. For example, Vogel (1979) points to the fact that there are positive benefits of REMS deprivation in depressed individuals but the benefits only last until REMS resumes. The person who is depressed already has a low drive level and REMS only further reduces it. In the absence of REMS, drives in the depressed person are more activated and approach a more normal level.

It is thought that sleep is helpful for emotions because dreaming during REMS helps balance emotions, especially regulating negative ones. Included by some in this context (e.g., Webb 1983) is Freud's discharge model of dreams which states that dreams act as a safety valve for repressed drive. Others see this emotional function as due to REMS itself and not its accompanying dreams (see Sect. 11.1.2.4).

Other observations show an increase in REMS time after days of stress, worry, and intense learning (Greenberg 1981; Hartmann 1973). Generally, this increase will occur following a large variety of emotionally demanding events, both positive and negative, during the day. It can be seen in exaggerated form in variable length sleepers (see Sect. 4.3). Van der Helm and Walker (2011) posit that REMS provides affective modulation—we sleep to consolidate memories of emotional incidents yet also sleep to forget their severity. Research suggests that there is greater consolidation for emotional compared to neutral information especially after a night of sleep. Declarative memories that are intricate and contain strong emotions are more dependent upon REMS than are simpler and more neutral ones.

It has also been shown that circadian rhythm interacts with amount of prior wake to influence mood, but the interaction is not simple (Boivin et al. 1997). Depending on circadian phase, mood elevates, deteriorates, or remains the same with increasing duration of waking. This interaction is complex and nonadditive such that a slight change in timing of the sleep-wake cycle can have notable effects on mood.

11.1.2.5 Other Adaptive Aspects of REMS

The active rems while in REMS stand in contrast to the inhibition of other body muscles. One suggested function of these rems has to do with using two eyes for vision. Complex organization and neural processing is necessary in order for the brain to receive and properly process coordinated input from two eyes. During early maturation, the rems of REMS may facilitate the proper growth of the brain mechanisms for binocular vision. Later in life, they may sever to maintain function in these areas. Support for these related ideas is seen in the high REMS in species with a lot of crossing of the optic nerves, but much less in species with little crossing. There is also some evidence that binocular coordination is better at the end of REMS. However, it has been pointed out that there are many exceptions to this generalization, and there is REMS in species with few or no eye movements.

David Maurice, affiliated with the Columbia University Department of Ophthalmology, advanced the hypothesis that the rems of REMS are to stir the fluids in the eye to keep them from not stagnating (Maurice 1998). Experimental evidence shows that when the eyelids are closed and the eyes not moving, the fluid in the eye does become stagnant, but eye movements are sufficient to prevent the stagnation and oxygenate the fluids in the eye. Experiments in animals demonstrated that the cornea shows signs of disease when the eyeballs are prevented from moving for a few days.

11.2 NREMS–REMS Sequence

The fact that REMS most often follows NREMS suggests that something happens during REMS that is in response to something that happens in NREMS (Benington and Heller 1994). Support comes from the facts that REMS percent is related to amount of NREMS, not the amount of waking, and the interval between REMS periods is dependent on the amount of elapsed NREMS regardless of the amount of intervening waking. One possibility is that the cellular activity of REMS warms the brain after a period of cooling during NREMS (Wehr 1992).

On the other hand, REMS may provide a regularized system check that can, in part, help determine the adequacy of repair done in NREMS and locate where more maintenance is needed during the subsequent NREMS episode (McGrath and Cohen 1978). Early in the night, the need is for macro restoration and adjustment that requires only brief testing; thus, NREMS is long and REMS is short. Later, however, the restoration and adjustment become more and more refined and delicate—a kind of micro restoration—that requires longer and more detailed evaluation that is possible only in REMS. For this reason, late in the night, NREMS is shorter and REMS is longer.

REMS may also be randomly testing the rest of the nervous system beyond the brain, resulting in the bodily concomitants of REMS such as irregular activation of the respiratory system, cardiovascular system, and other functions controlled by the automatic nervous system. In this case, it is important, for safety's sake, to prevent the muscles of movement from being activated while their nervous system controlling units are being tested.

Another possibility is that REMS helps to maintain a sufficient level of arousal in the cortex to compensate for the low level of arousal during NREMS (Vertes and Eastman 2000). REMS may provide a periodic respite from NREMS as a stand-in for wakefulness (Horne 2000; Rial et al. 1997). This serves to reduce the vulnerability of the sleeper to under arousal. NREMS is a time of brain quiescence that renders an animal less able to respond to challenges quickly. Periodic REMS reverses this state without the need for awakening. It also can serve to prepare the brain for awakening near the end of a period of sleep.

Horne (2009) proposes that REMS is neither sleep nor wake but more like when a computer goes into screen saver mode. It keeps the brain in a wake-ready state while helping to maintain the sleeping state. Put another way, it may be a wake substitute, or "pseudowake," rather than a state of sleep per se. In adults, REMS occurs at a time when an animal is not productive, stimulated, or endangered. Arousal is easier from REMS in the presence of stimuli indicating danger or other emotional significance. Greater amounts of REMS near the end of sleep or when sleep is extended may substitute for wakefulness when NREMS cannot be sustained, yet it is desirable to remain asleep rather than to wake up. However, research shows that allowing unlimited NREMS during the day in humans, which reduces NREMS at night, has no effect on REMS the following night. If REMS is a "filler", then there should be more of it in this situation. Put another way (Horne 2006), REMS is not so much sleep being on as it is wakefulness being switched off. In this sense, REMS can be thought of as a state of 'non-wakefulness'. Unlike NREMS, it can rapidly and easily be reversed to wakefulness. A further discussion of this interesting notion can be found in Jim Horne's book, *Sleepfaring* (2006).

Horne, in a review of the literature, concludes that in the end there is no solid evidence that REMS provides any unique, positive benefits (Horne 2000). REMS seems expendable in some animals such as those highly subject to predation or other dangers (Horne 2009). Sea lions sleep one side of the brain at a time with no REMS for weeks at a time when in the ocean, then show no REMS rebound when back on land. Humans deprived of REMS as a side effect of medications show neither obvious deficits nor much REMS rebound when the medication is discontinued. He concludes that the benefits of sleep come from NREMS, not REMS. Obviously, more research on the functions of sleep is needed.

Box 11.2 Is REMS Phylogenetically Older than NREMS?[3]

Reptiles, amphibia, and fish sleep (see Sect. 2.4). However, unlike birds and mammals, their sleep is of only one kind that leads to an important question: "Is this one kind of sleep comparable to REMS, NREMS, or neither?" Whatever the answer to this question, another logically follows: "what are the evolutionary steps between this unified primitive sleep in lower vertebrates and the multiple types of alternating sleep of higher vertebrates?"

A widely held view is that NREMS is older. Most of the support comes from studies of brain waves during sleep in reptiles that, to some, closely resemble only NREMS. It is only higher animals that also have REMS, thus NREMS must be older and REMS a later development during evolution.

Others hold that REMS is older. First, they see the brain wave data from sleeping reptiles as indicating a kind of REMS, not NREMS. They also point to the fact that the first sleep in infant mammals is REMS and that NREMS only gradually supplants much of it with maturity. Additionally, Rial and colleagues (1997) point to the fact that the control for REMS is in the brainstem, SWS (N3 in humans) in the midbrain, and waking in the cortex. This progression is the order of development of the brain during evolution. Thus, they maintain that REMS is older than SWS. Further, they continue, REMS is equivalent to waking in primitive animals, such as the lancet, SWS is equivalent to waking in more advanced animals, but true waking came along only later in evolution in the most advanced animals.

A third view, developed by Karmanova (1982), holds that neither REMS nor NREMS is oldest but that both emerged together out of older, sleep-like states. Ida Gavrilovna Karmanova has a doctorate in biological sciences and is retired director of the Laboratory of Wake-Sleep Evolution at the I. M. Sechenov Institute of Evolutionary Physiology and Biochemistry in St. Petersburg, Russia. Based on her decades of study of sleep in various phylogenetic levels of animals, she believes that both NREMS and REMS evolved somewhat simultaneously out of more primitive rest states that she calls "sleep-like states." From these primitive states, she has traced the evolutionary development of sleep from "primary sleep" in fish and amphibians through "intermediate sleep" in reptiles to "true sleep" in birds and mammals by studying some remnants of these stages in currently living

---

[3] Adapted and updated from Moorcroft (1993) with permission of the publisher.

animals. Siegel (e.g., 1997), based on his studies of the primitive echidna (see Sect. 2.4), comes to a similar conclusion that both NREMS and REMS evolved from a primitive mixture of the two.

Obviously, there is currently no consensus as to which type of sleep is the oldest. Perhaps someday with further research, we shall know the answer.

11.3 The Functions of Dreaming

Why do we spend so much time dreaming? Why does our mind put forth the effort to create dream, after dream night after night? Surely there must be good purpose for such an endeavor. Through the ages, there have been many ideas about what dreams are (see Sect. 8.1). Some of these ideas are related to functions. Rather than review all of these ideas, we shall focus our attention here on theories that give primary importance to dream function and that are also in the forefront of current consideration.

At the beginning of the twentieth century, Freud changed the focus of the function of dreams with his publication of *The Interpretation of Dreams* (1900). Prior to Freud, the prevailing notion was that the source of dreams came from outside the individual. Because of Freud much of the Western world came to believe that dreams were internal functioning as an individual's emotional drive or instinct relief valves. Pent-up pressure from basic drives and wants that could not be manifested while awake because of personal and societal constraints could be released during dreams in disguised forms. It was believed that if this pressure was not released, then severe psychological problems would result. During this time, there were others, collectively known as post-Freudians, who accepted Freud's basic foundation but modified his details (see Sect. 9.1.3).

The discovery of REMS in the middle of the twentieth century led to the rapid demise of the Freudian and related post-Freudian views, for it was found when people were deprived of sleep, or specifically REMS, hence major dreaming, they did not go crazy. Subsequently, there were a number of new putative functions for dreams, but all in the realm of the internal and the personal. As of yet, there is neither convincing evidence nor consensus about the correctness of any one of the theories of dream functioning. It may be, as with sleep itself, that several functions of dreaming coexist. The leading candidates today are that dreams benefit the emotions of the dreamer, generate creative solutions to problems, and/or play a role in consolidating memories.

Essentially, what many of these theories say is that we dream about things that are important to us, in the sense of being emotionally arousing or significant (Fiss 1979). The process is adaptive, since we focus on our problems and seek solutions (Cartwright 1990). These solutions may subsequently be assimilated into existing memory structures (Cartwright 1990) and may be of help for waking behaviors. Dreams, then, are involved in the processes of self-regulation and self-reflectiveness (Moffitt 1987). They function like a gyroscope to keep the self on a steady course in the face of the vicissitudes of daily life. Other theories, or corollaries to the main theories, conclude that dreams are for play, rehearse responses to potential threats, and/or distract our attention while asleep.

Still, there are many who believe that dreams have no functions; they are merely epiphenomena[4] generated as the brain is performing some other function (e.g., Domhoff 1985; Flanagan 1995, 2000; Foulkes 1999; Stickgold et al. 2001). In this regard, dreams are similar to the noise the heart makes when it pumps blood. The noise does not have a function; it does not help pump blood. It is a by-product, or, more properly, an epiphenomenon, of the pumping activity of the heart. Similarly, dreams are seen as a by-product of the activity of the brain as it goes about its other (real) functions during sleep. Many theories of dreams that come out of cognitive neuroscience are of this type, such as the activation-synthesis theory and Foulkes's cognitive theory of dreaming.

Others counter that dreams are much more organized than disorganized, have too much temporal progression, and focus too much on the dreamer in the world for them to be meaningless random epiphenomena (Revonsuo 2000). The Hall-Van de Castle analyses of series of dreams show there is consistency in dreams, hence meaning. Additionally, studies of the experiences that result when the brain is randomly stimulated, such as epileptic seizures of the temporal lobe, are quite different from those of dreaming. They contain varying perceptions that do not form a coherent world, no story-line and poor perceptual detail. Dreams contain all of these aspects.

It should be noted that many speculations about the functions of dreams do not differentiate between the dreams of REMS and the mentations of NREMS. Some theories are specific to only REMS. There appear to be no noteworthy theories that specifically focus on NREMS mentation.

Several aspects of REMS dreams have been influential in formulations about their functions including:

- Emotional content: Many dreams have noticeable emotional content, more often negative.
- Bizarreness: Many aspects of dreams are frequently bizarre including characters, settings, and activities, as well as the sequential flow.
- Personalness: Much of what a person dreams about is recognizable to the dreamer including characters, settings, and objects. For the most part, they are things that are a part of the individual's current life but also include things that are a part of the individual's biographical memory. They are mostly first person experiences.
- Lack of voluntary control: The dreamer is typically not in control of its content even while other cognitive processes are maintained.
- Realistic: While we are dreaming, the things in the dream seem very realistic and we unquestioningly accept what is in them.

---

[4] Something that secondarily occurs because of some primary event.

- Story-like: Dreams have a narrative structure.
- Single mindedness: There is a complete involvement in the experience while we are dreaming. This experience differs from waking when we are often distracted by other stimuli or thoughts.
- Dreams occur between two periods of waking: The contents of our dreams are influenced by our recent waking experiences and can have an effect on our subsequent waking.
- Number of dreams: We have many more dreams than we remember.

Before we explore the putative functions of dreaming in more detail, we need to keep a couple of things in mind. It is difficult to test the veracity of many of the theories of the functions of dreaming. First, as mentioned in the introduction to Part III, our only access to the content of people's dreams is through their description of what they remember of their dreams. The dream report may not be entirely accurate. Also, there may be whole categories of dreams that seldom, if ever, reach waking consciousness. As a result, we cannot be sure that our theories of functions of dreams are accurate and complete.

Second, it is necessary but difficult to show that dreams make a difference. One way to do so is to provide an adequate control group when doing dream research. Ideally such a control group might be people who do not dream or dream differently than the experimental group. However, there are practical problems in accomplishing this. There are people who say they never dream, but in most cases what really is happening is that they do not spontaneously remember their dreams. There are those with damage to specific areas of the brain who, as far as can be determined, do not dream (Solms 1997), but any differences between them and people who dream might be primarily caused by the brain damage itself rather than the lack of dreaming. Thus, the theories of dreams tend to be even more speculative, relying more heavily on logic and intuition than theories involving other aspects of sleep. That is, the fact to assumption ratio is often quite low, and the research attempting to test one or another of these theories has provided only weak support or contradictory results (Cartwright 1989). Without an adequate control group, it is difficult to separate any effect of dreaming from sleep itself. Nevertheless, many of the contemporary theories are interesting, instructive, and seem to have at least elements that are plausible.

The leading proposed functions of dreaming include: (1) dreaming facilitates emotional adaptation; (2) creativity occurs during dreaming; (3) play can occur during dreaming; and (4) there are cognitive benefits of dreaming. Other less prevailing theories about the functions of dreaming include: dreams act to distract the brain's attention to keep us from waking up; dreaming provides for, or results from, necessary stimulation of the brain from within, compensating for the loss of stimulation from the environment during NREMS or complementing waking stimulation; and when we dream, we rehearse perceptions of threats and ways to avoid them.

11.3.1 Dreaming Facilitates Emotional Adaptation

Dreams are best viewed as occurring between two periods of wake (Fiss 1979; Kramer 1987, 1990). The preceding period of wake can affect the mood of the dream as well as its contents. But the dream then affects the subsequent period of wake as a kind of mood regulator or sometimes as a mood disruptor.

The fact that dream content is heavily emotional leads to the notion that dreams play some kind of a role in emotional adaptation. In other words, dreaming helps individuals cope with the turmoil of their current waking life. This popular view has its origin in Jung's notion that dreaming helps maintain psychic balance, as well as Adler's view of a personal problem-solving function in dreaming (see Sect. 9.1.3.1). More recent studies, using functional imaging of the brain during sleep, lend some support. These studies show activation during REMS of the brain areas involved with emotions, suggesting that emotions may be important in shaping the content of dreams (Hobson et al. 2000).

One way that dreaming might provide emotional adaptation is by preserving our identity (Cartwright 2010). Dreams retell who we are. They act like an emotional gyroscope making corrections to try to keep us on an even emotional keel (Kramer 1987). They bring a balance into our lives. They can also act like a safety valve allowing us to relieve built-up emotional pressure.

There is an advantage in dealing with emotions in dreams, for there is an absence of inhibition from logic and no fear of ridicule. We can relate our waking stresses to past memories of a similar nature without being disturbed by the interruptions that are frequent when we are awake. We are then freer to try out different solutions, because we are free from the consequences and social constraints of waking life (Koulack 1991). We are also freer to mix ideas while dreaming than when we are awake. So, unlike when awake, our mind can work more directly on the emotional problem on its own terms. In the end when our dreams are working well, we can assimilate the emotional problem into our psyche in a way that promotes overall well being. Laboratory studies have shown that there is a measurable change in certain aspects of mood after dreaming—what Kramer calls the mood regulatory hypothesis (Kramer 1993). He finds that mood is generally better and less variable following dreaming. Furthermore, behavior is changed as a result. These studies have also shown that it is the dream content, especially the characters in the dream, that is related to the mood change (Nielsen and Lara-Carrasoco 2007). This is best seen following major events in the life of the dreamer such as the death of a loved one, making and breaking of new friendships, conflict with family partners, and birth of a child. And, while some aspects of mood are affected by sleep such as "clear thinking", others seem to be only affected by the dreaming such as "unhappiness."

As a test of Kramer's mood regulatory hypothesis, Cartwright and associates (Cartwright et al. 1998) studied the dreams of 61 volunteers undergoing divorce. Subjects were awakened in the sleep lab several minutes into each REMS period for dream collection. Those undergoing divorce that were not depressed had a low percent of negative dreams throughout the night. Those who were depressed at the time of the divorce, but were not a year later, had a lot of negative dreams early in the night, but fewer as the night went on suggesting that dreams helped to work through the depression. Those who were depressed both at the time of the divorce and a year later had a few negative dreams early in the night, but more as the night went on. In this last group, the dreaming process may have failed because the negative mood was too intense or possibly some other reason.

Cartwright and colleagues (Cartwright et al. 1998) also did similar research with a nondepressed group of "normal" people. A total of 60 students, 30 males and 30 females, were selected from a group of volunteers because of having no current or past major depression. Before and after each night of sleep, they filled out a mood scale. On the second night in the lab, they were awakened after several minutes into each REMS period and asked to report what they had been experiencing. The first dreams of the night were influenced by the presence of negative mood before sleep. They contained more negative emotion and less positive emotion early in the night, with the negative diminishing and the positive increasing as the night went on, suggesting a "working through" of the problems by the dreams. This pattern was not seen if the dreamer did not start the night with negative mood. Those who showed a moderate amount of depressed mood at bedtime showed better mood after dreaming. Cartwright's conclusion from these data is that a function of dreams appears to be to modulate mood when negative mood is moderate. Dreams especially strive to downregulate disruptive negative emotions from new experiences. They do this by linking the new with the old and thereby attempt to maintain and integrate our concept of ourselves. This helps to function better when awake. But for really big problems, the process may extend over more than one night.

In a related theory, Ernest Hartmann, Professor of Psychiatry at Tufts University School of Medicine and retired Director of the Sleep Disorders Center at Newton-Wellesley Hospital, in Boston, maintains that dreams are guided by our emotions and emotional concerns and then help us deal with these emotions (Hartmann 1998). This function is most easily seen in people who have experienced psychological trauma, since it is much clearer what emotion is involved with the dreams. However, Hartmann believes the same process occurs with all emotions, even ones we may not be consciously aware of. What dreams do is make emotions into visual metaphors. These metaphors help explain things better. Minor parts of the dream are used to connect the metaphors by weaving together similar traumas, stresses, and life events to make them into new material. In this way, new neural networks are created.

Cartwright, Hartmann, and others conclude that dreams thus help us by providing relief of the current trauma or emotion, and at the same time, prepare us for future trauma, stress, and problems of life all within the safety of the dream. Also, when sleeping, the brain is able to broadly reach out more easily to make the new connections than is possible when awake. In this way, dreaming can be therapeutic. Dreams are a kind of "built in psychotherapy" that occurs in a safe place. And, it all happens whether we remember the dream or not.

It is also possible that REMS and dreaming both are beneficial for our emotions. Each might act on different aspects of our emotions during the night (LaraCarrasco et al. 2009). Dreams bring access to our store of relevant memories that may not occur in REMS alone.

Modern thinkers have seen the relationship of dreams to the dreamer's waking life in one of two ways—complementary or continuous (Cartwright, 1978). Complementary dreams contain things that compensate for or are supplementary to what has recently occurred in waking life in an attempt to bring overall balance or harmony. For example, when Paul had been severely criticized for making an error at work, which he believed may have jeopardized his chances for promotion, he subsequently dreamed that he was competing in preOlympic track trials and was doing quite well and was "still in the running." Jill during the day had been bragging about being selected as one of 10 finalists in a contest by a popular teen magazine for a modeling feature. That night, her dreams contained an image of a group of strangers pruning rose bushes that is "cutting them down to size."

Continuous dreams, on the other hand, are those in which the themes, concerns, and events of waking life are taken up again in our dreams. Jerry had recently been working nights and weekends at his job, hoping to make a good impression and be rapidly promoted. After an argument with his wife about his "never being home", he had a dream that he was in a hot air balloon race in which he was "rising fast but on a collision course with a house that looked like mine".

Which is correct? Do our dreams take an active role in attempting to compensate for our waking lives in an effort to bring balance to our psyche? Or, is the focus of our dreams continuous with the cares and events of our waking lives? Probably, both are correct. Our mind may choose one or the other depending on current need, or perhaps the created dream may contain an element of each. The choice seems to depend upon where the greatest need exists in a person's life at the moment. However, research shows that continuous dreams are more prevalent. Seldom are they direct replays of the day's events. Rather they focus on more general personal concerns and interests such as family, friends, and work plus the way people think. People with aggressive dreams may not be aggressive in waking life but have a lot of aggressive thoughts.

On the contrary, according to Revonsuo (2000), the empirical evidence for the emotionally adaptive function of dreaming is only correlational and relatively weak. While the evidence is clear that much of the reported content of dreams is related to current emotional problems of the dreamer, there is little convincing evidence that dreaming of such problems has a salutatory effect on our waking psyche, since, he maintains, few causal relationships between dream content and waking adjustment have been established. Revonsuo also states that if this is indeed the function of dreaming, it is strange how often it fails given the high proportion of negative dreams that amplify the negative experiences, rather than those that overtly comfort and heal.

11.3.2 Creativity Occurs During Dreaming

Dreams are by their nature creative. Every night each of us produces several very original and unique dreams, which is a very creative process. The results carry over into our waking lives in several ways. Our dreams may subtly suggest solutions to our everyday personal problems (Koulack 1987) or solutions to matters that have been puzzling us. They do so because dreams are not restrained by logic or realism (Cartwright and Lamberg 1992). Thus, they allow less constrained associations between memories and cognitive processes than are allowed when awake (Stickgold et al. 1999), and they provide access to our recent and remote memories tying them to alternate cognitive strategies all followed by assimilation or accommodation into our existing memories and/or personality (Cartwright 1990).

Stickgold and associates (1999) awakened people from REMS or NREMS and immediately gave them a semantic priming task while the brain was thought to be functionally organized, as it was during the preceding stage of sleep. In this task, subjects were shown a series of words mixed with nonwords one at a time and had to identify as quickly as possible whether or not they were seeing a word. Before each word (for example "wrong") or nonword ("wronk") was shown, a word called a prime was displayed. The primes were either unrelated to the word ("paper"), weakly related ("thief"), or strongly related ("right"). The results showed that following NREMS awakenings, strong primes were very effective, but weak ones were not. However, the opposite is true following REMS awakenings, showing that associations are more remote, allowing more creativity. Creativity in our dreams, it seems, comes about because weak associations are facilitated during REMS.

The creativity in dreams can also help us with our personal, emotional problems. In dreams, we can creatively relate our current stresses to similar ones in our past experience, and then we are freer to try out different solutions (Koulack 1991). We are free from the interruptions that occur during wakefulness, free from social constraints, and freer to mix ideas than when awake. During dreams, we are also free from self-criticism allowing us to deal with our waking experiences creatively (Strauch and Meier 1996). In dreams we easily and unconsciously engage in novel experiences and playfully deal with the world.

But, there seem to be natural constraints on the solutions derived from dreams. First, we must be working on the problem or in some other way have the need for such a dream during our waking life. Second, we need to be able to recognize that the dream is offering a solution. Third, such dreams appear to be rather unpredictable, meaning that we cannot pick and choose when they will occur and that we have to be ready to record and use them when they do come. The following dream excerpt is an example:

> Before this dream, I'd been having trouble deciding how to work out a color scheme on a particular woodcut for art class. In my dream I somehow worked out an idea and woke up knowing what I was planning to do next.

Watt's lead shot dream presented in Sect. 7.9 is another excellent example of all of the factors involved with creative dreams. It was an important problem that he had been working on during his waking life, yet he had to have the dream several times before he recognized what it was saying to him. We can only wonder what new discoveries have been lost, because dreamers did not pay attention to what their dreams might have been trying to tell them.

Yet, this research is not conclusive (e.g., Revonsuo 2000). Achieving waking creative solution, which may be correlated with a dreamed solution, does not indicate a causal relationship. It is just as likely that the solution was arrived at when awake, and the dream simply reflects this.

11.3.3 Play Can Occur During Dreaming

Several investigators of dreams, such as Bulkeley (1999), have likened the function of dreams to that of play. Play is fanciful, yet important. It is enjoyable, but also useful. It can be creative and exploratory. It is done for its own sake in a semireal realm of its own making. Play involves strong emotions. Play tends toward exaggeration, variation, and nonsensical yet is governed by some rules that often differ from that of nonplay behavior. It is free, unpressured experimentation with possibilities and potentials. Play enables trying out various possibilities of experience. It allows safe experience with different skills and behaviors. It gives us the opportunity to experience events and social relationships differently from our serious life. In play, there may be exaggerated, bizarre imagery. We are free to explore and interact differently than we are in real life. In all of these ways, play can result in our enhanced flexibility and prepare us for the future. So in dreams, we can sometimes play. This idea encompasses both the emotion and creativity aspects of dreaming. It can be important.

11.3.4 Cognitive Benefits of Dreaming

Earlier models of dream function such as those of Freud and Jung have not been scientifically verified. In their place new models derived from research in cognitive neuroscience are coming to the fore. More and more evidence points to the idea that dreaming is the experience of mechanisms in the brain that are implementing emotional and memory reprocessing while asleep and then consolidating, assimilating, and even actively repealing changes that were acquired when awake. Rather than exact replay of what occurred when awake, dreams are made up of portions of several recent episodes mixed with older memories, information, and sensorimotor memories.

Just like REMS, dreaming is thought to facilitate memory reorganization and maintenance. It has been hypothesized that during dreaming, memories are reorganized by associating and integrating the past with the present (Hobson 1989). Dreaming also helps us master new experiences by assimilating them into the structure of preexisting memories helping keep our memories more efficiently organized (Scrima 2011). A related idea is that dreams are important for reprocessing waking experiences that are important for our survival (Winson 1990). For animals, the survival value of dreams involves memories such as where to obtain food or where to escape from predators. In this way, dreams are biologically relevant. For humans, the survival value is more involved with the complex interrelationships of humans and the complexities of human personality.

An experiment from Stickgold's lab elucidates what happens (Wamsley et al. 2010). Subjects worked on a three-dimensional virtual maze, then had an opportunity to nap 1½ hours or remain awake. Those subjects who reported that they had dream content related to the task later showed better performance on the maze. However, those who did not report any task-related imagery while napping or who remained awake and thinking about the maze showed no improvement.

Box 11.3 The Tetris Experiments: NREM Mentation After Intensively Playing Video Games

A series of experiments done at Harvard looked at NREM mentation content after intensively playing video games for 2 hours each day for a few days (e.g., Smith 2010; Wamsley and Stickgold 2011). One study used the video game Tetris—a tile match game with game pieces composed of four square blocks arranged in geometric shapes that have to be fitted together to form a larger, solid wall with no empty spaces. When subjects were then awakened shortly after falling asleep, 64 % reported images clearly related to the game such as seeing falling puzzle pieces. When Alpine Racer—a downhill skiing arcade game—was used 30 % of early sleep NREM mentation contained "visual and kinesthetic sensations of skiing down the hill." Experienced skiers reported images from their past skiing experiences, especially those where they recall crashing. The researchers concluded that NREM mentation that occurs early in sleep often involves a "reactivation of waking experience" that is possibly involved in memory consolidation. This was not a simple reiteration of the task but a melding of aspects of the recent learning experience with similar matter taken from existing memories. If awakened after 2 hours of sleep, the subjects from Alpine Racer game said they experienced mental imagery that was more remote such as "falling down a hill" or "moving through some kind of forest" suggesting the associations during NREM mentation had become weaker.

Scenes of Dr. Stickgold with a subject doing the Alpine Racer game are at http://www.pbs.org/wgbh/nova/body/sleep.html from 4:00–5:38).

Foulkes (1983) also focuses on a memory function of dreaming. He was struck by the parallel between cognitive development in children and the development of their dreams (Sect. 9.2.4). To him dreams help integrate our knowledge—especially that knowledge available to conscious recall. This integration occurs both within types of memory and between types of memory, such as semantic and episodic, recent and distant, and verbal and visual-spatial. To Foulkes, the integration occurs even though we do not remember much of our dreams. As a result, we are left with: (1) an increase in the range of our experiences that even includes unrealistic things, (2) greater reality testing, since when we awaken, we know that much of what we dreamed was not real, and thus we can more easily recognize that our minds are capable of creating images that are not real; and (3) better self-knowledge because of combining motor memories with recognition memories, giving us more flexibility.

Then again, perhaps the association of dreams with memory processes is more apparent than real. Siegel (2001) doubts that dreams reflect the consolidation of recent waking events, because so little of dream content is related to recent experiences, even a recently intensive learning task. And those dreams that do seem to incorporate experiences from recent waking seldom are an exact rehearsal of the experiences or learned tasks, but more about the situation related to the experience or learning. It is possible that dreams are epiphenomena of brain processes as they activate and then recombine memories and emotions (Stickgold et al. 2001), and the dreams themselves do nothing to aid in the process.

Ernest Hartmann maintains that dreams do not simply replay our waking lives but always make new connections (Hartmann 2010). For example, he notes that of the 440 dreams he studied after 9/11, none contained anything like images of planes hitting tall buildings although the dreamers had seen the 9/11 events many times on TV, and was an emotional experience for them. Likewise, he has studied recurrent and repetitive dreams and found that most are not exact replicas of something that happened but center around a theme, and the actual content changes over time. He says that dreams are hyperconnective because "the connections are broader and looser than in waking," which is an important function of dreaming. That is, to combine the new with what is already in memory, always directed by emotion.

Hartmann admits that he has "no direct experimental proof for this" but believes that this can be seen "on a clinical level" in a sequence of dreams, especially those that follow a traumatic event. The initial dreams in the series picture parts of the actual events, but with some changes. Subsequently, the emotion, such as fear or helplessness, may be represented in a strong dream represented by something like a tidal wave. After this dreams begin to integrate the actual trauma with pictorial representations of the emotion and images of similar events that bare an emotional connection. After a few months, the dreams gradually return to their pre-event pattern. Thus the functions of dreaming are to gradually connect and integrate new experiences with existing memories. That is, dreams help us to shape and reshape meaningful emotional systems of memory, which are the foundation of our unique selves.

11.3.5 Other Benefits of Dreaming

There are a few other theories related to the functions of dreaming that deserve to be noted in passing. One is that dreams act to distract the brain's attention to keep us from waking up (Freud 1900; Horne 2000). Horne (2006) puts it this way. While we are in REMS there is some awareness of our surroundings such that our brain can decide whether to awaken. Usually, we do not awaken because while in REMS our cortex is also showered by copious simulated sensations due to activation from the brainstem. The brain does its best to make some sense of all this activated sensation by what we experience as dreams. The content of our dreams keeps strangely and unexpectedly skipping from one thing to another because during REMS the frontal cortex is not exerting its executive function to control things in a sensible and orderly way. Nor is the frontal cortex doing its job of testing reality; thus, we unquestionably accept whatever is happening in our dreams while in REMS. Perhaps it is this acceptance of the strange sequence of events that renders our dreams more captivating, which distracts us from needlessly waking up. This process intensifies as the end of the sleep period gets nearer.

Another theory is that dreaming provides for, or results from, necessary stimulation of the brain from within, compensating for the loss of stimulation from the environment during NREMS or complementing waking stimulation.

Revonsou (2000) views the functions of dreams from an evolutionary standpoint. In order to understand the primary function of dreaming, we have to take into account that the environment in which our ancestors lived was full of threats. Anything that gave a survival advantage allowing for the increased possibility to reproduce would eventually tend to be favored by eons of evolution. Revonsou maintains that, when we dream, we rehearse perceptions of threats and ways to avoid them. These processes may be "threat scripts" from our ancestral past or in response to recently experienced threats during waking. This response is a safe way to enhance the probability of surviving such threats, thus being able to produce offspring. In this way, dreaming became established during evolution. Rather than alleviating emotional problems and thereby contributing to mental health or comfort, they aid reproductive success in much the same way that pain and suffering do. They do so, even if not remembered.

Revonsou (2000) supports this theory with a thorough and comprehensive review of the dreaming literature backed up by relevant information from psychology, evolutionary biology, and cognitive neuroscience. He focuses on the normative content of dreams, children's dreams, recurrent dreams and nightmares, PTSD dreams, and REM Behavior Disorder. He includes the dreams of people in hunter-gatherer societies of today that are filled with the kinds of threats that our ancestors would have experienced in their waking lives, but have far fewer of the experiences of modern humans. He finds that our dreams more often contain negative content such as misfortunes, aggression, and threatening strangers and animals, and less often pleasant experiences. Largely absent are experiences our evolutionary ancestors would not have had, such as working at a computer, reading, or calculating. He also points out that the areas of the brain that for emotional and perceptual experience are activated during REMS.

This theory has been said to be too narrow (Moorcroft 2000). While it seems adequate to explain the primal function of dreaming, it does not allow enough latitude of other functions that may be applicable today. Also, it begins with the questionable assumption of the veracity of the relatively new field of behavioral biology to explain the source of all behavior. Flanagan (1995, 2000) also takes an evolutionary approach to the function of dreaming but concludes that dreaming is an epiphenomenon without function. At this point in time, it is premature to accept fully the exclusiveness of the explanations of behavioral biology and the theories of dreaming by Revonsou and Flanagan.

11.3.6   Conclusion to the Functions of Dreaming

Most of the theories of the functions of dreaming emphasize the importance of emotions in the determination of dream content. Memory consolidation often involves memories that have an emotional component to them. Even the creative and play dreams can be said to involve emotions. Creative dreams involve things that are important to or necessary for the dreamer—things in which the dreamer has invested much of his or her recent waking life. Play can be a good emotional release. The behavioral biology based theory of Revonsou also focuses on emotions. This point is important in understanding dreams. Regardless of whatever else they may be, they have an emotional focus or core.

If the dreams are successful in fulfilling many of the proposed purposes, the dreamer awakens better able to cope and be more productive. But not all dreams successfully accomplish what they were intended to do (Cartwright 1991). Some fail, some are trivial, and some are noxious. "Just as not all sleep is physiologically restorative, so not all dreams are necessarily psychologically restorative" (Fiss 1979, p. 64).

11.4   Conclusion

Sleep and its accompanying dreams probably have many functions rather than a single overriding function. Some of these functions may be accomplished only during sleep. Other functions may also be undertaken when awake but are done more efficiently or effectively during sleep. While some functions of sleep may be found in all animals or at least all mammals studied to date, there is no conclusive evidence for what the functions of sleep are. It is possible that some functions of sleep are found only in some, but not all, animals or only at certain stages of an animal's life because of their unique circumstances or phase of development.

Likewise, the functions of dreams and dreaming are not conclusively understood. Certainly, humans dream and dream a lot, leading to the conclusion that dreams and dreaming must have important functions. It is not certain if animals dream, but it is likely. However, many of the proposed functions of dreams and dreaming do not easily apply to animals.

There are two dominant theories of the functions of sleep, dreams, and dreaming. In humans, sleep and probably dreams are important for cognition. They may support or compliment cognitive operations that occur during wakefulness (Walker 2011). In a similar way, sleep and dreaming are beneficial for our emotions. Both cognitive and emotional functions of sleep and dreams are beneficial for our subsequent waking lives.

References

Benington, J. H., & Heller, H. C. (1994). Does the function of REM sleep concern Non-REM sleep or waking? *Progress in Neurobiology, 44*, 433–449.

Boivin, D. B., Czeisler, C. A., Dijk, D.-J., Duffy, J. F., Folkard, S., Minors, D. S., et al. (1997). Complex interaction of the sleep-wake cycle and circadian phase modulates mood in healthy subjects. *Archives of General Psychiatry, 54*, 145–152.

Borbély, A. A. (1986). *The secrets of sleep*. New York: Basic Books.

Bulkeley, K. (1999). *Visions of the night*. Albany: State University of New York Press.

Cartwright, R. (1990). A network model of dreams. In R. Bootzin, J. Kihlstrom, & D. Schacter (Eds.), *Sleep and cognition* (pp. 179–189). Washington: American Psychological Association.

Cartwright, R. D. (1974). Problem solving: Waking and dreaming. *Journal of Abnormal Psychology, 83*, 451–455.

Cartwright, R. D. (1978). *A primer on sleep and dreaming*. Reading: Addison-Wesley.

Cartwright, R. D. (1989). Dreams and their meaning. In M. Kryger, T. Roth, & W. Dement (Eds.), *Principles and practice of sleep medicine* (pp. 184–190). Philadelphia: Saunders.

Cartwright, R. D. (1991). *Who needs dreams? The upper midwest sleep society meeting*. Minnesota: St Paul.

Cartwright, R. D. (2010). *The twenty-four hour mind*. New York: Oxford University Press.

Cartwright, R. D., & Lamberg, L. (1992). *Crisis dreaming: using your dreams to solve your problems*. New York: HarperCollins.

Cartwright, R., Luten, A., Young, M., Mercer, P., & Bears, M. (1998a). Role of REM sleep and dream affect in overnight mood regulation: a study of normal volunteers. *Psychiatry Research, 81*, 1–8.

Cartwright, R., Young, M., Mercer, P., & Bears, M. (1998b). Role of REM sleep and dream variables in the prediction of remission from depression. *Psychiatry Research, 80*, 249–255.

Cohen, D. B. (1980). The cognitive activity of sleep. *Progress in Brain Research, 53*, 307–324.

Corner, M. A., Mirmiran, M., Bour, H. L., Boer, N. E., van de Poll, H. G., van Oyen, M. A., et al. (1980). Does rapid-eye-movement sleep play a role in brain development. In P. McConnel, G. Boer, H. Romijn, N. van de Poll, & M. Corner (Eds.), *Adaptive capabilities of the nervous system* (pp. 347–356). Amsterdam: Elsevier.

Crick, F., & Mitchinson, G. (1986). REM sleep and neural nets. *Journal of Mind and Behaviour, 7*, 229–250.

Davenne, D., & Adrien, J. (1987). Lesion of the ponto-geniculo-occipital pathways in kittens. I. Effects on sleep and on unitary discharge of the lateral geniculate nucleus. *Brain Research, 409*, 1–9.

Domhoff, G. W. (1985). *The mystique of dreams*. Los Angeles: University of California Press.

Ellman, S.J., & Weinstein, L.N. (1991). REM sleep and dream formation: A theoretical integration. In S. Ellman, & J. Antrobus (Eds.), *The mind in sleep: Psychology and psychophysiology, 2*, 446–488. (New York).

Fiss, H. (1979). Current dream research: a psychobiological perspective. In B. Wolman (Ed.), *Handbook of dreams* (pp. 20–75). New York: Van Nostrand Reinhold.

Flanagan, O. (1995). Deconstructing dreams: The spandrels of sleep. *The Journal of Philosophy, 92*, 5–27.

Flanagan, O. J. (2000). *Dreaming souls: sleep, dreams, and the evolution of the conscious mind*. New York: Oxford University Press.

Foulkes, D. (1983). Cognitive processes during sleep: evolutionary aspects. In A. Mayes (Ed.), *Sleep mechanisms and functions in humans and animals: An evolutionary prespective* (pp. 313–337). Berkshire: Van Nostrand Reinhold.

Foulkes, D. (1999). *Children's dreams and the development of consciousness*. Cambridge: Harvard University Press.

Freud, S. (1900). *Interpretations of dreams*. New York: Modern Library.

Greenberg, R. (1981). Dreams and REM sleep: An intergrative approach. In W. Fishbein (Ed.), *Sleep, dreams, and memory* (pp. 125–133). New York: Spectrum.

Hartmann, E. (1998). *Dreams and nightmares: The new theory on the origin and meaning of dreams*. New York: Plenum Trade.

Hartmann, E. (2010). The dream always makes new connections: The dream is a creation, not a replay. *Sleep Medicine Clinics, 5*, 241–248.

Hartmann, E. L. (1973). *The functions of sleep*. New Haven: Yale University Press.

Hobson, J. A. (1988). *The dreaming brain*. New York: Basic Books.

Hobson, J. A. (1989). Dream theory: A new view of the brain mind. *The Harvard Medical School Mental Health Letter, 5*, 3–5.

Hobson, J. A., Lydic, R., & Baghdoyan, H. A. (1986). Evolinge concepts of sleep cycle generation: From brain centers to neuronal populations. *Behavior and Brain Science, 9*, 371–448.

Hobson, J. A., Pace-Schott, E. F., & Stickgold, R. (2000). Dreaming and the brain: Toward a cognitive neuroscience of conscious states. *Behavioral and Brain Sciences, 23*, 793–842.

Horne, J. (2006). *Sleepfaring*. New York: Oxford University Press.

Horne, J. (2009). REM sleep, energy balance and 'optimal foraging. *Neuroscience and Biobehavioral Reviews, 33*, 466–474.

Horne, J. A. (1988). *Why we sleep*. New York: Oxford University Press.

Horne, J. A. (2000). REM sleep—by default? *Neuroscience and Biobehavioral Reviews, 24*, 777–797.

Jouvet, M. (1998). Paradoxical sleep as a programming system. *Journal of Sleep Research, 7*(Supplement 1), 1–5.

Karmanova, I. G. (1982). *Evolution of sleep: Stages of the wakefulness-sleep cycle in vertebrates*. Basel: Karger.

Kavanau, J. L. (2001). Commentary: Brain-processing limitations and selective pressures for sleep, fish schooling and avian flocking. *Animal Behavior, 62*, 1219–1224.

Koulack, D. (1987). *Dreams and adaptation to contemporary stress*. Copenhagen: Fifth International Congress of Sleep Research.

Koulack, D. (1991). *To catch a dream: Explorations of dreaming*. Albany: State University of New York Press.

Kramer, M. (1987). *The mood regulatory function of dreaming: The dream as selective affective modulator*. Copenhagen: Fifth International Congress of Sleep Research.

Kramer, M. (1990). Nightmares (dream disturbances) in posttraumatic stress disorder: Implications for a theory of dreaming. In R. Bootzin, J. Kihlstrom, & D. Schacter (Eds.), *Sleep and cognition* (pp. 190–202). Washington: American Psychological Association.

Kramer, M. (1993). The selective mood regulatory function of dreaming: An update and revision. In A. Moffit, M. Kramer, & R. Hoffmann (Eds.), *The functions of dreaming* (pp. 135–195). Albany: State University of New York Press.

Kryger, M. H., Roth, T. R., & Dement, W. C. (Eds.). (2011). *Principles and practice of sleep medicine* (5th ed.). St. Louis: Elsevier.

Kryger, M. H., Roth, T., & Dement, W. C. (Eds.). (1989). *Principles and practice of sleep medicine*. Philadelphia: Elsevier.

LaraCarrasco, J., Nielsen, T., Solomonova, E., Levrier, K., & Popova, A. (2009). Overnight emotiona adaptation to negative stimul is altered by REM sleep deprivation and is correlated with intervening dream emotions. *Journal of Sleep Researchj, 18,* 178–187.

Lavie, P. (1989). To nap, perchance to sleep: Ultradian aspects of napping. In D. Dinges & R. Broughton (Eds.), *Sleep and alertness: Chronobiological, behavioral, and medical aspects of napping* (pp. 99–120). New York: Raven Press.

Maurice, D. (1998). An ophthalmological explanation of REM sleep. *Experimental Eye Research, 66,* 139–145.

McCarley, R. W., & Massaquoi, S. G. (1992). Neurobiological structure of the revised limit cycle reciprocal interaction model of REM cycle control. *Journal of Sleep Research, 1,* 132–137.

McGrath, M. J., & Cohen, D. B. (1978). REM sleep facilitation of adaptive waking behavior: A review of the literature. *Psychological Bulletin, 85,* 24–57.

Mirmiram, M. (1986). The importance of fetal/neonatal REM sleep. *European Journal of Obstetrics, Gynecology, and Reproductive Biology, 21,* 283–291.

Moffitt, A. (1987). *Experimental studies of individual differences in dream recall and the question of dream function*. Copenhagen: Fifth International Congress on Sleep Research.

Moorcroft, W. H. (1993). *Sleep, dreaming, and sleep disorders: An introduction* (2nd ed.). Lanham: University Press of America.

Moorcroft, W. H. (2000). Sorting out additions to the understanding of cognition during sleep. *Behavioral and Brain Sciences, 23,* 972–974.

Morrison, A. R., & Reiner, P. B. (1985). A dissection of paradoxical sleep. In D. McGinty, R. Drucker-Colin, A. Morrison, & P. Parmeggiani (Eds.), *Brain mechanisms of sleep* (pp. 97–110). New York: Raven Press.

Morrison, A. R., Ball, L. D., Sanford, G. L., Mann, G. L., & Ross, R. J. (1990). Orienting can be elicited by tones in paradoxical sleep without atonia. *Sleep Research, 19,* 23.

Nicolau, M. C., Akaarir, M., Gamundi, A., Gonzalez, J., & Rial, R. V. (2000). Why we sleep: The evolutionary pathway to the mammalian sleep. *Progress in Neurobiology, 62,* 379–406.

Nielsen, T., & Lara-Carrasoco, J. (2007). Nightmares dreaming and emotion regulation: A review. In D. Barrett & P. McNamara (Eds.), *The new science of dreaming* (pp. 253–284). Westport: Praeger.

Oskenberg, A. (1987). *Sleep and sleep function in mammalian development: REM sleep and CNS development in the visual system of the kitten*. Copenhagen: Fifth International Congress on Sleep Research.

Oswald, I. (1980). Sleep as a restorative process: Human clues. *Progress in Brain Research, 53,* 279–288.

Prinz, P. N. (1980). Sleep changes with aging. In C. Eisdorfer & W. Fann (Eds.), *Psychopharmacology of aging* (pp. 1–12). Jamaica: S P Medical & Scientific Books.

Revonsuo, A. (2000). The reinterpretation of dreams: An evolutionary hypothesis of the function of dreaming. *Behavioral Brain Science, 23,* 877–901.

Rial, R. V., Nicolau, M. C., Gamundi, A., Rossello, C., & Akaarir, M. (1997). The evolution of waking states. In O. Hayaishi & S. Inoué (Eds.), *Sleep and sleep disorders: From molecule to behavior* (pp. 99–112). Tokyo: Academic Press.

Scrima, L. (2011). Dreaming epiphenomena of narcolepsy. *Sleep Medicine Clinics, 5,* 261–275.

Shaffery, J. P., Sinton, C. M., Bissette, G., Roffwarg, H. P., & Marks, G. A. (2002). Rapid eye movement sleep deprivation modifies expression of long-term potentiation in visual cortex of immature rats. *Neuroscience, 110,* 431–443.

Siegel, A. (2001). *A mini-course for clinicians and trauma workers on posttraumatic nightmares.* Retrieved September 24, 2011, from http://www.asdreams.org/magazine/articles/ seigel_nightmares.htm.

Siegel, J. M. (1989). Brainstem mechanisms generating REM sleep. In M. Kryger, T. Roth, & W. Dement (Eds.), *Principles and practice of sleep medicine* (pp. 104–121). Philadelphia: Saunders.

Siegel, J. M. (1997). Sleep in monotremes; implications for the evolution of REM sleep. In *Sleep and sleep disorders: From molecule to behavior* (pp. 113–128).

Siegel, J. M. (2005). Clues to the function of mammalian sleep. *Nature, 437,* 1264–1271.

Smith, C. (2010). Sleep states, memory processing, and dreams. *Sleep Medicine Clinics, 5,* 217–228.

Snyder, F. (1966). Toward an evolutionary theory of dreaming. *American Journal of Psychiatry, 123,* 121–142.

Solms, M. (1997). *The neuropsychology of dreams: A clinico-anatomical study.* Laurence: Erlbaum.

Stickgold, R., Hobson, J. A., Fosse, R., & Fosse, M. (2001). Sleep, learning, and dreams: Off-line memory reprocessing. *Science, 294,* 1052–1057.

Stickgold, R., Scott, L., Rittenhouse, C., & Hobson, J. A. (1999). Sleep induced changes in associative memory. *Journal of Cognitive Neuroscience, 11,* 182–193.

Strauch, I., & Meier, B. (1996). *In search of dreams. Results of experimental dream research.* Albany: State University of New York Press.

Turek, F. W., & Zee, P. C. (1999). *Regulation of sleep and circadian rhythms.* New York: Marcel Dekker, Inc.

van der Helm, E., & Walker, M. P. (2011). Sleep and emotional memory processing. *Sleep Medicine Clinics, 6,* 31–43.

Vassalli, A., & Dijk, D.-J. (2009). Sleep function: Current questions and new approaches. *European Journal of Neuroscience, 19,* 1830–1841.

Vertes, R. P., & Eastman, K. E. (2000). The case against memory consolidation in REM sleep. *Behaval Brain Science, 23,* 867–876.

Vogel, G. W. (1979). A motivational function of REM sleep. In R. Drucker-Colin, M. Shkurovich, & M. Sterman (Eds.), *The functions of sleep* (pp. 233–250). New York: Academic Press.

Walker, M. P. (2009). REM, dreams and emotional brain homeostasis. *Frontiers in Neuroscience, 3,* 442–443.

Walker, M. P. (2011). Sleep, memory and emotion. *Progress Brain Research, 185,* 49–68.

Wamsley, E. J., & Stickgold, R. (2011). Memory, sleep, and dreaming: Experiencing consolidation. *Sleep Medicine Clinics, Sleep Medicine Clinics, 6,* 97–108.

Wamsley, E. J., Tucker, M., Payne, J. D., Benavides, J. A., & Stickgold, R. (2010). Dreaming a learning task is associated with enhanced sleep dependent memory consolidation. *Current Biology, 20,* 850–855.

Webb, W. B. (1983). Theories in modern sleep research. In A. Mayes (Ed.), *Sleep mechanisms and functions in humans and animals: An evolutionary prespective* (pp. 1–17). Berkshire: Van Nostrand Reinhold.

Wehr, T. A. (1992). A brain-warming function for REM sleep. *Neuroscience and Biobehavioral Reviews, 16,* 379–397.

Winson, J. (1990). The meaning of dreams. *Scientific American, 263,* 86–96.

Zohar, D., Tzischinsky, O., Epstein, R., & Lavie, P. (2005). The effects of sleep loss on medical residents' emotional reactions to work events: A cognitive-energy model. *Sleep, 28,* 47–54.

Part V
Problems with Sleeping and Dreaming

Up to this point, we have concentrated on the normal processes of sleeping and dreaming, but these processes do not always operate as designed. In this section, we will explore problems and difficulties of sleeping and dreaming. Chapter 12 discusses problems with sleep that are less severe in that they do not usually present themselves at a sleep disorders treatment center but are nevertheless problems of inconvenience, discomfort, and sometimes problems of great concern. In Chap. 13 we will take a look at more severe problems that typically come to the attention of one of the many sleep disorders treatment centers located in the United States and increasingly in the rest of the world.

In the 1970s, a new aspect of medicine evolved—sleep disorders. Previously, physicians as well as lay people knew that sleep could be problematic. However, knowledge of the kinds of problems people could have with sleep and the extent to which people suffered from them was limited, as was the knowledge of effective treatment for these problems. Insomnia, for example, has been known for centuries, but knowledge of the number of different contributing factors to insomnia was minimal, and treatment consisted primarily of prescribing sleeping potions.

As researchers in sleep laboratories around the world began to learn more and more about normal sleep, interest in abnormal sleep grew. Thus, during the decade of the 1970s, sleep disorder centers were developed in many medical centers for the purposes of learning more about the disorders of sleep and providing clinics for accurate diagnosis and effective treatment.

Classification of Sleep Disorders (American Academy of Sleep Medicine, 2005)

People show up at sleep disorders centers with one or a combination of three kinds of complaints: not being able to sleep, excessive sleepiness, or abnormal events that occur during their sleep. However, sleep disorders are classified and discussed by designations based on the patient's symptoms (e.g., insomnia), their physiological problem (e.g., a malfunction of the circadian alertness rhythm), and the body system involved (e.g., breathing disorders during sleep). This classification system is necessary because sleep problems are so varied and because the underlying physiological problem is not always well understood. There are 85 recognized sleep disorders. The common groupings of the more frequently occurring disorders are:

The *insomnias* include recurring problems with sleep initiation, length, consolidation, or quality despite adequate opportunity for sleep that result in daytime impairment. Also included is the person's perception that sleep is not restorative.

Hypersomnia is the condition of excessive sleepiness not apparently caused by some other sleep disorder designation.

Circadian rhythm sleep disorders are primarily related to a problem with the timing of sleep in the nychthemeron (see Sects. 3.2, 3.3). Examples range from sleep problems due to jet lag, shift work, and other problems where the internal circadian rhythm is not sufficiently synchronized with the cycle of day and night.

Sleep-related breathing disorders involve a problem with breathing during sleep. Most notable is sleep apnea. These disorders typically cause excessive daytime sleepiness.

Generally speaking, *parasomnias* are occurrences during sleep that are undesirable. They are not primarily problems with sleep or wake processes or may be a co-problem with another sleep disorder. They include bedwetting, nightmares, sleep walking, acting out of dreams, and rhythmic movements during sleep.

The *sleep disorders associated with medical or psychiatric disorders* occur in cases where sleep is a major component of the problem but is not the primary problem. Included in this category are people with major mental disorders such as schizophrenia, depression, anxiety, and alcoholism; neurological disorders such as Parkinsonism, Alzheimer's, and Huntington's disease; or other medical problems such as sleeping sickness, peptic ulcers, and emphysema. We will not review these disorders, since the sleep problem is secondary to the medical or psychiatric disorder that goes beyond the scope of this book.

Currently, evolving is an official classification of *childhood sleep disorders*. Some are similar to what is seen in adults but others are unique to children such as sleep onset association disorder and limit setting problems.

A World of Caution

A word of caution is in order here. As we examine these disorders, you may recognize some of these problems as occurring in yourself or someone you know. Indeed, your observations may reflect a genuine sleep disorder that should be evaluated by professionals at a sleep disorder clinic. However, more often than not, you may be suffering from the medical student syndrome. Medical students sometimes begin to see in themselves and others many of the diseases and disorders they are studying, although in reality there is no problem. This experience happens because often there is no clear distinction between health and disease, but rather the difference between them is a matter of degree. So, too, with sleep disorders. Almost everybody has had trouble sleeping at times or has had occasional sleepiness during the day without having a sleep disorder. Only when the problems become excessive and debilitating do they become sleep disorders.

Reference

American Academy of Sleep Medicine. (2005). The International Classification of Sleep Disorders, Revised. Westchester, Illinois.

Chapter 12
Some Difficulties That People May Have with Sleep

Contents

12.1 Problems with Getting Enough Quality Sleep

Sleep is like food for the brain, yet getting enough quality sleep is a problem for many people. Some of these problems are the fault of the sleeper's circumstances, others are due to choices made by the sleeper, while others are the result of what happens to the sleeper during sleep. First, we will explore problems people have with getting enough sleep. Then we will turn our attention to some of the things that happen during sleep that are a problem for some people.

Portions of this chapter have been adapted from Moorcroft 1993 with permission of the publisher. Specific references to statements in this chapter that can be found there and in multiple, widely available sources are not included in the text. A selection of these sources is listed below and can also be consulted for verification or more detail (Kryger et al. 2011; Lee-Chiong 2011; Cartwright 2010; Lee-Chiong et al. 2002).

W. H. Moorcroft, *Understanding Sleep and Dreaming*,
DOI: 10.1007/978-1-4614-6467-9_12,
© Springer Science+Business Media New York 2013

12.1.1 Sleep Need and Sleep Debt

Many people in the Western world do not get sufficient sleep through their own choice or demands imposed upon them. The National Sleep Foundation (2001, 2002, 2011) and the Centers for Disease Control and Prevention (2005, 2011) regularly conduct surveys of sleep and sleeprelated habits of people in the United States. Results showed that most adults do not get enough sleep during weekdays and the situation is even worse for teenagers. The surveys also show that these tendencies have further deteriorated over the last few decades. Nearly two-thirds of people report having or having had difficulty sleeping at some time. Almost 4 out of 10 people said they involuntarily fell asleep at least once during the most recent month. The greater the number of hours worked during the workweek, the less sleep obtained. Additionally, those caring for others and people with children report averaging slightly less sleep than do noncaregivers. As a counterpoint to these statistics, almost 90 % of those surveyed said they believe that obtaining good sleep is important to enhance their lives.

For most people, an insufficient amount of sleep is preventable through changes in lifestyle choices or through treatment for sleep disorders (see Chap. 13), but also through extensive changes in societal elements such as the smarter use of technology and better workplace guidelines (Centers for Disease Control and Prevention 2011).

Box 12.1 The Effect of Music on Sleep

Some people like to fall asleep to music. This fact prompted Ramiro Sanchez, while an undergraduate at Northwestern University under the direction of sleep researcher Richard R. Bootzin, to study the effect that different kinds of music have on sleep (Sanchez and Bootzin 1985). Forty eight students took a two-hour evening nap while listening to white noise that is like static when an AM radio is tuned between stations, classical music, soft rock, or hard rock. Those who slept with white noise averaged 15 min to get to sleep and slept for 103 min. Those who slept to classical music slept for 66–73 min. Soft rock listeners averaged a total sleep time of 38 min. The hard rock listeners did not get much sleep, only 5.4 min. Comparison data for those listening to nothing were not provided.

The researchers posited that music disrupted sleep to the extent that the sound was unpredictable. Those who choose to fall asleep to music with screaming guitars and drum solos or similar sounds are cheating themselves out of a good night of sleep.

12.1.2 Effects of Accumulated Sleep Debt

Charles Czeisler of Harvard University (personal communication) has compared sleep need to a semitrailer with a circadian driver that accumulates its load as the wakefulness goes on. The load is unloaded twice as fast during sleep. But without enough sleep, the trailer is only partially unloaded. When insufficient sleep happens night after night, the load accumulates and the speed and efficiency of the semitrailer suffers. For some people even a little sleep deprivation results in great performance impairment, but others may show little impairment until the sleep deprivation becomes severe. Older adults show more resistance to the effects of sleep deprivation than do younger adults.

Sections 3.1.2–3.1.4 and 12.1. detail the negative effects of insufficient sleep. Here we explore how these effects can make a difference in people's lives. Although most people often misjudge and minimize the effects of chronic insufficient sleep, the affects have been shown to be quite substantial including physiological, behavioral, cognitive, and emotional decrements resulting in "chronic diseases, mental disorders, health-risk behaviors, limitations of daily functioning, injury, and mortality" (McKnight-Eily et al. 2011). Many people accept being continually sleep deprived as normal, because it is the only experience they have. Additionally, it is not only the quantity of sleep that is insufficient but too often also the quality (Nowakowski and Ancoli-Israel 2011) (see Sect. 4.2).

12.1.2.1 Effects of Insufficient Sleep on Mood

The National Sleep Foundation poll published in 2001 yielded these details. People who sleep less and have more daytime sleepiness were less likely to have positive feelings such as a sense of peace, satisfaction with life, and feeling full of energy. They were more likely to have negative moods such as anger, stress, pessimism, and fatigue. Almost two people out of every five said that their sleepiness also interfered with their activities at least a few times a month, and one in six said the interference occurred a few days every week. Respondents who said they got less than 6 h of sleep on weekdays felt sleepier during the day than those who got more than 8 h. They said they were more likely to get impatient or irked by common irritations on days when they were sleepy. They also said they had problems getting along with others and experienced negative effects on the ability to communicate with others because of flattening of voice, problems retrieving words, and shorter and less frequent utterances.

Other studies have shown that insufficient sleep also causes problems with: controlling negative moods, causing excessive euphoria, inhibiting immature or inappropriate behaviors, keeping the lid on emotional outbursts, being empathetic, anticipating the range of possible consequences, having insight into one's own performance, and being more susceptible to argument and suggestion.

12.1.2.2 Brain Functioning Changes with Insufficient Sleep

Studies using functional imaging of the brain show that people who have lost one night of sleep have noticeable differences in brain activity (Drummond et al. 1999, 2000, 2001). Sleep deprivation causes a change in the distribution of activity in the brain when doing specific tasks such as arithmetic problems. Depending on the task some areas may become more active, others less active, and others, not typically used in well-rested people, are recruited in an effort to accomplish the task. The more difficult or complex the task the greater is the compensatory activation of other brain regions after sleep deprivation. Yet even when there is greater brain effort, there are still deficits in performance.

Many of the effects of insufficient sleep are the result of less than a fully functioning prefrontal cortex. While some effects of insufficient sleep, such as general arousal of the brain, are lessened by caffeine, the functions dependent on the prefrontal cortex are not lessened.

12.1.2.3 Effects of Sleep Debt on Performance[1]

There appears to be no effect of insufficient sleep on some kinds of tasks such as those that are based on rule, involve logical deduction or critical reasoning, have high intrinsic interest, are relatively short, less than 10 min, are strongly externally motivated, such as by money rewards, or are well practiced. New research coupled with informed speculation suggests that these findings have helped perpetuate the myth that sleep is not really all that necessary. It is now known that the effects of insufficient sleep are much broader than previously understood.

Years of research has shown that insufficient sleep has a very negative effect on long, dull, repetitive, and monotonous psychomotor tasks as well as reaction time, short-term memory, and other aspects of visual and auditory memory. The greater the monotony of these tasks, the more quickly the negative effects of insufficient sleep are manifested. Especially affected are those tasks that are not routine and higher level cognitive skills are required, such as innovation and flexibility. Problems also occur when great amounts of information need to be quickly assimilated, there are competing distractions that need to be sorted through to determine what needs attention and what can be ignored, and the big picture needs updating. Insufficient sleep can increase errors of omission, increase errors of commission, and decrease time spent on task. Sleepy people are more likely to make mistakes. Especially prevalent are the number of people who say that sleepiness impairs their performance at work, increases their chances of injury, and makes it more difficult to make decisions.

As mentioned in Sect. 3.1.2 sleep debt can result in lapses in attention due to both microsleeps. However, general perceptual, cognitive, and psychomotor

---

[1] The primary references for this section are Dinges (2002) and Harrison and Horne (2000).

inefficiency plus loss of capacity and alertness also occur (Dinges 1989; Harrison and Horne 1999; Hauri 1979; MacLean et al. 1990; Thomas et al. 1990). During a microsleep the person appears to stare off into space and to cease whatever they were doing. Lapses due to microsleeps are especially prevalent during the absence of external stimulation. Their occurrence is unpredictable, and as loss of sleep mounts up, the frequency of lapses increases and their duration can increase from about half a second to 10 s or longer.

An example of research on insufficient sleep involved military personnel in simulated or real operations for 48–80 h without sleep (reviewed in Harrison and Horne 2000). Performance noticeably deteriorated at 36 h when the individuals had problems keeping track of critical tasks, failed to update using new information, and put off tasks that required immediate attention. They became less flexible when generating possible responses to unpredictable problems. They became more docile, more resigned to their situation, yet more focused on personal survival rather than on the overall tasks at hand. Planning ahead was reduced, and behavior sometimes became disinhibited. In some cases leadership deteriorated. Communication became less accurate or misinterpreted.

Several other real-world studies have looked at the effects of accumulated sleep deprivation on the performance of medical interns (reviewed in Patton et al. 2001). Medical interns have work schedules that require them to be available for 24 h at a time, sometimes longer. It is not unusual for them to get little sleep during this time. Although they are apparently able to do things like grasp technical information from medical journals, studies have concluded that sleepdeprived interns show greater hesitancy in decision making, are not as well focused in their planning, not as innovative, and have impaired verbal fluency.

Another research approach has been to put people into game-like situations in the laboratory to see the effects of sleep debt. Harrison and Horne (1999) used their Masterplanner game for this purpose. This game simulates marketing strategy for managers and business students where greater innovation in the face of changing events increases potential sales. The game becomes more and more difficult as it progresses. After 36 h without sleep, it was apparent that players were no longer able to do what was required for success in the game, and their "sales" results deteriorated as they increasingly relied on solutions that were no longer successful. Nonsleep deprived participants did much better in comparison. The critical reasoning ability of the participants was concurrently tested showing both groups equally able to digest and comprehend large amounts of printed information. What the sleep deprived participants eventually lacked was the ability to use this information in new, useful ways.

Many of these findings are based on single bouts of sleep deprivation of 24, 36, or more hours. And the studies have typically used young adult males, mainly college students or young soldiers. Subsequent research has broadened the approach. Results have shown that the effects are "dose dependent." That is, the greater the degree of sleep deprivation, the greater the degree of negative effects. Likewise, recent research is showing that accumulation of partial sleep deprivation over a number of days may have similar effects to a night or two of continuous sleep deprivation (see Sect. 3.1.3).

The effects of lack of sleep on performance are more akin to an overworked automobile engine rather than a battery running down (Dinges and Powell 1989; Horne 1988). The overworked engine loses some peak horsepower as well as the occasional misfiring of a spark plug, causing the engine sometimes to sputter. Giving the engine more gas can compensate for these engine deficits early on but soon becomes ineffective. Similarly, a person can temporarily reduce the effects of sleep deprivation by exerting extra effort, stretching, or splashing cold water on their face, but eventually even these actions fail.

More research is still needed to show how age and gender influence these kinds of effects of sleep deprivation. For example, a couple of older studies that used simple types of performance tasks showed middle-aged subjects believed they were less affected by sleep deprivation than did younger subjects. But actually they did worse on tasks involving persistence and attention, meticulousness, and mental processing. Finally, more attention is beginning to be paid to individual differences in susceptibility to sleep deprivation.

> **Box 12.2** The Effect of Sleep Habits on Academic Performance
> A random sampling of 200 on-campus students at a large private university showed that sleep habits, especially wake-up times, correlated with grade point averages (Trockel et al. 2000). Specifically, later awakening times were correlated with lower average grades. This correlation was greater than for any other factor studied, including exercise, eating habits, mood states, perceived stress, time management, social support, spiritual or religious habits, number of hours worked per week, gender, and age.
>
> Other research has shown that university students who averaged less than 7 h of sleep per night averaged twice as many visits to physicians and reported two times as many infections than those who averaged more than 7 h (Coren 1998).
>
> When high school students forgo some sleep time in order to have more time to study, they report having greater difficulty understanding what is taught the next day in class and are more likely to have difficulty with an assignment or test (Gillen-O'Neel et al. 2012).
>
> In contrast, Gray and Watson (2002) found little evidence that sleep quality or quantity impacts academic performance, but being a regular early riser does have a positive effect.

12.1.2.4 Awareness of Sleepiness

Many people are not aware of just how sleepy they are. They may say they do not feel sleepy most of the time, especially if they are active and busy. What is really happening though is that arousing activities and situations mask their sleepiness

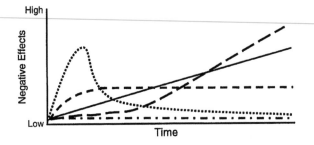

Fig. 12.1 Hypothetical trends showing how different people think insufficient sleep will affect them. The line with *small dashes* represents people who think that they will suffer effects for a few days but then "get used to it". The *dotted line* characterizes people who think that they will suffer for a while but then will adapt and actually do as well as they would with more sleep. The line with big dashes exemplifies those who believe they can do okay for a while, but eventually "it will catch up" with them. Finally, there are those represented by the dash–dot line who think there are no effects of sleep deprivation. The objective truth is shown as the solid line, a continually worsening linear trend

(see Sect. 3.1.2). A better indicator of whether you are sleepy or not is what happens when these masking stimuli are not present.

According to the 1999 National Sleep Foundation poll (2001), 58 % of the respondents mistakenly said they believed that people can learn to sleep less (see Sect. 3.1.3). There are four common beliefs about the pattern of the ability to adjust to sleep deprivation (refer to Fig. 12.1). There are those who believe that (1) they will suffer effects for a few days but then "get used to it"; (2) they will suffer for a while but then adapt and actually do as well as they would with more sleep; (3) they can do okay for a while, but eventually "it will catch up" with them; and finally (4) there are no effects of sleep deprivation. The objective truth is a continually worsening linear trend.

> **Box 12.3** Sleeping With Pets[2]
> John Shepard, former medical director of the Mayo Clinic Sleep Disorders Center, had a patient tell him that she often had to get up in the middle of the night to let her dog out. She had to wait up to 15 min before getting back to bed with her pet. Curious about how common this experience was, he asked the next 300 patients at the Mayo Clinic Sleep Disorders Center about how often and to what extent their sleep was affected by their pet. Of the 157 who said they had pets, mainly cats and dogs, almost 60 % said their pet slept in their bedroom. Fifty percent of the pet dogs slept in the bed. An even greater percent of cats were allowed to sleep in the bed. Over one-half of the pet owners said

---

[2]   Science Daily 2002.

their pet disrupted their sleep in some way every night, but only 1 % said the disruption averaged more than 20 min. Twenty one percent of the pet dogs were reported to snore, as were 7 % of the pet cats!

12.1.2.5 Managing Sleepiness

Most sleep debt can be alleviated by simple changes:

- Recognizing the importance of sleep and making sleep a high priority by allowing enough time for it every nychthemeron.
- Following good sleep hygiene (see Box 6.4).
- Taking steps to manage stress.
- Taking planned short naps. A short nap in the afternoon will help to keep you alert without disrupting your evening sleep schedule.
- Avoiding stimuli before bedtime such as caffeine, and TV in order to promote deeper sleep.
- Getting regular exercise to help you sleep more deeply.

Fulfilling our sleep quota leaves us more energetic, alert, happy, creative, productive, motivated, and healthy (Maas 1998). Some people may have difficulty obtaining enough sleep or have a sleep disorder that requires seeking professional help from a sleep disorders treatment center (see Chap. 13).

12.2 Problems Involving the Circadian Rhythm of Sleep

As reviewed in Sect. 3.2, sleep is affected by the circadian clock located in the brain. Here we will review several of the less serious problems with the clock that can cause problems with sleep. The more serious problems will be covered in Chap. 13.

12.2.1 Jet Lag

Jet lag occurs when there is a disparity between internal circadian clock time and environmental time following rapid travel east or west across several time zones. The result is sleep and wake problems. Additionally, sleep is often short and discontinuous before and during a trip that compounds matters with sleep deprivation. Travel to the north or south may cause some fatigue, but not jet lag per se. When traveling east the circadian rhythm of the body is behind that of local time, causing problems falling asleep at local bedtime, then difficulty awakening in the morning. It needs to be phase advanced. The opposite occurs when traveling west—sleepiness in the early evening and waking too early in the morning—requiring phase delaying. For example, the body may think it is morning, but according to local time it is the middle of the night.

One-third of people do not seem to be affected by jet lag. For the rest, it can range in severity from mild to strong. As a rule of thumb, it takes one recovery day for each time zone crossed when traveling to the west but one and a half recovery days for each time zone crossed when traveling toward the east for the effects of jet lag to completely remit. But for some people jet lag can last for weeks. In all cases, if several time zones have been crossed, adaptation is more rapid in the first few days before gradually tapering off. Symptoms include fatigue and sleepiness when awake yet difficulty getting to sleep when having traveled eastward or awakening too early when traveling westward. Additionally, gastrointestinal problems are frequent because of trying to eat at a time when the body is not biologically prepared for digestion. Other jet lag problems include headaches, reduced concentration, slower reaction times, irritability, and general disorientation.

Jet lag is usually worse depending on (1) if traveling eastward, (2) if there is a greater number of time zones crossed, and (3) increasing age. For example, professional baseball teams lose more games when they have just traveled from the west to the east than when traveling east to west. This difference occurs because the body's internal circadian rhythm is slightly longer than 24 h and thus tends toward phase delaying. When traveling east, this natural tendency must be opposed. However, it is not unusual for some people at some times to find traveling east easier than traveling west.

Countermeasures may be applied to attempt to assuage the effects of jet lag or to speed recovery. Some aim at improving the quality and quantity of sleep while others aim at more quickly resynchronizing the circadian rhythms of the body to local time. Some do both simultaneously.

Although at the time of this writing the U.S. Food and Drug Administration (FDA) had not approved any medication to treat jet lag, many people have found that using a short acting prescription sleeping medication can improve sleep while traveling and upon arrival at the destination. En route, you should try to time when you take the sleeping pill so that you sleep when you would be sleeping at the destination and be able to awaken when you would awaken there. On the other hand, research shows that even if sleep is improved with such medications, it does not seem to improve ensuing wakefulness.

Even more tentative are suggestions for taking melatonin[3] or a drug that mimics melatonin such as ramelteon to both reduce sleep deprivation and speed resynchronization of circadian rhythms. There is much research indicating positive

---

[3] Not enough is known about optimal doses, individual differences in sensitivities, interactions with drugs, or long-term effects of melatonin. Additionally, melatonin is not regulated in the United States, and the purity or amount may not be as indicated on the label. In some countries, it is illegal to possess it without a prescription. Also, be aware, since it can produce sleepiness, you should not drive or engage in other potentially dangerous activities that may require your full alertness.

results from taking melatonin to aid recovery from the effects of jet lag. However, timing is critical. It should be taken before bedtime to phase advance for eastward travel. However, it is not practical to use it to adjust to westward travel because it would have to be taking later in the sleep period and could result in sleepiness when subsequently awake. Note that this is just the opposite of when to seek light, since melatonin and light move the circadian clock in opposite directions.

It also helps to optimize the sleeping environment by reducing noise and light and improving body comfort as much as possible. Altering the environment can be done on the plane by using earplugs, eyeshades, and a c-shaped pillow at the back of the neck. Avoid alcohol and big meals while traveling and drink coffee only at the time you would do so at the destination, but continuously drink a lot of water. One additional bit of advice: when possible, leave early in the day when traveling east, but in the evening when traveling west.

Once underway try to go to sleep at your destination bedtime but stay awake otherwise even on the plane. However, brief naps of 15–20 min in flight and at destination can be helpful. If you traveled to the east, bright light and activity upon awakening can be helpful. If you traveled to the west, bright light and activity before bed can be helpful. Caffeine can also help relieve feelings of sleepiness. Regardless of these countermeasures, driving while experiencing jet lag can be risky.

Trying to adapt to the new time zone prior to the travel can help attenuate the symptoms of jet lag although it is not always convenient or possible to do so. This includes earlier bedtime and waking time for a few days before eastward travel or later bedtime and waking time before westward travel. Bright light upon awakening and dim light or wearing dark glasses before bedtime for eastward travel, but bright light before bedtime and dim light or wearing dark glasses upon awakening for westward travel, can supplement this schedule.

More detailed but more effective instructions can be obtained from *How To Travel the World Without Jet Lag* (Eastman and Burgess 2009).

12.2.2 Daylight Savings Time

Related to jet lag is a phenomenon experienced by many in the United States and other parts of the world who have Daylight Savings Time (Coren 1996). Every spring on a given date there is a 23-hour nychthemeron ("spring forward") requiring you to phase advance and every fall on a given date there is a 25-hour nychthemeron ("fall back") requiring you to phase delay. It is as if you and everyone else took a jet trip one time zone east in the spring and one time zone west in the fall. Because of this many people suffer for a day or so from mild jet lag symptoms. There are beneficial effects on mood at awakening and the perception of sleep quality for about a week after going off daylight savings time in the fall but opposite effects on mood in the spring when going on daylight savings time (Monk and Alpin 1980). Also, there is about a 7 % increase in traffic accidents the day after the time change in the spring, but about a 7 % decrease in them in the fall. There are similar changes in hospital admissions for other kinds of accidents.

12.2.3 Shift Work

Shift work loosely means working anytime other than between 7 am and 6 pm. It also can refer to rotating between working during the day and at other times. Shift work presents a challenge for employees. Currently, at least 20 % of the workforce in the Western world but higher if those with sporadic shifts are counted in getting enough good quality sleep. Shift work is even more difficult for people over 50 years of age, morning types (see Sect. 4.4), long sleepers (see Sect. 4.3), those with chronic illnesses, or those who have a sleep disorder (see Chap. 13). It is estimated that 20 % of employees cannot tolerate shift work (Coren 1996), but even those who can experience significant problems with mood, health, mental skills, and performance (Harrington 1994). Additionally, 12-hour shifts are becoming more popular, especially in certain industries and professions such as nursing (Coren 1996). The buildup of sleepiness, accompanied by feelings of fatigue and decreased alertness, is greater during a 12-hour shift than an 8-hour shift. This buildup tends to accumulate as the workweek goes on. The result has been found to be the occurrence of errors in work and judgment.

There are three interacting sources of problems for shift workers—poor quality/ quantity of sleep, disrupted circadian rhythms, and domestic/social problems.

Shift workers typically do not get enough sleep or good quality sleep because of trying to sleep when their circadian rhythm says they should be awake. The result is symptoms of insomnia (see Sect. 13.8) and excessive sleepiness. The average shift worker in the United States and Europe gets 5–7 h less sleep per week than their nonshift working counterparts. Sleep may also be difficult because of inter- ferences from light and noise. The sleep that is obtained is of poorer quality, because it is fragmented (see Sect. 4.2) by arousals. Research studies have shown that N3 is less affected than are N2 and REMS by shift work. An interactive on sleep when doing shiftwork can be found in a portion of http://healthysleep. med.harvard.edu/interactive/sleep_lab.

Rotating shift workers may, at best, get their circadian rhythms synchronized to their current shift for a few days before rotating to the next shift. Most of those who permanently work a non-day shift without rotating may be frequently de- synchronized, because on their days off they often assume a diurnal pattern of daytime waking and nighttime sleeping in order to take part in social/domestic activities. Since the many different body functions resynchronize at different rates, bodies of shift workers are operating like different instruments in a band playing the same song but at various notes ahead or behind the others. It takes longer, up to a week, to resynchronize to working at night and sleeping during the day, because humans are biologically organized for night sleep.

Shift workers are forced to cope socially and domestically with a world that is diurnally oriented. They often need to be awake during the day on days off, requiring them to sleep at night. A weekend of night sleep can quickly cause resynchronization that again needs to be reset during the work week. This pattern is especially true for women shift workers who are expected to continue to run the household on a "normal" schedule. But it can also affect men in their roles as a sex partner, social companion, and father. In addition, religious, recreational, and entertainment functions are mainly oriented toward a diurnal cycle. Shift workers are like salmon trying to jump waterfalls to get upstream, finding that it is hard to advance but easy to fall back.

As a result of disruptions to their sleep, circadian rhythms, and social/domestic lives, shift workers often experience more problems than their day working counterparts. They frequently struggle to remain awake when working. About 75 % of shift workers experience sleepiness every shift, and at least 20 % fall asleep at work (Coren 1996). An increasing amount of research shows there is lower productivity and more mistakes and accidents on the job among shift workers during the nightshift. Shift workers typically have less job satisfaction and more absenteeism. They have a 50 % higher than average number of car accidents when driving home from work. They report more negative moods and have more emotional problems. They complain of social isolation, more family problems, and have 57 % higher divorce rates. They have higher incidences of sleep disorders, stomach and intestinal problems, cardiovascular illnesses, and cancer. They also have higher mortality rates.

A special problem that some shift workers experience is "night shift paralysis." It is the inability to move for several minutes (Coren 1996). It has been observed in flight controllers, especially when working successive night shifts, and in those with the most sleep deprivation. It has also been observed in nurses on 12-hour shifts. In some people, the problems with shift work are so severe that they are labeled as having shift work sleep disorder.

While there are several possible remedies for the problems of shift work, none are completely successful or totally practical. One is slower rotations; however, in Europe more rapid rotations are favored, such as every two nychthemerons, with the idea that the person will not even try to resynchronize. Another suggested remedy is rotating "with the clock" from day to evening to night and back to day rather than, what is all too common, in the opposite direction. Also helpful is more light during the shift but avoidance of bright light immediately following work by wearing dark glasses, and when trying to sleep by having a very dark bedroom. Permanent night shift has not been shown to result in fewer problems even when maintaining a night shift schedule on nonwork days. Other recommendations include brief naps during breaks, the judicious use of caffeine or the newer arousal drugs that help mitigate the effects of sleepiness on the job, and having two 4-hour sleep periods—one that is the same every day such as 8 am to noon and the other taken whenever possible. Research on how to improve things for shift workers is continuing (e.g., Smith and Eastman 2008). Even when shift work is discontinued, sleep problems and daytime sleepiness may continue for a long time.

12.2.4 Additional Problems with Sleepiness in the Workplace

Sleepiness in the workplace is a serious problem. A poll by the Centers for Disease Control and Prevention (2012) found that 30 % of workers said they get less than six hours of sleep per nychthemeron. Some of the sleepiness is due to the job, and other aspects are due to the employee. The sleepiness employees bring to work causes them to perform worse on a variety of tasks and have less healthy interpersonal relationships (Patton et al. 2001) as well as affect other aspects of their lives including at home and when driving.

Some of the National Sleep Foundation annual polls have also looked at the effects of sleepiness in the workplace (National Sleep Foundation 2001). In 1997, it was found that sleepiness cost employers in the U.S. about $18 billion per year due to lost productivity. When mistakes, damage, and health problems caused by sleepiness were included, the costs were even greater. One out of every seven employees surveyed said they were sometimes late for work because of sleepiness. For young adults, it was over one in five. Close to one in five employees reported sometimes making mistakes at work due to sleepiness. Respondents said sleepiness made concentration harder (65 %), stress was more difficult to handle (65 %), solving problems and making decisions was more difficult (58 %), and listening to others on the job was harder (57 %).

A variety of factors in the workplace contributes to employee sleepiness. These factors include schedules of working such as shift work, long hours, and overtime, nature of the tasks including prolonged vigilance, and high stress, and the physical nature of the workplace, for example, lack of bright lights or poor temperature control. The effects of accumulated sleep deficits because the demands of the job that often leave their employees inadequate time to sleep has been the focus of a lot of research attention in long haul truck drivers, airline personnel, military, and medical interns among others.

Unfortunately, there are no perfect solutions to these problems (Rosekind et al. 1996). Yet, there are many things employees can do for themselves to improve their sleep and sleep time to minimize sleepiness (see Sect. 4.2 and Box 6.4). Likewise, there are things employers can do to help minimize the employee sleepiness including education and training, improving work schedules, and improving the workplace.

For more information on sleepiness in the workplace, see a chapter I helped write, Krauss et al. (2003).

12.3 Sleep Difficulties with Advanced Age[4]

Advanced age has several effects on sleep that can cause problems. In fact, more than half of those over age 65 report disturbed sleep. One cause is the natural change

---

[4] Primary sources for this section are from Carrier 2001 and American Academy of Sleep Medicine 2001.

in circadian rhythms in adults. As adults age, they tend to phase advance their internal circadian rhythms. But there is evidence that the rhythms also begin to flatten, so there is less difference between the low point and the peak, plus the response to zeitgebers gets a bit weaker. Additionally, the amount of slow wave sleep diminishes with age in adults, as does the release of melatonin and growth hormone. The net result is that it can be more difficult to get to sleep and stay asleep by retirement age and the sleep obtained is shorter, shallower, and more fragmented. Yet, it is easier to doze off more during the day when engaged in quiet activities. Many of these changes occur sooner in males than females. Additionally, as people age, they are more likely to develop sleep disorders (see Chap. 13) and chronic medical illnesses that can affect sleep. The sleep changes develop gradually during adult life. Some changes begin to manifest themselves earlier than others. For example, beginning in their forties or fifties, some people may have more trouble adapting to jet lag or shift work because of the weakened response to zeitgebers.

12.4 Problems That Occur During Sleep

Some problems occur during sleep rather than with sleep itself such as snoring, sleepwalking, and nightmares.

12.4.1 Snoring[5]

Mark Twain called snoring "sleeping out loud". Others have called snoring "sound sleeping". Snoring, however, can indicate serious problems and may cause some of those problems. Snoring occurs when there is less room for the air to travel through the upper airways during sleep. The air has to move faster through the space and causes vibrations of the soft tissue of the throat, like a flag flapping in a stiff breeze. Anything that constricts the upper airway passages or results in there being more flaccid tissue in the throat can contribute to snoring, including relaxation of the throat muscles that normally contract when inhaling, excess tissue, inflammation, inherited differences in the shape of the upper airways, and diminished elastic content of the tissues with age. Allergies, infection, respiratory irritants, and smoking can cause swelling of these tissues. Alcohol and some drugs can cause the muscles of the throat to relax. Lying on the back can cause the tongue and other throat tissue to be pulled back by gravity. Large tonsils and adenoids may constrict the size of the throat. Nasal congestion may force more mouth breathing. Even depression, stress, or anxiety can cause changes in blood flow to the nose, causing swelling.

---

[5] The primary source for information in this section is from Lipman 1996.

There is general agreement that snoring is common, males snore more than females, and the incidence of snoring increases with age after 20 years of age. 70 % of children snore occasionally, but 7–10 % do so every night. There are thought to be over 40 million people who snore in the United States.

There are degrees of differences in snoring, ranging from occasionally mild to what has been called heroic. The latter group snores virtually every night and can be heard by others in distant rooms or even by neighbors! Loud and frequent snoring can be a sign of obstructive sleep apnea (Sect. 13.1), but not all people who snore have apnea although snoring can progress to apnea over time. However, snoring can occur in all sleep stages but can be more common in N2 and N3. It may be more common in some families because predisposing characteristics of the upper airway may have a genetic basis.

Snoring has long been recognized as being a problem for sleeping partners and others nearby. However, more recently, snoring, even without apnea, has been linked to a number of medical and behavioral problems in many people. Persistent daytime sleepiness, tiredness, problems with concentration, subtle cognitive deficits, and declines in performance all have been found in some people who snore. To a lesser extent, headaches, increases in blood pressure, increased sympathetic nervous system activation, cardiac disease, cerebrovascular disease, and hormone problems have also occurred in some people who snore. Some of the behavioral problems seem to arise because snoring causes fragmented sleep resulting from the increased effort needed to breathe. The heart and vascular effects are thought to be related to the increase in chest pressure caused by the constriction of the upper airways.

There is a long and continuing history of various treatments for snoring, many of which did not work or were even dangerous. Even today there are claims made for various treatments that are questionable and could be dangerous if they keep people from seeking medical treatment for sleep apnea. These include devices that hold the mouth closed under the mistaken idea that the sole cause for snoring is breathing through the mouth. Recently throat sprays that are said to reduce snoring have been advertised, but their effectiveness is unproven. An acceptable treatment sequence starts with lifestyle changes, moves on to oral appliances, then CPAP, and, finally, to surgery if necessary. Lifestyle changes may include weight loss to reduce the excess tissue in the throat, reduction of the use of alcohol or medications that cause the muscles of the throat muscle to relax, cessation of smoking, avoidance of irritants to the upper airways, and not sleeping on the back. Oral appliances are mouthpieces that keep the tongue forward or advance the lower jaw. CPAP is explained in Sect. 13.1. Surgeries to the throat or nose may enlarge the upper airways and/or remove soft tissue. The treatments beyond lifestyle changes need to be made by qualified medical personnel.

Fig. 12.2 Schematic
diagram representing the
overlap of the three states of
being (modified from
Mahowald and Schenck
1992)

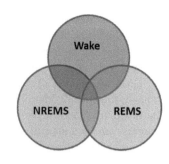

12.4.2 Parasomnias

Parasomnias are undesirable and usually unpleasant experiential or behavioral occurrences primarily or exclusively during sleep. Common examples are sleep walking, sleep terrors, and bed wetting. Many are exclusive to NREMS, others to REMS, and a few to either stage of sleep. Most are much more common than generally thought but are treatable.

Parasomnias occur because waking, NREMS, and REMS are not all-or-none unitary states. Rather each is a condition in which various components in the brain usually function together and operate in a coordinated fashion. However, in some people one or more of these components can break away at times and operate independently of the rest. Put another way, components of one state can intrude into another state (see Fig. 12.2). A common example is sleepiness where elements of sleep are occurring during wakefulness. The mechanisms of parasomnias are not always clear, but both genetic and environmental factors are thought to play a role. It is important to emphasize that, contrary to popular belief, parasomnias are not often related to psychopathology.

12.4.2.1 NREMS Parasomnias

The NREM parasomnias occur when the brain is in NREMS but also partly awake. That is, the brain is sufficiently awake to carry out very complex, and often lengthy motor or verbal behaviors while still being primarily asleep. There is no conscious awareness while performing these behaviors. The most common NREM parasomnias include confusional arousals, sleep walking, sleep terrors, sleep-related eating, sleep sex, and sleep starts or hypnic jerks.

Confusional Arousals

Confusional arousals occur when waking up (Mahowald et al. 2012). They are more common in children (16 %) but also occur in adults (around 4 %). Typically there may be confusion, lack of responsiveness, inconsolable crying, and/or unacceptable behavior in bed that may range from flailing to violence lasting 5–15 min. There is no subsequent memory of what happened. Sleep inertia (see Sect. 4.10) may be a variant if there is greater waking but with lingering elements of sleep. Relatives of people with confusional arousals may also have them. Treatments involve avoiding sleep deprivation and even obtaining more sleep, scheduled awakenings, and medication.

Sleepwalking

Sleepwalking is not what most people think it is (Pressman 2012). At one time many parasomnias, including sleepwalking, were thought to be due to demons or other supernatural phenomena. Subsequently sleepwalkers were thought to have a mental disorder. Today many people assume that sleepwalkers are acting out their dreams. This is not true. However, people with REM Behavior Disorder do act out their dreams (see Sect. 13.7). Sleepwalking begins during NREMS, not REMS, typically occurs in the first half of the night, results in little if any dream recall, and can be induced in people who are predisposed to sleepwalking by forced arousal. It occurs when the brain does not fully awaken from a deep sleep.

Sleepwalking begins with the person moving about in bed and then suddenly sitting up with a glazed look on their face and in their eyes. Next, they may repeatedly engage in stereotyped behaviors such as picking at their covers, undressing, and dressing. Simultaneously, they may mumble or make other sounds. The event may end at this point as they lie down and resume normal sleeping. Or the next step may be for them to get out of bed and walk around the room. Sometimes, they may walk to nearby rooms, the yard, around the neighborhood, or even further. The frequency of these components diminishes the greater the distance from the bed. A person who is sleepwalking may be anywhere between calm and agitated. Most instances last from less than a minute up to 15 min but sometimes last an hour or more.

Movements during sleepwalking appear purposeless and tend to be clumsy. The person may trip, bump into things, or knock things over. Injuries can occur, but violent acts are rare. Yet, at other times, they may do something very complex like prepare a meal, play a musical instrument, or even drive a car. They may vocalize or even have conversations, yet screaming is highly unusual. However, full mental abilities such as memory, planning, and interacting with others are greatly or entirely lacking (Dev Banerjee and Nisbet 2011). Responsiveness to the environment, including to their own name, may be greatly reduced. Because a person who is sleepwalking does not have conscious awareness, they are not held responsible for their actions, even criminal ones (Pressman 2012; also see Box 12.4).

Several things contribute to the occurrence of sleepwalking (Ohayon et al. 2012). About 33 % of sleepwalkers have an immediate family member who also sleepwalks or has sleep terrors. Studies of twins show a pattern of genetic inheritance. People who sleepwalk are more likely to talk in their sleep, wet their beds, and have confusional arousals or sleep terrors. Sleepwalking is most common in children, with up to 30 % having done it at least once, and 3–4 % frequently. The onset of sleepwalking is typically from 4–6 years of age, with the peak occurrence at 11–12 years of age. It most often abates by 15 years of age, but 10 % continue through adolescence. By adulthood, 3.6 % report sleepwalking once a year and 1 % report it happens two or more times per month. Eight out of every 10 adults who reported sleepwalking say it has been going on for years. It usually continues from adolescence but is rare in the elderly.

Sleepwalking is not associated with any psychological pathology in children but tends to occur more in children who sleep very deeply. Most sleepwalking in adults is not a sign of psychiatric or psychological conditions, yet it is more likely in people with obsessive–compulsive, mood, or anxiety disorders or with those taking certain medications, including over-the-counter sleeping compounds, and those abusing alcohol. It is also more common in people with other sleep disorders (see Chap. 13). Sleep deprivation is the most common precipitating factor; others include an irregular sleep–wake schedule, fever, stress, a full bladder, or noise.

There are several things that can be done for people who sleepwalk. Awakening a person who is sleepwalking is difficult and may be met with resistance or even violence. It is sometimes possible and more successful to gently lead them back to bed without awakening them. By all means, the sleepwalker should be kept out of harm's way. Since most children outgrow sleepwalking, the best thing for parents to do is simply to wait for the child to grow out of it. While waiting, they can try to reduce the things that trigger sleepwalking events, such as sleep deprivation and stress. Encouraging good sleep hygiene (see Box 6.4) is important. Making the bedroom and the rest of the house safer is also advisable. Scheduled awakenings—waking the person briefly about 15–30 min before the time of the typical occurrence—may be helpful. However, if the sleepwalking is intense, frequent, potentially dangerous, or occurs in adulthood, then one of the following might also be tried: relaxation therapy, stress management skills, hypnosis, medications, or treatment of any causal psychological problems.

Box 12.4 Sleep-Related Violence[6]

Mr. Parks was a young married man in Canada who had fallen asleep on the couch, then in the early morning hours got up from the couch, put on his shoes and jacket, and drove his car for about 20 min along 14.5 miles of a well-traveled road with turns and traffic lights. Upon arriving at the home of his in-laws, he carried the tire iron in from the car and retrieved a knife from the kitchen, killed his mother-in-law, and attempted to kill his father-in-law. After testimony by sleep disorder specialists based on their examination of Mr. Parks and the circumstances of the incident, the court acquitted him of responsibility for the murder on the basis that he was sleepwalking.

---

[6] The primary sources of information for this box are Kryger et al. 2000; Shapiro and Smith 1997; Mahowald et al. 2011.

There are other well-documented cases of other sleep-related violence and aberrant behaviors including attempted suicides, self-injury, damage to objects, and indecent exposure. These cases have been found to be due to sleepwalking, sleep inertia, REMS behavior disorder (see Box 6.4), jet lag, or sleep disorders such as narcolepsy (see Sect. 13.2) and sleep apnea (see Sect. 13.1). Elements common in such cases include sleep deprivation, chronic stress, and, occasionally, use or overuse of sleep medications and caffeine. In many cases violent sleepers got shortened, fragmented sleep. Such incidences are more common than might be expected and generally thought to involve 2 % of adults. However, individuals rarely repeat these behaviors.

Such cases are examples of automatisms—complex behaviors that occur without conscious awareness or voluntary intention, and therefore the person is not held responsible and punished, because in some countries such as the United States a person must "knowingly intend to commit the crime". Instead, they may be required to get treatment for their sleep problems.

Yet, many skeptical people have asked how a person who is asleep can perform behaviors complex enough to commit a crime. Disbelief occurs because of the assumption that sleep is an all-or-none phenomenon. However, as presented in Sect. 12.4.2, this is far from the truth. A person can be asleep but have elements of wakefulness occurring. These elements of wakefulness can be sufficient to perform automatic complex behaviors.

A number of people accused of crimes have tried to use sleep walking and other sleep disorders as their defense. Some were genuine but many were faking. Since 2000, there have been well-established criteria and sleep lab methods to determine if a person is a sleepwalker or has other sleep disorders that may have been active during the criminal incident. When the lab evidence is negative, the person is not able to use the sleep behavior defense. But while some people have been acquitted because they were sleeping when they committed the crime, many more who should have been acquitted have been convicted because the evidence from the sleep lab has not yet been authorized as a legally valid diagnostic tool.

More extended discussion of this issue can be found in Mahowald et al. 2011.

Sleep Terrors

Sleep terrors differ from nightmares and bad dreams in several significant ways and are associated with children. Typically, the child partially arouses suddenly from N3 in the first third of the night and emits a piercing scream that awakens parents who rush into the room to see the child sitting up with a terrified facial expression and maybe thrashing about. This may be followed by getting out of bed and running around, sometimes even out of the house. Injury or property damage may result. The child may be sweating, have a racing heart, and be breathing rapidly with wide open eyes. Although not apparent, the child may also have an elevation in blood pressure and a decrease in skin resistance. The attempts of the parents to soothe the child are unsuccessful and the child may become physically hostile toward the comforter, for the child is in a dazed state and not readily responsive to them. After about 1–5 min, the child usually does calm down a bit and returns to sleep, but other times may frantically run around with what can only be described as a glassy-eyed expression. The next morning, the child has very little or no recall of the incident and little or no dream recall. If there is recall, it is only of an image of something like a monster or a wall closing in.

Sleep terrors are generally considered to be benign and are usually outgrown, much to the relief of the parents. They occur in about 3 % of children, peaking at 3–5 years of age with most ceasing by adolescence. Their occurrence in adults at 4–5 %, especially males, is more common than generally thought. They tend to be found in others in the family and may overlap with sleepwalking. Sleep deprivation, emotional stress, and fever may increase their frequency, but there is no relationship with psychopathology. Treatment consists of scheduled awakenings, stress reduction, hypnosis, or avoidance of precipitating factors. Severe cases that do not remit over time may be successfully treated with prescribed medications.

Sleep-related Eating Disorder[7]

Frequent eating or drinking while asleep occurs in some people with their fully realizing it the next morning until they discover the remains of their meal. They may consume food, often highly caloric, or inappropriate even inedible substances, such as buttered cigarettes, often in bizarre quantities. The result can be negative consequences for health such as poor sleep and weight increase. Sleep-related eating disorder is not associated with real hunger or waking eating disorders but can occur in people with restless legs syndrome (Sect. 13.4), periodic limb movements during sleep (Sect. 13.5), or obstructive sleep apnea (Sect. 13.1). Sleep-related eating disorder has been reported to occur in a small but noteworthy percent of people using the sleeping medication Ambien. It is more frequent in females. Treating any underlying sleep disorder can help, as well as taking steps such as reducing poor sleep hygiene, stress, and mood disorders. Sometimes medication is necessary.

Sleep Sex[8]

Although not common, sleep sex describes a variety of sexual behaviors, often inappropriate, that repeatedly are performed during sleep without conscious awareness. It can range from masturbation to intercourse. An episode may occur in

---

[7] The primary source for information in the section if from Howell 2011.

[8] The primary source for information in this section is from Buchanan 2011.

the sleeper's bed or may begin with sleepwalking to another bedroom in the house or even a different house. It occurs in both genders, although it seems more common in males than in females. It can happen anytime during the night.

Treatment consists of reassurance that this is usually benign, does not have psychological implications, and tends to fade over time. Advice is also given to avoid recreational drugs and sleep deprivation. Additional treatment is usually not necessary unless there is a history of disturbing or injuring others. In such cases psychotherapy, teaching relaxation methods, hypnosis, or medication treatment may be necessary. Additionally, sleeping in separate beds or different bedrooms or even in a sleeping bag that is fully zipped-up has been found to be useful.

Sleep Starts (Hypnic Jerks)

Most people, probably including you, have experienced a sudden jerk of a leg or arm when falling asleep. This is called a sleep start or hypnic jerk and may awaken you or your bed partner. In some people it may instead be a flash of light or other brief hallucination, a loud bang or snapping noise that is also called exploding head syndrome, or a sensation in the body such as tingling, pain, or floating. Sleep starts are considered benign and are treated with explanation and reassurance.

12.4.2.2 REMS Parasomnias

The major REMS parasomnias include sleep paralysis, hypnagogic and hypno-pompic hallucinations, and nightmares. They all tend to occur during the second half of the sleep period because REM sleep is relatively more common then (Fig. 1.8). The related sleep problems, REM behavior disorder and narcolepsy are discussed in Chap. 13.

Isolated Sleep Paralysis

You, like most other people, have probably experienced waking up but unable to move, maybe accompanied by a hallucination. This experience, typically lasting about a minute, is called sleep paralysis. Although it is a component of narcolepsy (see Sect. 13.2), it is also very frequent, especially during adolescence, as an independent occurrence. It is the continuance into wakefulness of the paralysis that is a part of REMS. Sleep deprivation, an irregular sleep schedule, and lying on the back can make it more likely to occur. It is benign and no treatment is necessary. Coming out of it can be speeded by moving the eyes back and forth, then extending these movements to the face and the rest of the body.

Hypnagogic and Hypnopompic Hallucinations

Sometimes upon awakening or when just falling asleep people have a vague experience such as an indistinct person or creature in the room. These are called hypnopompic and hypnagogic hallucination respectfully and are quite common. They may be accompanied by sleep paralysis. They are benign and no treatment is necessary.

Nightmare Disorder[9]

The term *nightmare* comes from night + maere (Old English for goblin or demon). It originally referred to a specific kind of occurrence when persons would awaken with what seemed like a demon, also called an incubus, sitting on their chest causing a feeling of suffocation. In the last century, nightmares came to include other negative, upsetting sleep experiences including all sorts of bad dreams. While there are similarities between the experiences we commonly group together as nightmares, there are important differences among true nightmares and bad dreams, post-traumatic stress disorder nightmares, and sleep terrors.

The official definition of nightmares is "coherent dream sequences that seem real and become increasingly disturbing as they unfold. Emotions usually involve anxiety, fear, or terror … or other negative feelings" (American Academy of Sleep Medicine 2005). The person having a nightmare often abruptly awakes. Upon awakening there is full alertness frequently with a moderate increase in heart rate and breathing rate and immediate, good recall of the content of the nightmare. They usually occur after at least 10 min into a REMS episode during the last half of the sleep period.

Nightmares and Bad Dreams

Bad dreams, also known as *anxiety dreams*, are sometimes distinguished from nightmares by the fact that the person does not awaken during the dream but recalls the disturbing content upon awakening later. However, this distinction does not matter. More important is how distressing they are to the person when awake and if they result in functional impairments and sleep disturbance (Lee-Chiong 2006). Some people are greatly distressed by them, but an equal number are very little, if at all, distressed. Some people look upon their nightmares and bad dreams as creative, interesting, and fascinating and even enjoy them much as they would enjoy a horror film. Others simple dismiss and ignore them. Some experts believe that the important factor is whether the nightmare or bad dream has a negative effect on waking life, not whether the person has nightmares or bad dreams.

---

[9] From Cartwright and Lamburg 1992; Krakow and Neidhardt 1992.

Almost everyone can recall at least one nightmare or bad dream during their lifetime, but recalls are more frequent among those who are generally better at recalling their dreams (Lee-Chiong 2006). Many children experience nightmares and bad dreams with a peak occurrence between 3 and 10 years of age. As many as one out of every four college students report having one nightmare or bad dream per month with 5 % reporting them once per week. This number declines to 1–2 % in adults and the elderly. They usually become less frequent in adults but with a greater number of females experiencing them. From another perspective, 4–8 % of all people report that nightmares and bad dreams are a "current problem", and another 6 % say they were a past problem. Yet, retrospective self-reports under-estimate nightmare and bad dream frequency when compared to daily logs by a factor of at least 2½ in young adults and by a factor of 10 in the elderly.

Bad dreams are often spontaneous but can be triggered by other sleep disorders, fevers, ingestion of or withdrawal from drugs and alcohol, and trauma. Nightmares and bad dreams are more frequently reported during times of personal crisis, loss, and trauma. Persistent nightmares and bad dreams can cause insomnia, daytime sleepiness, and anxiety.

According to some, bad dreams and nightmares are a failure of the dream function (Cartwright 2010), while others see them as a normal response to psychological trauma and can help us recover from it (Hasler and Germain 2009). When they help, nightmares or bad dreams change over time and then seem to gradually fade away. But they may return in the future when some new experience revives memory of the trauma that originally precipitated the nightmare or bad dream. Sometimes the content of the nightmare literally reflects the precipitating event, but the terror and vulnerability triggered by the event can also be meta-phorically represented by nightmares and bad dreams of tidal waves and big whirlwinds, for example. The nightmares and bad dreams occurring soon after the trauma may result in a lot of terror and fear, sometimes accompanied by feelings of great vulnerability. Survivor guilt, and sometimes grief and anger, may follow. Nightmares and bad dreams can also be caused by general stress, normal child-hood fears and problems, illness and fever, and be a side effect of some medications.

Contrary to widespread belief, nightmares and bad dreams are not necessarily a sign of mental disorder, although there may be psychiatric, personality, and bio-logical links. Nightmares are also more frequent in people who have suffered trauma or abuse. If anything, it is the concern about them that contributes to anxiety, depression, and other psychological problems. Those who suffer from nightmares and bad dreams often share the psychological trait of what psychiatrist Ernest Hartmann calls "thin boundaries" (Hartmann 1998). People with thin boundaries are more open, sensitive, and responsive to their internal and external environments, and as a result, view more events as more personally traumatic than do most people. Nightmare and bad dream distress has also been found to be more likely in those who are creative and absorbed in fantasy and esthetic experiences. But there are also people who have nightmares who fit none of these categories.

Often reassurance is the best therapy for most people and children who have nightmares, but for more serious cases cognitive behavior therapy such as relaxation techniques, systematic desensitization, or a drug that suppresses REMS may be necessary (Hasler and Germain 2009). In contrast, traditional psychotherapy has not been shown to be effective for treating nightmares and bad dreams. The most effective treatment has been the use of imagery rehearsal (IRT) (Krakow and Zadra 2006) that has sufferers write, talk, paint, or draw about their nightmares and bad dreams; then to change one or several of their components in some way when awake; and followed by frequently rehearsing the new scenario (Hasler and Germain 2009). In the context of a safe and supportive relationship with a psychotherapist, sufferers may also be encouraged to adopt a more playful attitude toward such dreams and to be aware that the content of the dream cannot really hurt them. Sometimes persons are encouraged, when awake, to converse with the characters in their nightmares and bad dreams. Other approaches encourage sufferers to become lucid during the nightmare or bad dream and change it then. For some people, hypnosis has proven to be effective.

Parents can help their child who is particularly distressed by their nightmare by taking the child to a soothing location and having the child describe it (Horne 2006). If the child becomes distressed during the relating, try to calm them down, yet not reinforce this upset by giving the child too much comfort or cuddling. The key is to disconnect the emotion of the nightmare from the images. Handle the emotion in a more 'matter-of-fact' manner. Repeat this later as much as necessary until the fear of the dream is gone.

Post-traumatic Stress Disorder (PTSD) Nightmares

Following a harshly menacing traumatic experience, a small but noteworthy number of people will develop PTSD. Ninety percent of them will have nightmares that are a repetitive re-experiencing of the traumatic event, although not always an exact depiction of trauma. This kind of nightmare is intense, emotional, distressing, beyond present waking experience, and easily recalled (Ameen et al. 2002). People with a history of nightmares prior to the trauma are more likely to have more severe PTSD. They can start at any age and may persist.

PTSD nightmares can occur during any stage of sleep, although they are more likely to occur during REMS early in the night, and are more emotionally intrusive and anxiety causing than most nightmares. It is as if the normal, beneficial dream process gets stuck and the normal function of dreams is not occurring. They also are a cause of sleep disruption including more awakenings, fear of sleep, and various changes in REMS. Gross body movements and activation of the autonomic nervous system accompany the nightmare and subsequent awakening. When aroused from the nightmare, the person will be confused and anxious but not always remember the entire nightmare.

Treatment for PTSD nightmares can be complex and difficult, but recent new approaches are showing much promise. The treatment has to be individualized

Table 12.1 Some common repetitive metaphorical elements reported in dreams

Being chased	Being trapped
Appearing naked in public	Large-scale disasters such as floods and tornadoes
Falling	Being paralyzed and unable to move
Ghosts returning from the dead	
Being kidnapped	Being endangered
Rejection, humiliation	A violent attack
Losing teeth	An out-of-control vehicle

because of related psychological and medical conditions. The cognitive-behavioral techniques used with other nightmares and bad dreams, especially IRT, can also be helpful with PTSD nightmares, but additional psychotherapy, psychosocial therapy, and medications are also often helpful.

Other information concerning nightmares can be found at http://www.youtube.com/watch?v=9nmVzXxdUeU&NR=1&feature=endscreen part 41:04–49:28.

Recurrent Dreams and Repetitive Nightmares

Recurrent dreams and repetitive nightmares range from virtual duplication of the entire dream or nightmare to the recurrence of themes or components in various dreams. They have a negative quality and often involve only the dreamer. Also typical are recurrences of metaphorical depictions of conflicts or stress such as tidal waves, tornados, and hurricanes. They are more frequent in childhood. Their occurrence correlates with increases of waking anxiety, depression, stress, or personal adjustments. Resolution of a waking situation usually is accompanied by less frequent repetitive elements in dreams (Table 12.1) or their compete disappearance.

12.4.3 Miscellaneous Problems That Occur During Sleep

There are other parasomnias, not always well understood, that are not always directly or specifically related to REMS or NREMS. The most prominent among them are bruxism, enuresis, rhythmic movement disorder, and sleep talking.

12.4.3.1 Teeth Grinding (Sleep Bruxism)

Ten to twenty percent of people may grind or click their teeth frequently during sleep, but it is most prevalent in adolescents. For the vast majority of these people, bruxism is not serious, but it can cause damage to the teeth or cause sore jaw muscles for some. While bruxism has not been shown to be associated with any psychological problems, it may be more prevalent during times of stress. Bruxism occurs most frequently during N2 sleep and REMS but has also been observed during other stages of sleep. It may be accompanied by a partial arousal, yet the sleeper has no awareness of it and seldom awakens. Other body movements and an increase in heart rate frequently accompany it. Dentists can treat bruxism by fitting the sleeper with a guard worn over the teeth during sleep.

12.4.3.2 Bedwetting

Bedwetting (enuresis) is considered an annoying but otherwise typically benign problem. It is much more common than generally realized but is usually outgrown. It can occur during NREM or REM sleep, usually earlier in the night, but the sleep is otherwise normal. Thirty percent of 4 year-olds wet the bed, more so in males than females, but the percent decreases with age after that. For some children, neurological control of the bladder sphincter can even come as late as 12–15 years of age. Yet up to 2 % of 18 year-olds still wet the bed as do 0.5 % of adults, more so in females than males. It is better not to make a big issue out of bedwetting that occurs in children under 6 or 7 years of age if they have never been dry for more than a few successive nights. The reemergence of wetting the bed after a number of dry months or years can indicate urinary tract problems, psychological problems, or even neurological problems such as epileptic seizures and should be brought to the attention of a medical doctor. Bedwetting tends to run in families but seems unrelated to behavioral or psychological problems. The most effective treatment (70 %) involves placing a pad that is sensitive to wetness under the child. The wet pad causes a bell to ring awakening the child. Eventually, the child learns to associate the pre-urination sensations with self-awakening in time to get up and go to the toilet to urinate. Drug therapy is an alternative, especially when control is needed on specific nights such as sleepovers. Psychotherapy is usually ineffective.

12.4.3.3 Rhythmic Movement Disorder

Some young children have stereotyped movements such as rhythmic head-banging. It is usually self-limiting and not considered serious unless it is severe enough to cause injury. It rarely persists into adulthood. It can run in families. It can occur when falling asleep or in any stage of sleep. The only known treatment is medicinal.

12.4.3.4 Somniloquy (Sleep Talking[10])

Sleep talking is often related to sleepwalking and is most common in children, but also occurs in adults. Estimates of people who have sleep-talked one time or another range from 20 % to nearly 100 %. Most often, sleep talking consists of a

---

[10] The primary source for the information in this section is from Arkin (1981).

few mumbles to, occasionally, a few understandable words to, more rarely, a hundred or so intelligible words. People have been known to sing, laugh, and make other kinds or utterances. Most often sleep talking lasts for only a few seconds. Although you may have heard accounts of two-way conversations with a sleep-talker, verification of this occurrence in the sleep lab has only been partially successful. Although occasionally used in literature, such as Othello being convinced by Iago's relaying the supposed sleep talking of Cassio, secrets are seldom spoken.

While sleep talking can occur during any stage of sleep at any time during the night, most of it occurs during N2 sleep and only 10–20 % during REMS. Although sleep talking during REMS tends to be more grammatically correct and more emotional, it usually is without reference to the person's surroundings. Rarely has it been shown to be related to the content of the ongoing dream, and attempts to use it as a play-by-play narration of the dream have failed because the speech is too frequently garbled or nonsensical.

Sleep talking tends to occur more frequently in related family members but is considered benign and therefore not treated. There is only one reported case of serious consequences resulting from sleep talking; a firefighter who frequently talked in his sleep in the fire station dormitory was in danger of losing his job because he was keeping other firefighters awake!

There are several other parasomnias, most of which are quite rare, that are not covered here other than mentioning two with noteworthy names—nocturnal groaning (catathrenia) and painful nocturnal erections.

12.5 Conclusion

Many people would find improvement in their quality of life if they regularly got the amount of sleep that they truly needed. It begins with realizing that sleep is important and necessary and then making adequate time for it. But sometimes sleep is not easily achieved because of problems involving the circadian clock. For others it is the unusual things that happen during their sleep that cause problems for them such as bedwetting, snoring, sleepwalking, and nightmares. In most cases there are solutions available for these people. Problems that occur with the sleep itself are covered in Chap. 13.

References

Ameen, S., Ranjan, S., & Nizamie, S. H. (2002). *The reinterpretation of dreams*. Retrieved June 13, 2011, from Mental Health Reviews: http://www.psyplexus.com/excl/dicp.html.

American Academy of Sleep Medicine. (2001). *Sleep as We Grow Older*. Rochester, Minnesota: American Academy of Sleep Medicine.

American Academy of Sleep Medicine. (2005). *The International Classification of Sleep Disorders, Revised, 155*. Illinois: Westchester.

Arkin, A. M. (1981). *Sleeptalking: Psychology and Psycholphysiology*. Hillsdale: L. Erlbaum Associates.

Buchanan, P. R. (2011). Sleep sex. *Sleep Medicine Clinics, 6*, 417–428.

Carrier, J. (2001). Sleep in the later years of life. *Sleep Review, 2*, 48–50.

Cartwright, R. D. (2010). *The Twenty-four Hour Mind*. New York: Oxford University Press.

Cartwright, R. D., & Lamberg, L. (1992). *Crisis Dreaming: Using Your Dreams to Solve Your Problems*. New York: HarperCollins.

Centers for Disease Control and Prevention. (2005, September 23). *Percentage of Adults Who Reported an Average of < 6 Hours of Sleep per 24-Hour Period, by Sex and Age Group— United States, 1985 and 2004*. Retrieved from http://www.cdc.gov/mmwr/preview/ mmwrhtml/mm5437a7.htm.

Centers for Disease Control and Prevention. (2011, March 4). *Unhealthy sleep-related behaviors—12 states, 2009*. Retrieved http://www.cdc.gov/mmwr/preview/mmwrhtml/ mm6008a2.htm?s_cid=mm6008a2_w.

Centers for Disease Control and Prevention. (2012, April 27). *Short sleep duration among workers—United States, 2010*. Retrieved http://www.cdc.gov/mmwr/preview/mmwrhtml/ mm6116a2.htm.

Coren, S. (1996). *Sleep Thieves*. New York: The Free Press.

Coren, S. (1998). Sleep deprivation, psychosis and mental efficiency. *Psychiatric Times, 15*. Retrived from http://www.psychiatrictimes.com/display/article/10168/54471?pageNumber=1.

Dev Banerjee, D., & Nisbet, A. (2011). Sleepwalking. *Sleep Medicine Clinics, 6*, 401–416.

Dinges, D. (2002, June 10). What it means to be awake. President's address given at the annual meeting of the Associated Professional Sleep Societies. Seattle, Washington.

Dinges, D. F. (1989). The nature of sleepiness: Causes, contexts, and consequences. In A. Stunkard & A. Baum (Eds.), *Eating, Sleeping, and Sex* (pp. 147–180). Hillsdale: Erlbaum.

Dinges, P. F., & Powell, J. W. (1989). Sleepiness impaires optimum response capability—it's time to move beyond the lapse hypothesis. *Sleep Research, 18*, 366.

Drummond, S. P., Brown, G. G., Gillin, J. C., Stricker, J. L., Wong, E. C., & Buxton, R. B. (2000). Altered brain response to verbal learning following sleep deprivation. *Nature, 403*, 655–657.

Drummond, S. P., Brown, G. G., Stricker, J. L., Buxton, R. B., Wong, E. C., & Gillin, J. C. (1999). Sleep deprivation-induced reduction in cortical functional response to serial subtraction. *NeuroReport, 10*, 3745–3748.

Drummond, S. P., Gillin, J. C., & Brown, G. G. (2001). Increased cerebral response during a divided attention task following sleep deprivation. *Journal of Sleep Research, 10*, 85–92.

Eastman, C. I., & Burgess, H. J. (2009). How to travel the world without jet lag. *Sleep Medicine Clinics, 4*, 241–255.

Gillen-O'Neel, C., Huynh, V. W., & Fuligni, A. J. (2012, August 20). To study or to sleep? The academic costs of extra studying at the expense of sleep. *Child Development*. Retrieved from http://onlinelibrary.wiley.com/doi/10.1111/j.1467-8624.2012.01834.x/full.

Gray, E. K., & Watson, D. (2002). General and specific traits of personality and their relation to sleep and academic performance. *Journal of Personality, 70*, 177–206.

Harrington, J. M. (1994). Shift work and health–a critical review of the literature on working hours. *Annals Academy Medicine Singapore, 23*, 699–705.

Harrison, Y., & Horne, J. A. (2000). The impact of sleep deprivation on decision making: A review. *Journal of Experimental Psychology: Applied, 6*, 236–249.

Harrison, Y., & Horne, J. A. (1999). One night of sleep loss impairs innovative thinking and flexible decision making. *Organizational Behavior and Human Decision Making Processes, 78*, 128–145.

Hartmann, E. (1998). *Dreams and Nightmares: The New Theory on the Origin and Meaning of Dreams*. New York: Plenum Trade.

Hasler, B. P., & Germain, A. (2009). Correlates and treatments of nightmares in adults. *Sleep Medicine Clinics, 4*, 507–517.

Hauri, P. (1979). What can insomniacs teach us about the functions of sleep? In R. Drucker-Colin, M. Shkurovich, & M. Sterman (Eds.), *The functions of sleep* (pp. 251–271). New York: Academic Press.

Horne, J. (2006). *Sleepfaring*. New York: Oxford University Press.

Horne, J. A. (1988). *Why we sleep*. New York: Oxford University Press.

Howell, M. J. (2011). Sleep eating. *Sleep Medicine Clinics, 6*, 429–439.

Krakow, B., & Neidhardt, J. (1992). *Conquering bad dreams and nightmares: A guide to understanding, interpretation and cure*. New York: The Berkley Publishing Group.

Krakow, B., & Zadra, A. (2006). Clinical management of nightmares: Imagery rehearsal therapy. *Behavioral Sleep Medicine, 4*, 45–70.

Krauss, D., Chen, P., DeArmond, S., & Moorcroft, W. (2003). Sleepiness in the workplace: Causes, consequences, and countermeasures. (Eds.),. New Yor. In C. Cooper, & I. Robertson (Eds.), *International Review of Industrial and Organizational Psychology*. New York: Wiley.

Kryger, M. H., Roth, T. R., & Dement, W. C. (Eds.). (2000). *Principles and Practice of Sleep Medicine*. Third Edition (3rd ed.), New York: W.B. Saunders Company.

Lee-Chiong, T. (Ed.). (2006). *Sleep: A comprehensive handbook*. Hoboken: Wiley.

Lee-Chiong, T. (2011). *Somnology 2*. Seattle: Amazon.

Lee-Chiong, T. L., Sateia, M. J., & Carskadon, M. A. (Eds.). (2002). *Sleep medicine*. Philadelphia: Hanley and Belfus, Inc.

Lipman, D. S. (1996). *Snoring from A to ZZZ : proven cures for the night's worst nuisance*. Portland, Ore: Spencer Press.

Maas, J. B. (1998). *Power sleep: The revolutionary program that prepares your mind for peak performance*. New York: Villard Books.

MacLean, A. W., Reiz, W. A., Austin, P., Coulter, M., Brunet, D. B., & Knowles, J. B. (1990). Psychophysiological correlates of lapses: Power spectral analysis of the EEG. *Sleep Research, 19*, 120.

Mahowald, M. W., & Schenck, C. H. (1992). Dissociated states of wakefulness and sleep. *Neurology, 42*, 44–52.

Mahowald, M. W., Cramer Bornemann, M. A., & Schenck, C. H. (2012). State dissociation: Implications for sleep and wakefulness, consciousness, and culpability. *Sleep Medicine Clinics, 6*, 393–400.

Mahowald, M. W., Schenck, C. H., & Cramer Bornemann, M. A. (2011). Parasomnias and sleep forensics. In C. Chokroverty & P. Sahota (Eds.), *Acute and emergent events in sleep disorders* (pp. 93–129). Oxford: Oxford University Press.

McKnight-Eily, L. R., Liu, Y., Wheaton, A. G., Croft, P. G., Okoro, C. A., & Strine, T. (2011, March 4). *Unhealthy sleep-related behaviors—12 states, 2009*. Retrieved from http://www.cdc.gov/mmwr/preview/mmwrhtml/mm6008a2.htm?s_cid=mm6008a2_w.

Monk, T., & Alpin, L. (1980). Spring and Autumn daylight saving time changes: Studies of adjustment in sleeping timings, mood and efficiency. *Ergonomics, 23*, 167–178.

Moorcroft, W. H. (1993). *Sleep, dreaming, and sleep disorders: An introduction* (2nd ed.). Lanham: University Press of America.

National Sleep Foundation. (2001). *Sleep in Amerca polls, 1995, 1998, 1999, 2000, 2001*. Retrieved from http://www.sleepfoundation.org/publications/sleeppolls.html.

National Sleep Foundation. (2002, April 2). *2002 sleep in America poll*. Retrieved from http://www.sleepfoundation.org/sites/default/files/2002SleepInAmericaPoll.pdf.

National Sleep Foundation. (2011, March 7). Annual Sleep in America Poll Exploring Connections with Communications Technology Use and Sleep. Retrieved from http://www.sleepfoundation.org/article/press-release/annual-sleep-america-poll-exploring-connections-communications-technology-use.

Nowakowski, S., & Ancoli-Israel, S. (2011). Acute and emergent events in the sleep of older adults. In S. Chokroverty & P. Sahota (Eds.), *Acute and emergent events in sleep disorders* (pp. 247–263). Oxford: Oxford University Press.

Ohayon, M. M., Mahowald, M. W., Dauvilliers, Y., Krystal, A. D., & Léger, D. (2012). Prevalence and comorbidity of nocturnal wandering in the US adult general population. *Neurology, 78.*

Patton, D. V., Landers, D. R., & Agarwal, I. T. (2001). Legal considerations of sleep deprivation among resident physicians. *Journal of Health Law, 34,* 377–417.

Pressman, M. R. (2012). Common misconceptions about sleepwalking and other parasomnias. *Sleep Medicine Clinics, 6.*

Rosekind, M. R., Gander, P. H., Gregory, K. B., Smith, R. M., Miller, D. L., Oyung, R., et al. (1996). Managing fatigue in operational settings. 2: An integrated approach. *Behavioral Medicine, 21,* 166–170.

Sanchez, R., & Bootzin, R. R. (1985). A comparison of white noise and music: Effects of predictable and unpredictable sounds on sleep. *Sleep Research, 14,* 121.

ScienceDaily. (2002, February 15). *Dog tired? It could be your pooch.* Retrieved from http://www.sciencedaily.com/releases/2002/02/020215070932.htm.

Shapiro, C., & Smith, A. M. (1997). *Forensic aspects of sleep.* New York: Wiley.

Smith, M. R., & Eastman, C. I. (2008). Night shift performance is improved by a compromise circadian phase position: study 3. Circadian phase after 7 night shifts with an intervening weekend off. *Sleep, 31,* 1639–1645.

Thomas, M., Sing, H. C., Belenky, G., Shepanek, N., Thorne, D., McCAnn, U., et al. (1990). EEG changes following 48 hours of sleep deprivation in humans. *Sleep Research, 19,* 358.

Trockel, M. T., Barnes, M., & Egget, D. L. (2000). Health-related variables and academic performance among first-year college students: implications for sleep and other behaviors. *Journal of American College Health, 49,* 125–131.

Chapter 13
Disorders of Sleep

Contents

Portions of this chapter have been adapted from Moorcroft 1993 with permission of the publisher. Specific references to statements in this chapter that can be found there and in multiple, widely available sources are not included in the text. A selection of these sources is listed below and can also be consulted for verification or for more detail. (Kryger et al. 2011; Lee-Chiong 2011; Cartwright 2010; Horne 2006).

W. H. Moorcroft, *Understanding Sleep and Dreaming*,
DOI: 10.1007/978-1-4614-6467-9_13,
© Springer Science+Business Media New York 2013

The typical sleep disorders lab in many ways resembles the sleep lab described in Chap. 1, since it contains the facilities to measure the nighttime and daytime sleep of patients. The standard EEG (brain wave), EOG (eye movement), and EMG (neck muscle) measurements are used to assess the states of sleep, but other bodily functions during sleep are also measured to aid in the diagnosis of sleep disorders[1].

A sleep disorders clinic has technicians, just as the research lab does, and clinicians/researchers who are typically Ph.D.s and M.D.s. The Ph.D.s are most often psychologists or psychobiologists and the M.D.s are specialists in sleep medicine but also may include pulmonary physicians, neurologists, psychiatrists, internists, and other related specialists. In many clinics the team meets regularly to review and discuss patient histories and to confer on newly admitted patients about possible diagnoses and potential treatments. In addition, they usually meet once a week for about an hour with other interested professionals to discuss specific topics or patients in-depth. These case studies, or "grand rounds" as they are sometimes called, provide a forum for sharing knowledge and ideas among the participants. In this chapter, several of the major sleep disorders will be presented as grand rounds case studies followed by discussion of the disorder in general.

13.1 Sleep Apnea

R.P.[2] is a 43-year-old high school math teacher who came to the sleep disorders center—or rather was pushed here by his wife, his third—because of excessive snoring. During the interview he indicated that he had "always been a snorer." His snoring got worse in his late twenties, coinciding with a 40-pound weight gain. He says that he is never aware of snoring, because he is a very, very deep sleeper who awakens slowly and in a "fog." His wife reported that he sometimes snores so loudly that, even when she goes to another part of the house in a desperate attempt to get her own sleep, she can still hear him "through closed doors and with a pillow over my head." She said his snoring has a gagging, choking quality separated by a minute or so of silence. His wife also mentioned that he "flails around a bit" in his sleep, and he related that even in a cool room, he will wake up with sweaty pajamas.

While teaching he always has to be moving or standing at the blackboard in order to stay alert. Even during tests, he paces around. During teachers' meetings, he often has to fight off the urge to sleep by sitting in uncomfortable positions. When grading papers, he drinks a lot of coffee, gets up frequently, and sometimes splashes cold water on his face. He does not nap because naps have never been refreshing for him. He says that he does not attend movies, watch TV, or play cards, claiming to be bored by them. "They must be boring because I always fall asleep!" He avoids long drives because of accidents he has had from sleeping behind the wheel. He used to coach basketball but had to give it up.

---

[1] Some screening for sleep disorders can be done in the patient's own bed at their home. It is thought as technology improves there will be even more home screening for sleep disorders

[2] All of the names used in this chapter are fictitious. The case histories are based on real patient histories with embellishments and additions for clarity and completeness. Many of the case histories presented were derived by combining the case histories of more than one patient.

"The practices were O.K.—I could keep moving around, but during the bus trips, in the locker room, and even during the games, I would drift off to sleep!"

R.P. is overweight by about 50 pounds. He appears to have no neck; rather his head continues straight down to his shoulders. He has a history of high blood pressure and heart problems. Otherwise, he appears to be in good health.

R.P. reported trying several methods to stop snoring, including a special thick neck collar he purchased through the mail. Nothing helped. He also related that he had tried hypnosis. When asked if that had helped, he hesitated, showing a wry smile and replied, "Well, yes." When asked to elaborate, he continued, "The hypnotist gave me a post hypnotic suggestion—every time I would start snoring, I would turn over."

"And did it work?"

"Well, I spent the next three nights spinning!"

In the lab, R.P. fell asleep within 3 min of lights out (see Fig. 13.1) but awakened 62 s later with a gasping, snoring sound. This cycle continued throughout much of the rest of the night; as soon as he was in N1 or N2 sleep, his breathing ceased, and then he would awaken a minute or so later, gasping and snoring loudly. He woke 424 times in 433 min of the sleep period.

The profile of his sleep was very abnormal. In addition to the frequent arousals, he never reached N3 and had very little REMS. Most of his sleep was N1 with the rest N2. Time awake totaled about 1/5 of the sleep period. Sleep efficiency was low. Considerable body movements accompanied most of his arousals.

Additional data were included on the polysomnogram about his breathing by electronically measuring the air going into or out of his mouth and breathing movements of the chest, the amount of oxygen in the blood, and his sleep position.

These measurements confirmed that, although the chest was making breathing movements, no air was entering or leaving his body between the bouts of snoring. This condition is called *obstructive sleep apnea* (i.e., absence of breathing while sleeping) due to his upper air passages collapsing shut while he is asleep.

At other times the air passages were only partially blocked, allowing some air to move in and out of his body but at well below normal levels. This condition is called *sleep hypopnea* (i.e., partial breathing while sleeping). The average number of apneas plus hypopneas per hour was 57. His blood oxygen level was significantly low for a total duration of 108 of the 433 min of the sleep period.

Fig. 13.1 The record of sleep of R.P.—a person with obstructive sleep apnea

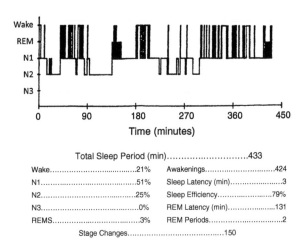

Total Sleep Period (min)............................433	
Wake...................................21%	Awakenings..............................424
N1.......................................51%	Sleep Latency (min).......................3
N2.......................................25%	Sleep Efficiency.......................79%
N3...0%	REM Latency (min)....................131
REMS.....................................3%	REM Periods.............................2
Stage Changes...150	

The next morning R.P. stated that he had a typical night of sleep for him and thought he had awakened maybe 8–10 times. He did not feel refreshed, and he had a headache. He asked if we could help him.

Treatment consisted of placing Mr. R.P. on a CPAP (i.e., continuous positive air pressure) machine. Each night, he placed a small, soft plastic breathing mask over his nose. This mask was connected to a specially designed air pump placed close to the bed that was carefully adjusted so that air pressure would keep the throat open to allow normal breathing. A check with Mr. R.P. a few days later revealed a dramatic change. He said he felt alert and rested during the day. Although sleeping with the mask on was a bit uncomfortable, he loved it because of the rest he was now getting. And his wife said he was no longer keeping her awake with his snoring.

A few months later, R.P. spent another night in the sleep lab while using the CPAP machine. This time his sleep was essentially normal for his age. He showed only few apneas and almost no oxygen desaturations. He stated his sleepiness during the day had almost disappeared. His blood pressure was also much improved.

Because of obstructive sleep apnea, people like R.P. wake up regularly throughout some or much of the night in order to breathe. Waking frequently results in very poor sleep with little, if any, N3 and reduced REMS and excessive daytime sleepiness. The breaths are frequently accompanied by loud snoring. Usually there is little awareness of the snoring and no awareness of the frequent awakenings during the night. Those who do complain of the awakenings tell of the choking or suffocating sensations at such times that may be accompanied by anxiety. Some patients show sleep apnea for only a part of the night or only in some sleep positions, such as on the back. An interactive website showing the sleep of a person with sleep apnea can be found within http://healthysleep. med.harvard.edu/interactive/sleep_lab. A video discussion of sleep apnea is located at http://medicalnewstoday.healthology.com/hybrid/hybrid-autodetect. aspx?content_id=2954&focus_handle=sleep-apnea&brand_name=medicalnewstoday.

One out of four adult males have obstructive sleep apnea but only one out of ten premenopausal females. Post-menopausal women have as frequent incidence of obstructive sleep apnea as men. Two to three percent of children suffer from obstructive sleep apnea with the incidence of obstructive sleep apnea increasing with age. It tends to run in families. Many, but not all, sufferers are overweight and have thick necks.

Sleep apnea is frequently accompanied in middle-aged patients by high blood pressure and various heart problems, especially arrhythmias. Sleep apnea gets progressively worse with time. The hypertension and heart problems may be caused, at least in part, by a fall in blood oxygen and a dramatic increase in blood pressure during the apneic episodes. Some people with years of obstructive sleep apnea are in danger of dying in their sleep from heart failure. On the other hand, following successful treatment, some people with obstructive sleep apnea show dramatic reductions of high blood pressure and heart problems.

People with untreated sleep apnea may complain of other problems such as blackouts, automatic behaviors, night sweats, and morning headaches. They frequently maintain that they sleep deeply and are hard to arouse, yet they often awaken disoriented and "foggy headed." They may complain that they gag easily and that naps are not refreshing. Almost half complain of insomnia. Alcohol, antihistamines, tranquilizers, and sleeping pills make their symptoms worse. Some individuals may show symptoms only after having several alcoholic drinks prior to going to sleep.

Because of the excessive sleepiness,[3] they frequently have a history of divorce, multiple car accidents, and employment problems. It is not unusual for them to become depressed and irritable and have diminished sexual desires. Many also complain of concentration, judgment, and memory problems, as well as changes in personality marked by irritability and hostility.

Obstructive sleep apnea occurs because the throat is constricted shut during sleep in patients with this disorder. The chest is moving, trying to inflate the lungs, but air cannot get through the throat. Snoring occurs because the throat does not completely open up during the brief awakenings causing the air and throat tissue to vibrate as the air is forced through the narrow passage.

CPAP, or one of its more recent variations, has become the most commonly prescribed treatment for obstructive sleep apnea. In some cases, other treatments are often tried first including avoidance of alcohol, certain sleeping pills, opioids, and muscle relaxants. Weight loss may be prescribed, especially in those patients who showed a dramatic gain in weight prior to the onset of the apnea. People who only have obstructive apnea when sleeping on their backs may be advised that sewing a tennis ball into the upper rear of their pajamas prevents them from sleeping in that position. Increasingly an oral appliance is used instead of CPAP. Some of these oral appliances resemble mouth guards worn by athletes when competing; others are more metallic and mechanical looking. The appliance holds the lower jaw or tongue forward, thereby opening the throat. A qualified dentist must fit them.

If these treatments are not successful, surgery such as enlargement of the throat can be considered. Abnormal constrictions of the respiratory passages are frequently found in children complaining of excessive daytime sleepiness or who show attention deficit/hyperactivity problems. Most often surgically removing the tonsils and adenoids corrects obstructive sleep apnea in children.

Obstructive sleep apnea is the most common of a group of *sleep disordered breathing* problems. Others include: (1) hypopneas and upper airway resistance when the throat is partially constricted during sleep allowing insufficient air through; (2) central sleep apnea when the brain does not send out breathing commands during sleep; and (3) a pattern of a one-half to two-minute cycle of increasingly deeper and occasionally faster breathing, followed by a gradual decrease in breathing depth and rate, sometimes up to the point of breathing cessation.

---

[3] Excessive daytime sleepiness is a common problem among people with sleep disorders. It has been found to occur in up to one out of every five people resulting in problems such as reduced quality of life, cognitive deficits, and even higher mortality (Ohayon 2006).

Box 13.1 Sudden Infant Death Syndrome (SIDS)[4]

The sudden death of an infant that is not explained by medical history, autopsy, or death scene investigation is labeled sudden infant death syndrome. One possibility is that it is a version of sleep apnea. However, SIDS may also be caused by cardiovascular failures, viral infections, over wrapping/overheating, and genetic sources. It may be that SIDS in any individual is caused by multiple, interacting factors. "Back to sleep" and avoiding soft sleeping surfaces and loose bedding or other soft items has reduced the incidence of SIDS. Additionally, use of a pacifier during sleep has been identified with reduced risk of SIDS, but such use has been criticized because of associated side effects.

13.2 Narcolepsy

L.I. is a 35-year-old female who said her symptoms first appeared as a teenager when she noticed a weakness in the knees especially when she laughed at something funny. Eventually she began to drop things she was holding, and her eyelids would often droop. Gradually the symptoms became more frequent and more intense. About the time she started college she noticed that she was increasingly sleepy during the day. Even after a long night of sleep, she would fall asleep in class, at movies, after dinner, and at other quiet times. These behaviors began to affect her functioning, especially in social situations. Her symptoms became worse if she became emotionally aroused; the example she gave was that a number of times she had "passed out" while kissing her date. She was obliged to take frequent naps, after which she felt refreshed. If she tried to "fight off" the need to nap, she would subsequently fall asleep in inappropriate places, such as the dinner table. She had tried "sleeping-in" in the morning but was unable to do so.

About once a week, usually when going to sleep, she experienced hallucinations that were strong and frightening such as someone in the room holding a knife about to stab her. The same thing also sometimes happened when awakening from sleep. Usually at these times she was unable to move for 1–2 min, even after awakening.

In the past, she experienced blackouts. She reported having periods of time when she had no memory of what she was doing. For example, she noted several instances of driving home, then suddenly becoming aware of having driven many miles past her home.

L.I.'s sleep was assessed in the lab for one night followed by an MSLT (see Sect. 3.1.1.2) the next day. Figure 13.2 shows the results of her night in the sleep lab. Comparisons with the typical night of sleep of the young adult (Fig. 2.8 and Table 2.1) revealed several characteristics. First, she reported a vague awareness of someone "lurking in the shadows" of the room and feeling very frightened but being unable to call out or move. Second, she fell asleep quickly after the second time the lights were turned out and went into REMS almost immediately, followed by a relatively normal cycle of REMS. Third, her sleep was fragmented with more N1 and less N2 and N3, as well as a high number of awakenings. This entire pattern resulted in low sleep efficiency for her age.

---

[4] Fleming and Blair 2007.

Fig. 13.2 The record of sleep of L.I.—a person with narcolepsy

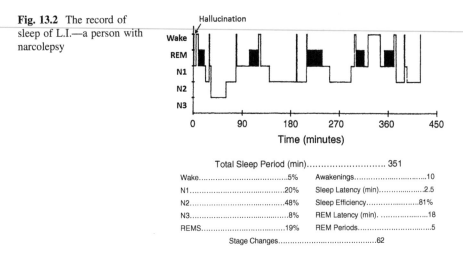

Total Sleep Period (min)............................ 351

Wake.....................................5%	Awakenings...................................10	
N1..20%	Sleep Latency (min)....................2.5	
N2..48%	Sleep Efficiency......................81%	
N3..8%	REM Latency (min). 18	
REMS.....................................19%	REM Periods.................................5	
	Stage Changes......................................62	

Her MSLT (Fig. 13.3) also was revealing. During each nap period, she fell asleep very quickly, in contrast to the normal pattern of averaging over 15 min to initiate sleep. In addition, during three of her five naps, she quickly went into REMS.

Overall, this case is fairly typical of narcolepsy. The most common complaints are those of excessive, seemingly perpetual, sleepiness. Less commonly, people with narcolepsy experience sleep attacks that are irresistible and occur without warning, even in arousing situations. The resulting nap may last up to an hour and be refreshing. The next most common complaint (60–90 %) is that of cataplexy, ranging anywhere from weakness in the limbs, face, or speech muscles to total, wilting collapse. Cataplexy is often triggered by emotions. During brief cataplectic attacks a person is conscious, but if prolonged to over 2 min REM sleep may occur.

Hallucinations at the beginning or end of sleep and sleep paralysis occur together, or singly, in almost one-half of people with narcolepsy. These hallucinations are vivid, brief, dream-like occurrences at entry to and from sleep, respectively, that sometimes leave the person with a sense of fear or dread but may also be reenactments of a part of the past few hours. They may be visual, auditory, tactile, or involve movement. Sleep paralysis is the inability to move that occurs

Fig. 13.3 The results of L.I.'s Multiple Sleep latency Test

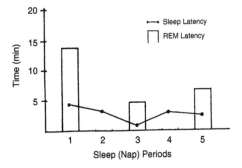

on awakening or when attempting to fall asleep. Hallucinations and paralysis can also occur in individuals without narcolepsy, especially children and sleep-deprived adults without narcolepsy. About half of people with narcolepsy report sometimes acting out their dreams while still asleep (see REM behavior disorder Sect. 13.7).

About one-third of all people suffering from narcolepsy report experiencing automatic behavior or blackouts (Sect. 3.1.3 and Box 12.4). Blackouts are probably similar to sleepwalking. During these episodes, persons may continue behavior typical of wakefulness but later have no memory of what they did. These episodes can last minutes or even hours. Naps, although inconvenient, are often refreshing to people with narcolepsy.

Narcolepsy appears to be a problem of components of REMS intruding on waking but also poor NREMS at night. Cataplexy and sleep paralysis are the muscle paralysis of REMS, while hypnogogic hallucinations are the dreams. REMS occurring soon after sleep onset that occurs in people with narcolepsy is not typical of normal adult sleep. Another factor is poor night sleep with frequent arousals and awakenings contributing to excessive sleepiness. Poor sleep may result from overactive REMS-on mechanisms in the brain (see Sect. 5.3.6) or from frequent awakenings, less N3, and fragmented REMS. People with narcolepsy, in contrast to those with normal sleep, fall asleep quickly during the MSLT and usually have two or more REMS onsets.

Typically, narcolepsy begins to appear in the teens or early twenties, although onsets in younger and older people do occur. Sleep attacks are usually the first symptoms. Gradually the sleep attacks worsen, then cataplexy and other symptoms begin to appear and become more frequent. However, 10–50 % have narcolepsy without cataplexy.

Overall, narcolepsy impairs a person's life, including their social life, as they cannot go to movies, concerts, dinner parties, play cards, or participate in other "quiet" activities. The sleepiness of persons with narcolepsy even affects their participation in more active events such as sports. Since cataleptic attacks are likely to be triggered by strong emotions, people with narcolepsy tend to guard their emotions, thus appearing dull and emotionally flat. Many have a history of being fired for falling asleep on the job, and people with narcolepsy frequently have had a number of accidents, both while driving automobiles and on the job. They also complain of problems with their memories, which may really be a problem of paying attention. As a result of these problems, they often are somewhat depressed, anxious, and frustrated. Others describe them as being unmotivated, withdrawn, and aggressive or believe they are lazy, bored, slothful, or depressed. Divorce is frequent, reflecting interpersonal complications caused by the symptoms.

Narcolepsy occurs in over 5 out of every 10,000 persons. There is evidence of predisposing genetic factors, but narcolepsy may also be caused by damage to the brain or from other medical conditions. People with narcolepsy plus cataplexy typically have reduced levels of orexin/hypocretin (see Sect. 5.1) resulting from a gradual die-off of cells that produce it and show other brain chemical defects.

Treatment includes improvement of sleep with good sleep hygiene and sleeping pills; control of waketime symptoms with scheduled naps and drugs such as a stimulant for the sleepiness and other drugs for the cataplexy; and avoiding potentially dangerous activities. Also important are psychological support and family therapy.

13.3 Idiopathic Hypersomnia[5]

Some people are always excessively sleepy. They are classified as having *idiopathic* (meaning not caused by something else) *hypersomnia* . There are two types: (1) when nocturnal sleep time plus nap time are not unusually long, or (2) when nocturnal sleep time plus nap time is unusually long and followed by lengthy sleep inertia. Both types of individuals with idiopathic hypersomnia sleep deeply and normally at night. Neither variation is common but striking when it occurs. It often begins for no apparent reason in adolescence or early adulthood. In both variants daytime naps can be resisted but when taken are only refreshing in the first variant. Those with the second variant may also experience automatic behavior, (See Sect. 3.1.3 and Box 12.4), blackouts, and microsleeps (see Sects. 3.1.2 and 12.1.2.3). Family members typically show a similar condition. The only treatment is emphasis on good sleep hygiene and use of simulant medications.

Idiopathic hypersomnia needs to be distinguished from the *long sleeper syndrome* as well as behaviorally induced insufficient sleep syndrome and recurrent hypersomnia. Long sleepers may arrive at the sleep disorders clinic complaining about many of the same things as people with idiopathic hypersomnia, but careful history taking and polysomnographic testing reveal differences. Long sleepers need 10 or more hours of sleep per night. If they try to get along on less, they show the effects of continuous partial sleep deprivation (see Sect. 3.1.3), including excessive daytime sleepiness, shown both by their own subjective reports of a constant struggle to stay awake, multiple napping, blackouts, and automatic behavior, and by a low average MSLT sleep latency. They usually report having difficulty arousing and often experience "sleep inertia" (Sect. 4.10). They are hard to awaken and can be abusive and aggressive if awakened, even when they themselves have requested it. If they do get the 10 or more hours of sleep per night they require, the daytime sleepiness and accompanying symptoms remit to normal levels.

Behaviorally induced insufficient sleep syndrome occurs in those people who voluntarily sleep deprive themselves. They typically sleep more on weekends and holidays but otherwise suffer the consequences of lack of enough sleep.

People with *recurrent hypersomnia* experience weeks of excessive daytime sleepiness, often around 10 times per year. Sleep, alertness, and cognitive functioning are normal during the intervening periods.

---

[5] Dauvilliers and Billiard 2006.

13.4 Restless Legs[6]

R.S. is a 59-year-old male Postal Service employee who came to the clinic complaining of a problem falling asleep. He said it has been getting worse . He said that he cannot be still in the evening because of feelings in his legs. The feelings go away while moving his legs but this makes it difficult to fall asleep. He said that he had tried "everything" including natural herbal sleep aids, hypnosis, and acupuncture, but none of them helped very much. He said that his inability to get to sleep easily was "getting to him." Even when he is just sitting still, he feels the discomfort inside his calves and must get up every 15 min to "walk it off." These sensations become more noticeable during the evening as bedtime approaches and are getting worse as he gets older. They are also worse when he is tired. His father may have had a similar problem because he couldn't stand deskwork and would rather have a job that kept him moving around. One of his brothers complains of problems similar to his.

Restless legs syndrome (*RLS*) is characterized by unpleasant, "creepy-crawly" sensations from deep in the legs, or in some people also in the arms, when stationary that may be relieved by movement temporarily or for up to an hour. Up to half describe the sensations as painful. It begins or worsens during times of rest or inactivity becoming especially worse at night. As a result, people with restless legs complain that they have trouble getting to sleep. Many also report experiencing excessive daytime fatigue or sleepiness but others do not report fatigue and maintain that they are completely alert during the day. It is thought that 5–15 % of the general population have restless legs with occurrence twice as often in females. RLS can begin at any age including children, often misdiagnosed as growing pains or attention-deficit/hyperactivity, but the highest incidence is in middle-aged and older people.

The evidence is strong for a genetic basis for RLS. Up to a third of cases may be caused by iron deficiency. A total of 15–40 % of people undergoing dialysis complain of RLS. Twenty percent of pregnant women temporarily experience RLS. Sometimes it is a side effect of medications. For some, RLS seems to be related to irregularities in the brain. However, in many cases no direct cause is apparent. Caffeine, warm rooms, and exposure to cold can intensify restless legs symptoms. Strangely, RLS has been reported to disappear with fever.

Treatment begins with encouraging good sleep hygiene and improving exacerbating circumstances such as stress or fatigue. If blood tests show that iron levels are low then iron supplementation can be helpful. For some people stretching, massage, or heat or cold will help as will moderate exercise, relaxation procedures, and avoiding alcohol in the evening. If none of these are sufficient, one of several different types of medication may be prescribed.

---

[6] Pigeon and Yurcheshen 2009.

13.5 Periodic Limb Movement Disorder[7]

E.C. is a 51-year-old woman who came to the clinic complaining of insomnia and serious sleepiness during the day . She reports that although she sleeps very deeply, she awakens not feeling refreshed or rejuvenated. Her husband reports that she often "shakes the bed" during sleep and kicks off the bedcovers.

E.C. reported trying many remedies for her "insomnia" including many drugs, both prescribed and over-the-counter, but to no avail. Likewise, 6 weeks off caffeine was of no help. She exercises on an Exercycle or plays tennis daily. She occasionally takes voluntary naps, but they are not refreshing. Her sleepiness has caused her to have a car accident and several near misses.

The polysomnogram showed that E.C.'s sleep was punctuated with many, usually brief, awakenings. Most of these awakenings were caused by leg kicks measured by placing a pair of sensors on the front of each leg half way between the knee and ankle. The kicks were very stereotyped, that is, identical to one another, abrupt contractions of certain lower leg muscles each lasting a few second that occurred every 42 s. The kicks tended to come in sets of 30 or more. Typically the early kicks in a series disturbed and lightened her sleep, with only the later jerks actually awakening her.

The quality and characteristics of her overall sleep pattern was not good, as can be seen in Fig. 13.4. Both the time to get to sleep and the REMS latency were very long. Note the high percentage of wake time and N1 accompanied by lowered amounts of N2 and N3. The number of awakenings is very high as are the number of movements and stage shifts. Sleep efficiency was a very poor 70 %. During the 425 min of the sleep period, she had 353 kicks with slightly more of them during REMS. The next morning she reported that her sleep was typical and that she felt tired and unrefreshed as usual. She had no awareness of the many awakenings or leg kicks during the night.

People with periodic limb movements (PLMs) go through spurts of jerking their legs or arms during their sleep. The movements are of short duration, 0.5–10 s and come at remarkably regular intervals in an individual ranging from 5 to 90 s. The

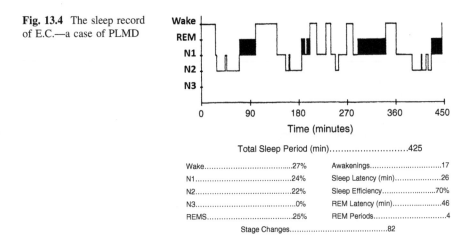

Fig. 13.4 The sleep record of E.C.—a case of PLMD

Total Sleep Period (min)...........................425

Wake.....................................27%		Awakenings................................17
N1...24%		Sleep Latency (min)....................26
N2...22%		Sleep Efficiency........................70%
N3...0%		REM Latency (min).....................46
REMS....................................25%		REM Periods..............................4
	Stage Changes...82	

---

[7] Pigeon and Yurcheshen 2009.

movements come in clusters lasting several minutes to hours. They are more likely to occur during the first half of the night. When there is an accompanying complaint of insomnia or excessive daytime sleepiness it is considered *periodic limb movement disorder*, yet many who have periodic leg movements have no sleep complaints of difficulties with daytime sleepiness or fatigue. About 5 % of the general population is thought to have PLMs, but it is much more common in middle-aged people and in up to one-half of older adults. Three-fourths or more of people with restless legs have PLMs and one-third of persons with PLMs have restless legs. PLMs also accompany many other sleep disorders such as narcolepsy, obstructive sleep apnea, and REM behavior disorder. There is usually no awareness of the movements during sleep and awareness of only a few of the multiple awakenings caused by them. However, the bed partner is very aware of them because of the bed shaking or being repeatedly kicked.

PLMD tends to run in families, where it is frequently associated with leg cramps. It tends to get worse with insufficient sleep, stress, or emotional upheaval. A person may have PLMD every night or only occasionally. Although often occurring spontaneously, PLMD may be precipitated or caused by other medical conditions or drugs.

Therapy for periodic limb movement disorder is similar to that for restless legs, but no treatment is required unless it causes daytime sleepiness or disturbs the bed partner.

13.6 Circadian Rhythm Sleep Disorders[8]

W.N. is a 20-year-old student living in the dorm at a nearby college. During the initial appointment, he was reasonably alert and energetic, yet looked tired. He was 20 min late for his 11 a.m. appointment.

He described his problem as insomnia. "I just can't get to sleep." The problem started midway through the first semester of his junior year, when he had to take a required course only offered at 8 a.m. He said he was lucky when he started college to have no early-morning classes. He could "take advantage of college dorm life" at night without having to worry about getting up early. As a result, he typically went to sleep between 3 and 4 a.m.—even later on weekends. After that he carefully selected his courses in order to avoid those that met early in the morning. This schedule worked well for him and he felt that he was getting sufficient sleep. All this changed this semester.

Because he could not get to sleep early enough at night, he had missed many of his 8 a.m. classes this semester, since he "just could not wake up." He had repeatedly tried going to bed at midnight, but just lay awake for several hours. He had tried "everything" including: warm milk and graham crackers, sleeping pills, herbal teas, exhaustive exercise, alcohol, a dull textbook, and, on the advice of a friend, facing his bed due north to get the "proper magnetic pull" on his brain. Nothing worked. He was desperate, because when he did get up after only a few hours of sleep, he was so "wiped out" that he got little out of

---

[8] Lack et al. 2009; Cvengros and Wyatt 2009.

the 8 a.m. lecture. He actually fell asleep in the class several times. He missed so many classes that his professor threatened to drop him from the course.

Upon questioning, he related how weekends and breaks were his salvation, because he slept in until mid-afternoon. When asked when he felt most alert, he immediately and emphatically stated "in the evening—once I make it past supper, I'm O.K." He also related that he is more moody in the morning and daytime than in the evening. He scored 15 on the morning type/evening type questionnaire (see Sect. 4.4), which classified him as a strong evening type. His psychological tests were within normal limits.

It is apparent that W.N.'s problem was not insomnia, but a sleep phase delay disorder (see Fig. 13.5). He can fall asleep only when his body is in its circadian primary sleepiness zone (see Fig. 3.8), which, for him, occurs after 3 a.m. His body stubbornly refused to advance that zone when he tries going to bed earlier, thus he was unable to get to sleep until much later. He has much difficulty arising before 10 a.m. but otherwise seems to get good sleep.

Circadian rhythm sleep disorders occur when there is a misalignment between the desired or necessary sleep schedule and the circadian sleep-wake rhythm. As shown in Fig. 13.5 the rhythm can be delayed, such as in this case, or advanced. Other types include non-24-hour sleep/wake rhythm, irregular sleep/wake rhythm, and the effects of shift work (Sect. 12.2.3) and jet lag (Sect. 12.2.1). Circadian rhythm sleep disorders can be chronic as in the case of W.N. or temporary as with jet lag or shift work. The most common is phase delay syndrome.

People with *delayed sleep phase syndrome* resemble people with insomnia in that they seem to have trouble getting to sleep. But unlike people with sleep onset insomnia (Sect. 13.8), they fall asleep about the same time every night. Thus, if they go to bed at this delayed time, they have no problem falling asleep, but if they go to bed earlier, they have trouble falling asleep quickly. Furthermore, they tend to have problems awakening until late in the morning or even early afternoon. Thus, they are on a stable 24 h rhythm and their primary sleepiness zone (Fig. 3.8) is during the same clock hours every nychthemeron. It is just that their primary sleepiness zone is delayed from what is desired or demanded by their situation.

People with delayed sleep phase syndrome can be considered extreme night owls. No amount of willpower or use of sleeping pills is able to help. These people show peak alertness and efficiency only late in the day. The primary cause seems to be a longer than average circadian sleep/wake rhythm that constantly exerts phase delaying pressure. The problem often starts in 2–15 % of adolescents,

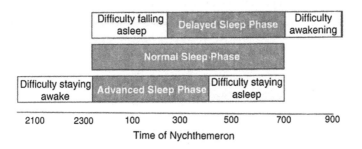

Fig. 13.5 Normally phased sleep, delayed sleep phase, and advanced sleep phase

perhaps aided by late-night study or social habits and exposure to light, such as from a computer or similar device screen, but sometimes for no apparent reason. Also, since the person feels most alert in the evenings the urge to stay up later is strong and doing so only strengthens the problem. Using caffeine to counter sleepiness may be another contributory factor. Severity may weaken during early adulthood. It does seem to run in families, suggesting that some people may be more prone to develop it.

There are relatively few reports of people with *advanced sleep phase syndrome*. These are people with the diminished ability to remain awake and alert in the evening and who typically go to sleep between 6 and 9 p.m., then awaken at about 2–5 a.m. and are unable to return to sleep. Otherwise their sleep is normal for their age. Like phase delay persons they are on a 24 h schedule, but they are unable to modify the placement of their sleep period during the 24 h. These people are true day larks. Advanced sleep phase syndrome is more common in middle-aged and older adults and thought to occur in about 1 % of them. The reason so few cases of sleep advance syndrome have been reported is unclear. Perhaps it is not as troublesome to job and school schedules, and no sleep loss occurs, so these people have no need to seek help. Or perhaps there truly are few of them, since the propensity in humans is to phase delay (see Sect. 3.2.2).

Non-entrained (free running) sleep/wake rhythm is characterized by progressively later sleep onset and arousal times; that is, a person's body is on slightly longer than 24 h sleep/wake schedule. For part of each month, things are relatively fine. They go to sleep and arise more or less as the world expects. But eventually they drift out-of-phase with the world—desiring sleep when the world is awake and wake when the world is asleep. The result is insomnia and excessive daytime sleepiness. However, as the clock setting continues to drift they will be more in-phase with the world and can sleep at night and feel awake during the day. This sequence repeats itself over and over again. Most people with non-24-hour sleep/wake rhythm are totally blind, showing how important light is in entraining the circadian clock (see Sect. 3.2.2). Chronotherapy or light therapy is used to treat these cases unless the person is blind in which case carefully timed administration of melatonin can be helpful (see below).

The final type of circadian rhythm disruption is the lack of any well-defined rhythm at all. In this less common condition the persons' nychthemeron consists of many daytime naps and shortened nocturnal sleep with no consistent pattern from nychthemeron to nychthemeron except that the total sleep time remains near-normal. Meal patterns also often become disrupted, and they simply eat whenever they feel like it. It most often occurs in older adults, especially those with diseases such as Alzheimer's and those residing in nursing homes. Weakness, languor, and many bodily complaints typically also occur. These people usually complain of insomnia, not realizing that the inability to sleep well at night is caused by their disordered schedules.

Treatment of circadian rhythm disorders involves selective use of good sleep hygiene, rigid sleep period scheduling 7 days per week, exposure to bright light at critical times, avoidance of bright light at other critical times, carefully timed use of melatonin, carefully timed exercise and other activities such as meals and a version of chronotherapy. Often, this treatment requires someone living with the person to be responsible for establishing routines until the person becomes synchronized.

Careful timing of exposure to and avoidance of bright light takes advantage of the fact that bright light is a major zeitgeber for human circadian rhythms (see Sect. 5.3.7).

Melatonin can also affect the setting of the circadian clock (see Sect. 5.3.7). It is important to point out that melatonin has not been approved by the U.S. Food and Drug Administration for use in this way.

Chronotherapy is the general term for adjusting the sleep period by a few minutes to a few hours every sleep cycle or every week until a more desirable sleep period is achieved. Advancing the circadian clock setting, that is, setting it to an earlier time, is generally more difficult. Thus, each advance is a matter of minutes. Delaying the circadian clock setting is generally easier and thus can be done in steps of an hour or more.

13.7 REM Behavior Disorder

R.D. is a 73-year-old male, retired librarian. He is a very pleasant, mild, and considerate person who came to us because of hitting, slapping, and even choking his wife "a couple of times a week" during his sleep. He has also bolted from the bed, breaking objects in the room and damaging furniture. He has injured himself. These incidents were often accompanied by yelling. During the most recent event, which resulted in his hospitalization and referral to our sleep/wake disorders clinic, he dove from the bed into a dresser, breaking his nose. He said that he thought he was diving out of the boat to escape ugly thugs who were making threats and pursuing him.

When questioned, he said that some of his dreams had become very vivid and violent in the last decade or so. His wife of 47 years said she could awaken him during these incidents but only after screaming his name many times for several minutes. When awakened, he reported vividly dreaming of protecting himself and/or her from a variety of threatening criminals and monsters. She also reported that he always jerked a lot during his sleep.

They both agreed that there were no marital problems or personality changes—only these sleep outbursts. His psychological tests showed no depression or pathology.

R.D. spent one night in the sleep disorders lab during which there were no incidents or vivid dream reports. His polysomnogram was normal except for (1) somewhat more N3, (2) high rem density, (3) random, irregular limb movements and twitches in all sleep stages, and (4) brief loss of muscle paralysis during REMS.

R.D. was diagnosed on the basis of these facts and findings as having *REM Behavior Disorder* (*RBD*).

(A video focusing on another person with RBD can be found at http://www.youtube.com/watch?v=9nmVzXxdUeU&NR=1&feature=endscreen from 6:52 to 11:12.)

RBD is very different from sleepwalking. It is a parasomnia characterized by occasional unusual dreams and nightmares whose content is vividly filled with a great deal of activity and violent confrontations. The behavior of the sleeper during the RBD event parallels the events of the reported dream or nightmare. Other dreams not accompanied by RBD are less active and less violent. Incidents occur 2–14 times per week and are much more frequent in the second half of the night. The sleeping person sometimes actually engages in complex, vigorous behavior including punching, kicking, grabbing, and leaping from bed, that are often accompanied by vocalizations. Usually the dreamer is experiencing fear, and the behaviors are defensive against what was reported to have been happening in the dream. Injuries to the dreamer and sleeping partner are common. The events tend to occur in the latter half of the night. Interestingly, unlike during sleepwalking, the eyes are usually closed during an RBD event.

Sleep laboratory studies confirm that these events occur during REMS. The characteristic EEG of REMS is present but rapid eye movements occur in greater frequency and muscle twitching in both arms and legs, occurring in both NREM and REM sleep, is common. During an event muscle tone is intermittent. There is no arousal from sleep during the event. There is more N3 than is typical. Other aspects of sleep are normal.

RBD occurs in 1 of 200 people, is more common in older males, and sometimes runs in families. The average age of onset is in the early sixties. However, it has been observed at other ages, including children. For the majority of patients, RBD appears to be an early sign of brain degeneration such as Parkinson's disease or Alzheimer's disease, often with a 10-year lag. For others it may be a side effect of a medication they are taking or a co-problem of some other sleep disorder such as narcolepsy (Mahowald et al. 2011) or temporarily as a result of alcohol or psychoactive drug withdrawal. In other cases, no psychopathology is associated with RBD. In fact, most sufferers are very pleasant when awake and tend to be happily married. It is almost always chronic and gets progressively worse over time.

There is striking similarity between RBD and cats with damage to specific parts of the brainstem (see Box 7.4). In these animals, just as in RBD humans, animated and violent behaviors occur during sleep. In RBD, it appears that the pontine REM-ON system (see Sect. 3.5.6) goes awry, such that the motor inhibition that is normally a part of REMS sometimes malfunctions. At the same time, cells that produce complex sequences of movement are activated, resulting in the behaviors. The cortex responds to these movements by synthesizing the dream content (see the Hobson-McCarley activation-synthesis model of dreaming in Sect. 9.2.1).

Effective treatment of both the vivid dreams and the behaviors has been achieved with low doses of medications, but avoidance of any precipitants is also important plus making the bedroom as safe as possible. Recent research suggests that a movement sensor that triggers a voice recording of a calming message can halt an injurious event and may be most useful when other treatments have been ineffectual (Howell et al. 2011).

Box 13.2 Sleep-Related Eating Disorder

Sleep-Related Eating Disorder is bizarre. A person with this disorder frequently gets out of bed while asleep, then finds something to eat. It usually occurs about an hour after sleep onset but can occur up to eight - times per night in some people. The preference is for eating high-calorie foods, and the result can be weight gain. Yet, over 80 % are unaware, or only somewhat aware, that they do it. The missing food, open refrigerator, or partially eaten food may be the most obvious clues. Sleep-Related Eating Disorder can be considered a disorder of arousal unrelated to nocturnal eating disorder in which the person is awake and consciously eats close to or during sleep time. The onset of Sleep -Related Eating Disorder is typically in the late teens to early twenties, and two-thirds of those with the disorder are female. It is unrelated to waking eating disorders or any kind of hunger. Eating prior to bed has little effect on its occurrence. A number of possible precipitating causes have been noted including medications, other sleep disorders, stress, and giving up smoking or alcohol. This disorder often responds to drug treatment.

13.8 Insomnia[9]

Instead of individual cases, for our study of insomnia, we will focus our attention upon a hypothetical symposium at SLEEP, the annual meeting of the Associated Professional Sleep Societies. During this symposium a panel of experts on insomnia from five different sleep clinics reviewed and discussed insomnia. The following is a summary of the symposium. A moderator is asking the questions.

13.8.1 What is Insomnia?

Essentially, insomnia is not being able to efficiently get enough quality sleep despite adequate opportunity to do so. It results in negative consequences during subsequent wake time. Insomnia has been likened to fever. Just as a fever may have many different causes, insomnia is a symptom resulting from any number of causes.

A further discussion of insomnia by two experts in the field can be found at http://medicalnewstoday.healthology.com/hybrid/hybrid-autodetect.aspx? content_id=2956&focus_handle=insomnia&brand_name=medicalnewstoday.

---

[9] Several Articles in Lichstein 2009.

13.8.2 How Prevalent is Insomnia?

Studies of insomnia in the Western industrialized world show around 30–50 % of all people report that they have at least mild or occasional insomnia, with about 6–10 % saying it is a serious problem. About 35 million Americans label themselves as people with serious insomnia. But this varies with age and gender, with almost no complaints of insomnia in 8–10-year olds, but serious complaints in 25–35 % of retirees. Overall there is a 1.5 times greater prevalence in females than in males. Insomnia occurs more often in people with depression, anxiety, sleep disordered breathing, substance abuse, and recurrent health problems. Insomnia has been called the "common cold" of sleep problems. Only 21 % of females and 25 % of males say that they never experienced insomnia in their lifetime (Bootzin 2012).

13.8.3 What Are the General Characteristics of Insomnia?

Figure 13.6a shows the typical sleep profile of people with *sleep onset insomnia*. They have difficulty initially falling asleep. They lie in bed at the beginning of the sleep period wanting to get to sleep but remaining awake for a considerable time.

Other people have no problem falling asleep but are unable to maintain sleep throughout the night. Such *sleep maintenance insomnia* is shown in Fig. 13.6b, with several relatively long wake episodes punctuating the sleep period. See also the interactive website at http://healthysleep.med.harvard.edu/interactive/sleep_lab.

Others awaken earlier than desired, as shown in Fig. 13.6c. In these people with *early awakening insomnia* sleep onset is reasonably rapid and sleep continuity is good, but awakening is earlier than desired resulting in an inadequate amount of sleep.

A fourth kind of insomnia, *sleep dissatisfaction,* is a very different insomnia. Here the complaint is not feeling refreshed even after a night of seemingly sufficient sleep.

Sleep-onset insomnia is slightly more common in younger adults, whereas sleep-maintenance insomnia is more frequent in older adults. In reality any individual may have any combination of these types of insomnia or may find that their type of insomnia changes over time. Also, good nights of sleep may be interspersed with poor nights. Most people with insomnia underestimate the amount of sleep they actually do get by around 50 %. Nevertheless, their complaint is real in that they are not getting enough good quality sleep.

13.8.4 So, is Insomnia a Problem with Sleeping?

Yes, but it is also a 24 h problem because, by definition, the person's waking quality of life must also be affected by the troubled sleep. Usually this means complaints of fatigue or of being washed-out, as well as a lack of concentration

Fig. 13.6 Sleep patterns of insomnia

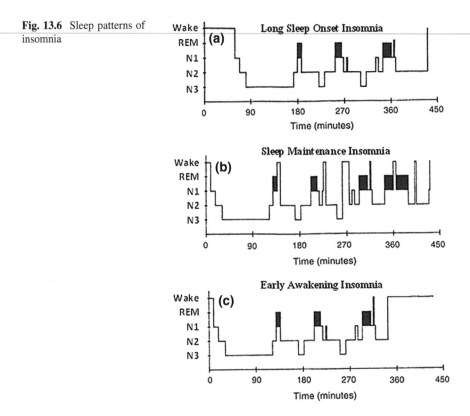

and alertness, plus poor memory and response time. It can cause physiological problems, is frequently reported to be mentally and emotionally distressing, and can lead to grave consequences, such as automobile accidents and interpersonal problems in the family, on the job, in school, and elsewhere. Also, many people with persistent insomnia have problems with depression or anxiety or an increased risk of developing them, or in adolescents, depression with suicidal thoughts. Insomnia can lead to alcohol or substance abuse. See http://medicalnewstoday. healthology.com/hybrid/hybrid-autodetect.aspx?content_id=2935&focus_handle= insomnia&brand_name=medicalnewstoday and http://medicalnewstoday.healthol ogy.com/hybrid/hybrid-autodetect.aspx?content_id=2938&focus_handle=depress ion&brand_name=medicalnewstoday for how some psychological problems are related to insomnia.

13.8.5 Is Anyone Who Meets These Criteria an Insomniac?

Yes, but the duration of these problems also needs to be considered. When the symptoms of poor sleep with waking consequences persist for more than three months, it is labeled *chronic insomnia*. People with chronic insomnia require and benefit from treatment. Other people may experience insomnia that lasts a few days or weeks. This may be caused by transient events such as stress or excitement, hospitalization, sleeping in a different bed, or interpersonal problems. Usually once the person adjusts to the stress or the loss, normal sleep returns.

13.8.6 Can You Be More Specific About the Most Common Diagnoses of Insomnia?

About 15 % of all cases of chronic insomnia have no apparent source. This is called primary or *idiopathic insomnia*. It usually begins early in life and tends to be a life-long condition if not treated. Memories of childhood are of long, lonely, sleepless nights followed by days of struggle, constantly fighting off fatigue. In many of these people neither sleeping pills nor stimulants are of much help. Although it is presumed to be caused by a malfunction of the sleep/wake mechanisms of the brain, extensive medical examination and testing do not uncover any physical or psychological problems causing the sleeplessness. Often these people show both onset and maintenance sleep problems, and the sleep they do get is light and not refreshing. That is, they are easily aroused with reduced N3 and reduced REMS.

Another 15 % of people with insomnia have *psychophysiological insomnia*. They are usually chronically hyperaroused. When awake, they tend to be restless, overactive, nervous, and apprehensive. It should not be surprising that such people also sleep poorly. Their physiological mechanisms in the brain and body that underlie arousal are more intense and persistent. Thus, they are over-aroused, resulting in greater wakefulness both at night and during the day (Roehrs et al. 2011). Many have higher levels of arousal hormones and higher body temperatures at bedtime.

People with psychophysiological insomnia describe themselves as light sleepers. In the laboratory, their sleep recordings often show higher than normal activity in their muscles, and their pulse rate tends to be high. They report and demonstrate numerous, sometimes prolonged awakenings later in the night that are often associated with worried thoughts and anxious dreams. They tend to persistently process sensory perceptions and information during their sleep. Often this sleep disturbance results in reduced REMS and N3. Additionally, they are likely to worry about and have unreasonable beliefs about need for sleep and unrealistic fears about effects of insufficient sleep. Their anxiety is often limited to issues concerning their sleep. They actually get more sleep than they think they do and do not show objective signs of being sleepy during the daytime. Their subpar performance at the workplace and in school is not due to sleepiness, as is often assumed, but to their hyper-arousal (Horne 2011).

These people are more fatigued than truly sleepy. They seldom nap, and when they do make attempts, they often fail to fall asleep. On the other hand, they tend to sleep better at the start of vacations. It is as if they feel they have permission to relax since they are on vacation. Psychophysiological insomnia usually is a chronic condition that may get worse over time if not treated.

Another 5–7.5 % of people classified with insomnia fall into the category of *paradoxical insomnia*, also known as sleep state misperception. They complain that they have insomnia and may even say that on some nights they get no sleep at all. They may describe themselves as light sleepers who hear every little noise. They are usually quite anxious about their sleep problem, yet they seldom report much impairment of daytime functioning. In spite of their complaints, their sleep length and sleep profile are entirely within normal limits. Some sleep disorders experts have speculated that paradoxical insomnia is real, but we have not discovered what to look for or how to measure it. It has been said that "they think all night long" and that such mental effort is fatiguing rather than restful. When people with paradoxical insomnia are treated their perception of their sleep usually greatly improves and their anxiety about it diminishes, even though such treatments may make little change in their actual sleep.

Short sleepers are worried because they have heard that healthy individuals need 7–8 h of sleep per night but they get much less. The key is that they do not suffer the waking symptoms typical of others with insomnia. Their short sleep is simply adequate for them. They are usually quite relieved when told this and their anxiety about their sleep ends.

13.8.7 Are There More Complex Insomnias?

Purely idiopathic insomnia, psychophysiological insomnia, and paradoxical insomnia account for slightly over one-third of all insomnias. Many other cases of insomnia coexist with medical or psychological disorders. In such cases the insomnia is considered to be *comorbid*. Additionally the effect of medications, illicit drug intake, or environmental factors can directly contribute to insomnia as pointed out in a chapter I helped write (Glidewell et al. 2010).

Some long-term illnesses cause persistent insomnia because of pain and discomfort. However, it is important to note that insomnia may continue even after resolution of the comorbid conditions that initially caused it. In these cases usually both insomnia and the comorbid condition need to be treated to alleviate the insomnia.

Over one-third to one-half of people seeking medical help for persistent insomnia have a psychological problem as the primary contributor or cause (Glidewell et al. 2010). Both mild and severe psychological problems may affect sleep. People with anxiety problems, phobic disorders, or those who are obsessive–compulsive tend to have sleep onset difficulties, as well as some sleep maintenance problems. People with adjustment problems like continuing marital or job stress may also experience sleep difficulties as do people with post-traumatic stress disorder. However, persons with schizophrenia often complain of sleep onset problems and generally poor sleep.

While about one out of five depressed people report hypersomnia, depression is the most common psychological problem causing persistent sleep maintenance but also early awakening insomnia. As a result they feel achy and washed-out although not really tired. Frequently, depressed people have shorter REMS latencies with longer REMS periods earlier in the night. They also show reduced N3. The reduced REMS latency is so dramatic in endogenously depressed individuals that it is considered a biological indicator for depression and may even be used as a very early sign of depression. Some of these disturbances of sleep tend to persist even when the behavioral indicators of depression are in remission.

There are also cognitive factors that can negatively influence sleep. A lot of people with insomnia have many detrimental negative thoughts and attitudes about sleep. For example, they may have exaggerated concerns about poor functioning the next waking day if "enough" sleep is not obtained.

Some people become dependent on sleeping pills. While taking the sleeping pills their sleep may still not be as good as they would like. But when they try to go without sleeping pills their sleep seems worse so they return to using the sleeping pills.

Alcohol is a common substance that can produce insomnia. While many people self-medicate with alcohol because it makes them sleepy, once asleep alcohol eventually disrupts sleep (see Sect. 6.2.7.2) because they toss and turn more frequently. Additionally, alcohol reduces the amount of REMS during sleep, with REMS rebound following cessation of intake. Alcohol, however, does increase total sleep time. Sleep will progressively disintegrate with continued, excessive alcohol use, resulting in a reduction of total sleep time, breaking up of REMS periods, and less REMS overall. Severe alcoholism can lead to a permanent, irreversible reduction of both REMS and N3. Sudden abstinence in alcoholics usually results in severe sleep onset problems, sharply reduced N3, and a dramatic increase in REMS. This withdrawal pattern is most severe for 10–14 days after the last bout of drinking. However, some insomnia symptoms can last for months or even years in alcoholics who are abstinent and are a risk factor for relapse (Glidewell et al. 2010).

People also use drugs such as amphetamines and substances such as caffeine to keep themselves awake and alert. Some weight reduction agents have the side effect of increased arousal. For any of these, depending on the amount used, length of use, and individual susceptibility, the user may suffer various degrees of sleep disturbance. These disturbances include sleep onset delays, less total sleep time, reduced N3 and REMS, and, with continued use, sudden daytime sleepiness. Some coffee drinkers are so sensitive to caffeine that even one cup in the morning may disturb their subsequent night of sleep.

13.8.8 What is the PPP Model of Insomnia?

An acute stressor such as a momentous life event, change in sleeping situation, or a sudden illness can sometimes result in chronic insomnia. For most people most of the time, sleep returns to normal with the end of the acute stressor or adaptation to it. However, for some people the insomnia persists. Spielman's PPP model (Spielman and Glovinsky 1991) explains this.

Some people are more likely than others to develop insomnia because of their psychological or biological characteristics. Such characteristics are the first P, *predisposing factors*. A family history or prior personal history of insomnia increases the likelihood of insomnia. Females are two to three times more likely to report having insomnia than males. Being over 50 years of age, of lower socioeconomic status, unemployed, divorced or widowed, or having poor health or a physical disability can increase the probability of developing insomnia. Another predisposing factor is hyper-arousal, as measured by elevated metabolic rate, greater activation of the sympathetic nervous system, increased activity in the stress system in the brain-hormone connection, and greater general cortical brain arousal. A weak or dysfunctional sleep drive component and/or a weak or temporally displaced circadian component may also predispose a person to insomnia.

Then an event or stress may temporarily made sleep onset more difficult, such as excessive noise, a stressful life occurrence, poor weather, or an acute illness. This is the second P, precipitating factors. For most people, this situation is temporary and normal sleep quickly returns. But sometimes, for some susceptible individuals, the poor sleep persists. It becomes self-perpetuating—the third P— because of acquired maladaptive coping behaviors such as staying in bed longer in the hope of getting more sleep or taking frequent or long naps. Additional factors include beliefs or thoughts such as the fear that poor sleep will ruin their life, belief that they may be losing their ability to sleep, and performance anxiety.

Another perpetuating factor that frequently occurs is unconscious learned negative associations with the bed and bedroom that interfere with sleep. For most of us, the bedroom stimuli become cues to sleep. They are always present just before we successfully fall asleep, so we learn that when these cues are present, we will soon fall asleep. For many people with insomnia, however, very often something goes wrong. They begin to unconsciously associate the bedroom cues with not sleeping. Then even after the original cause is long gone, the learned insomnia remains, and insomnia becomes self-perpetuating as the bedroom becomes more and more associated with cognitive, emotional, and/or physiologic arousal resulting in difficulty sleeping. So on and on it goes. Left untreated learned insomnia seldom disappears; rather it usually gets worse. Interestingly, people with learned insomnia often sleep better when not in their own bed and bedroom because the learned cues are weaker when the stimuli are different. An extreme example of this problem was a student who, while mountain climbing was forced to sleep on a narrow ledge tied to the rocks, yet had his best night of sleep in a year! He did so because the sleeping situation was so different from his bedroom that he did not have enough learned associations to keep him awake.

13.8.9 Are There Other, Less Common Insomnias?

Other much less common but interesting insomnias include temporary insomnia at higher altitudes because of breathing irregularities and insomnia caused by food allergies. Also see box 13.3.

> **Box 13.3** Fatal Familial Insomnia
> Fatal familial insomnia is a rare but dramatic disorder characterized by progressively worse insomnia that eventually results in the total inability to sleep within one or several years. People with this disorder experience vivid dreaming and sudden dreamlike stupor with movement. It is accompanied by other medical dysfunctions and disorders. It is hereditary. There is no known treatment.

13.8.10 Are There Factors That Affect Insomnia Regardless of the Type?

Yes. There are several factors that are thought to be involved in many, if not all, of the types of insomnia. One factor is the influence of lifestyle. Some people are their own worst enemy when it comes to sleep. For example, they may not practice good sleep hygiene, stay up late on weekend nights and then sleep the next morning, and over-consume substances that interfere with sleep. These contribute to and in some cases cause insomnia. It should be obvious by now that factors affecting insomnia are usually complex.

> **Box 13.4** Behavioral Insomnia of Childhood
> Excessive daytime sleepiness in children can contribute to their waking attention and behavior problems (Calhoun et al. 2012). Usually the problem is insufficient sleep at night either because of too little time in bed or insomnia. Insomnia in children older than six months of age most often is caused by a sleep-onset association problem or a limit-setting problem.

The *sleep-onset association* type involves problems with what the child needs in order to fall asleep. Common examples occur when the child becomes accustomed to being rocked to sleep by a caregiver or nursed until falling asleep rather than being left to fall asleep on their own in their crib. When these learned associations are not present, sleep onset is prolonged and the child often protests by crying, screaming, or otherwise fussing until attended to by a caregiver. Not only does this occur at the beginning of the night but also when the child wakes up during the night, as most do 3–5 times, resulting in problems "sleeping through the night."

The *limit-setting* type occurs when the child resists going to sleep because of inadequate enforcement of bedtime by caregiver. At an appropriate bedtime there is repeated stalling or refusal to go to sleep. For example, there may be requests for one more story, then a drink of water, then need to go to the toilet again, then another drink of water, then have the door opened, then the light turned on, and so on.

Treatment for both of these involves having parents and other caregivers change the situations that are causing these problems.

13.8.11 What is the Best Treatment for Insomnia in Adults?

Just like a good physician would not treat a patient with a fever simply by pre-scribing aspirin, insomnia should not be simply, reflexively treated with sleeping pills. The most effective and long-lasting treatment for insomnia changes the thoughts, emotions, and behaviors that cause and perpetuate insomnia. Thus, this approach is called *cognitive-behavioral treatment for insomnia*, or *CBT-I*. It has been shown to be as effective as several weeks of sleeping pills but superior to sleeping pills for subsequent months and years (Backhaus et al. 2001). It is con-sidered the first-line treatment for insomnia by the National Institutes of Health (NIH) Consensus Statement (National Institutes of Health 2005) and the British Association of Psychopharmacology (Wilson et al. 2010) and recommended by the American Academy of Family Physicians (Ramakrishnan and Scheid 2007).

CBT-I is effective in most people with any type of insomnia and even helps when comorbid conditions are present (see for example Manber et al. 2011). The goal of CBT-I is both alleviation of the perceived or actual nighttime sleep problems and relief from the daytime consequences of insufficient or poor sleep.

CBT-I begins with investigating what has gone wrong with the person's sleep and what may be contributing to their sleep problems including comorbid con-ditions. Throughout treatment the person keeps track of their sleep with a sleep log. Most sleep logs include space to daily record information such as bedtime, how long it takes to get to sleep, number and duration of awakenings during the night, quality of sleep, level of daytime sleepiness, and naps.

The CBT-I treatment resembles solving a jigsaw puzzle. When working on a jigsaw puzzle, one or maybe two pieces at a time are fitted into place. When enough interlocking pieces are in place the picture emerges. So too when treating insomnia. Several components need to sequentially and individually be given to the patient. These components work with one another, and when enough are in place, good sleep emerges. Which components are used and in what order depends on the nature of the insomnia in the individual patient. The goal is to improve the person's sleep so that it is compatible with their desires by changing those cognitions and behaviors that are incompatible with sleep and adding those that are beneficial but are missing.

For example, the most common complaint of people with insomnia that are seen in a CBT-I practice is, "I can't turn off my mind at night." Anything from worries and concerns to a repetitive song that is occupying their mind might be preventing sleep. In such cases, the patient can be taught to engage their mind with something that is compatible with falling asleep while leaving little room for other sleep disrupting thoughts. A method for attending to worries and concerns when awake can be added so that they are less likely to interfere with sleep at night. To complement these, a method to relax the patient's body and mind when wanting to go to sleep is helpful. This combination most often works and is available for the rest of their life to use to obtain good sleep.

CBT-I generally takes several weeks to complete although there are shorter variations that have shown some success. It has proven highly successful when done on an individual basis or in groups led by a medical or mental health professional trained in behavioral sleep medicine. More recently self-help CBT-I has become more available. This includes books and programs available on the Web. Research has shown that self-help CBT-I can be beneficial but the gains are only modest. CBT-I conducted by a professional is more successful because the components can be gradually introduced over the course of the treatment, motivation for the program maintained, and compliance and progress monitored with adjustments made as necessary.

13.8.12 What About the Use of Sleeping Pills?

We are now into the second and third generation of prescription sleeping pills that are much safer and have fewer side effects than the first generation. Generally they are shorter acting, so there is less carryover of sleepiness into the waking period. They have less disruptive effect on the components of sleep, especially less or no reduction of REMS. Some are much better for helping with sleep onset, while others are also effective for sleep maintenance. Like the first generation, their effectiveness may begin to diminish with continued use in some, but not all, people with insomnia. They can be very effective for transient or short-term insomnia but generally should not be used on a regular basis except in certain cases as determined by a specialist in sleep disorders. Also, many people with insomnia who have been using sleeping pills for a long time find that they are no longer effective or desirable. Prescription sleeping pills should not be used by people with certain medical or psychological conditions or who are employed in jobs that might require immediate response during sleeping hours. Also, numerous side effects and risks have been associated with continued consumption of sleeping pills including risks of dependence, higher risks of accidents and falls, and cognitive problems. A study in 2012 reported a much greater risk of death and cancer in those who regularly use sleeping pills (Kripke et al. 2012). Some other prescription medications are used as sleeping pills such as sedating antidepressives or antipsychotics, but there is a lack of adequate evidence regarding their effectiveness. Finally, even when any of these medications improve sleep, there is little evidence that they enhance daytime performance.

Discontinuation of the long-term use of medications to obtain sleep can be difficult (Belanger et al. 2009). Sleep most often returns to what it was before use of the medication or may be even worse for a while. Often then the person sees no alternative other than to return to using the medication regardless of its side effects or reduced effectiveness. Another factor has been posited for the continued use of sleep promoting medications. Many of them cause mild, temporary amnesia while in the person's system. Thus, they may think their sleep is better on the night when taking them because they do not remember the sleep difficulties that actually occurred.

Over-the-counter, non-prescription sleep aids are poor or ineffective in countering insomnia. In spite of the many different brand names and expensive advertising campaigns to convince us that each is unique and most effective, none is very powerful in producing sleep in any natural and consistent way. These sleeping pills usually contain some kind of antihistamine, which is often also one of the main ingredients in cough medicines and decongestants. In some, the main ingredient is combined with other ingredients such as aspirin. At best they produce some drowsiness in some people, but at worst they may produce troublesome side effects, including arousal that can actually make sleep worse. Their drowsiness effects often persist well past the sleep period. Numerous side effects are common with their use including confusion, dizziness, vision problems, urinary problems, and constipation. Most sleep professionals do not recommend over-the-counter sleep aids.

Most sleep professionals also do not recommend other kinds of aids promoted to obtain sleep. Alternative therapies, such as the use of magnets or herbs, including kava, passionflower, skullcap, and valerian, have been poorly studied. There is little or no objective evidence that they really work. None have been shown to be as effective as prescription sleeping pills much less CBT-I. Also, as discussed in Sect. 6.2.7.5, you cannot be sure of their purity or if the preparation actually contains the amount of active ingredient stated on the label. For a person who has enduring insomnia, such treatments are not likely to be of much help.

13.8.13 Can Sleeping Pills and CBT-I Be Combined?

To some extent prescription sleeping pills and CBT-I can be combined for greater effectiveness (Morin et al. 1999). The sleeping pills provide immediate relief while the person gradually acquires the long-term benefits of the CBT-I. However, the best long-term outcome is achieved if the use of the sleeping pills is gradually discontinued after the CBT-I is completed.

We now conclude the symposium on insomnia. Thanks to all of our participants. Your comments and questions have been very useful.

13.9 Conclusion

Sleep/wake disorders medicine has a relatively brief history. However, since the first sleep/wake disorders center opened in the early 1970s, increasing numbers of people have been assessed and treated. Many of these people were found to have serious sleep/wake disorders that were not even known to exist prior to research conducted at sleep/wake centers. Today, the majority of people with any kind of sleep complaint have a condition that is potentially diagnosable and, more importantly, treatable. Most people can now live better quality lives as a result. The likelihood is for even more improvement of life for countless numbers of people as they too are diagnosed and treated and as research finds out more about these disorders, how they affect our lives, and how they can be treated.

References

Backhaus, J., Hohagen, F., Voderholzer, U., & Riemann, D. (2001). Long-term effectiveness of a short-term cognitive-behavioral group treatment for primary insomnia. *European Archives of Psychiatry and Clinical Neurosciences, 251,* 35–41.

Belanger, L., Belleville, G., & Morin, C. M. (2009). Management of hypnotic discontinuation in chronic insomnia. *Sleep Medicine Clinics, 4,* 583–692.

Bootzin, R. (2012, June). Orgins and future directions of behavioral sleep medicine treatments for insomnia and sleep disturbance. Presentation at the inaugural meeting of the society for behavioral sleep medicine. Boston.

Calhoun, S. L., Fernandez-Mendoza, J., Vgontzas, A., Mayes, S. D., Tsaoussoglou, M., Rodriguez-Muñoz, A., et al. (2012). Learning, attention/hyperactivity, and conduct problems as sequelae of excessive daytime sleepiness in a general population study of young children. *Sleep, 35,* 627–632.

Cartwright, R. C. (2010). *The twenty-four hour mind.* New York: Oxford University Press.

Cvengros, J., & Wyatt, J. (2009). Circadian rhythm disorders. *Sleep Medicine Clinics, 4,* 495–505.

Dauvilliers, Y., & Billiard, M. (2006). Chronic hypersomnia. *Sleep Medicine Clinics, 1,* 79–88.

Fleming, P., & Blair, P. S. (2007). Sudden infant death syndrome. *Sleep Medicine Clinics, 2,* 463–476.

Glidewell, R. N., Moorcroft, W. H., & Lee-Chiong, T. J. (2010). Comorbid insomnia: Reciprocal relationships and medication management. *Sleep Medicine Clinics, 5,* 627–646.

Horne, J. (2006). *Sleepfaring.* New York: Oxford University Press.

Horne, J. (2011). The end of sleep: 'Sleep debt' versus biological adaptation of human sleep to waking needs. *Biological Psychology, 87 ,* 1–14.

Howell, M. J., Arneson, P. A., & Schenck, C. H. (2011). A novel therapy for REM sleep behavior disorder (RBD). *Journal of Clinical Sleep Medicine, 7,* 639–644.

Kripke, D.F., Langer, R.D., & Kline, L.E. (2012, February 27). Hypnotics' association with mortality or cancer: A matched cohort study. BMJ Open, 2:e000850. Retrieved from http://bmjopen.bmj.com/content/2/1/e000850.full.

Kryger, M. H., Roth, T. R., & Dement, W. C. (Eds.). (2011). *Principles and practice of sleep medicine* (5th ed.). St. Louis: Elsevier.

Lack, L., Wright, H., & Bootzin, R. (2009). Delayed sleep-phase disorder. *Sleep Medicine Clinics, 4,* 229–239.

Lee-Chiong, T. (2011). *Somnology 2.* Seattle: Amazon.

Lichstein, K. (Ed.). (2009). Sleep medicine clinics adult behavioral. *Sleep medicine. 4*, 473-610.

Mahowald, M.W., Schenck, C.H., & Cramer Bornemann, M.A. (2011). Parasomnias and sleep forensics. In Chokroverty C, & Sahota, P. (Eds.), *Acute and emergent events in sleep disorders* (pp. 93–129). Oxford: Oxford University Press.

Manber, R., Bernert, R., Suh, S., Nowakowski, S., Siebern, A., & Ong, J. (2011). Cbt for insomnia in patients with high and low depressive symptom severity: adherence and clinical out¬comes. *Journal of Clinical Sleep Medicine, 7*, 645-652.

Moorcroft, W. H. (1993). *Sleep, dreaming, and sleep disorders: An introduction* (2nd ed.). Lanham: University Press of America.

Morin, C. M., Colecchi, C., Stone, J., Sood, R., & Brink, D. (1999). Behavioral and pharmacological therapies for late-life insomnia: A randomized controlled trial. *JAMA, 281*, 991–999.

National Institutes of Health. (2005). NIH state-of-the-science conference statement on manifestations and management of chronic insomnia in adults. *NIH Consensensus State of the Science Statements, 22*, 1–30.

Ohayon, M. M. (2006). Epidemiology of excessive daytime sleepiness. *Sleep Medicine Clinics, 1*, 9–16.

Pigeon, W. R., & Yurcheshen, M. (2009). Behavioral sleep medicine interventions for restless legs syndrome and periodic limb movement disorder. *Sleep Medicine Clinics, 4*, 487–494.

Ramakrishnan, K., & Scheid, D. C. (2007). Treatment options for insomnia. *American Family Physician, 76*, 517–526.

Roehrs, T. A., Randall, S., Harris, E., Maan, R., & Roth, T. (2011). MSLT in primary insomnia: Stability and relation to nocturnal sleep. *Sleep, 34*, 1647–1652.

Spielman, A. J., & Glovinsky, P. (1991). The varied nature of insomnia. In P. HaurI (Ed.), *Case studies in insomnia* (pp. 1–15). New York: Plenum Press.

Wilson, S. J., Nutt, D. J., Alford, C., Argyropoulos, S. V., Baldwin, D. S., Bateson, A. N., et al. (2010). British association for psychopharmacology consensus statement on evidence-based treatment of insomnia, parasomnias and circadian rhythm disorders. *Journal of Psychopharmacology, 24*, 1577–1600.

Epilogue

As a way of summing up this book, I would like to present some of my views, especially those on the functions of sleep. But first, I would like to invite you to consider becoming a part of the exciting field of sleep and dreams.

E.1 Careers in Sleep and Dreams

In this textbook, you have seen that much has been learned about sleep and dreaming, especially since the discovery of REMS in 1953. Certainly, enough has been learned to fill a textbook such as this one. But the quest is not over. There is still a lot more to be learned, and in order to learn it, there is a need for more sleep and dream research and thus a need for more sleep and dream researchers. Perhaps you will want to be a part of this quest. Also knowledge has accumulated about how to treat problems with sleep. Perhaps you would like to help people with sleep problems. A background in the biological, chemical, or psychological sciences is an excellent preparation for any of these fields.

You could get started now. See if there is someone at your college, university, or local sleep disorders center who is doing sleep or dream research, then volunteer to help.

If you are interested in working in a sleep lab as a sleep technologist, start by looking at http://www.aasmnet.org/techresources.aspx.

If you are interested in basic research in sleep or dreams, begin to investigate professional or graduate schools. Many graduate schools have someone on the faculty who is doing sleep or dream research and can help you get special training in these areas. You can see who is publishing research in an area you might be interested in and contact them to see if they have a post-graduate program you might be able to join.

If treating people with sleep problems appeals to you, you will need a post graduate degree in medicine, psychology, or dentistry. Following this you will need specialized training in sleep disorders medicine, behavioral sleep medicine,

W. H. Moorcroft, *Understanding Sleep and Dreaming*,
DOI: 10.1007/978-1-4614-6467-9,
© Springer Science+Business Media New York 2013

or dental sleep medicine. More information on any of these fields can be obtained by going to http://www.aasmnet.org and clicking on "About AASM," then clicking on "Affiliated Sites."

E.2 Conclusion

Parts I and II of this book showed us that sleep is not just a passive shut down of the brain and body with nothing important going on other than to recharge our batteries. Rather, sleep is actively produced with many important things going on. Part III revealed that knowledge and understanding about dreams and dreaming has been more elusive compared to the knowledge and understanding about sleep. Nevertheless, knowledge has accumulated and we know that, like sleep, dreams are actively produced and important.

Part V reviews some of the more common problems people have with their sleep or dreams. Much has been discovered about these problems and how to treat them effectively. Today there are sleep disorder centers in almost every moderate sized city in the United States and growing numbers in other parts of the world, where people with sleep or dream problems can have these problems diagnosed and treated. This opportunity has led to great improvements in the quality of life and sometimes the longevity of life for many people. The National Sleep Foundation website http://www.sleepfoundation.org/articles/sleep-disorders is an excellent resource for professionals and non-professionals alike who would like to obtain more information about sleep and sleep disorders.

Part IV explored the functions of sleep and dreaming from a variety of perspectives. The search has been on for the primary function of sleep. It is thought, based on evolutionary theory, that this primary function of sleep gave its possessors an advantage that enabled them to live more successfully and reproduce, thus passing this trait on to their offspring. Later, additional functions were added to sleep (Sleep Research Society 1997), and they, in turn, may have added to reproductive success.

However, research to date has not convincingly found this primal function of sleep among all the possibilities so far advanced. It is possible that over the eons, the original function of sleep was lost and only the added functions remain. It is also possible that more than one function of sleep coevolved (Arden 1996; Nicolau et al. 2000). This view maintains that no single function by itself was advantageous enough to be the cause of the evolution of sleep, but several functions evolving collectively may have provided the advantage. Thus sleeping and dreaming evolved. Given our current state of knowledge, this idea of the evolving of several sleep functions seems the most plausible to me.

The well-known symptoms of sleepiness may not point the way to the functions of sleep. This is because they may be the way that the body encourages sleep that is useful for another, less obvious purpose (Rechtschaffen 1998). This concept is similar to the symptoms of hunger, such as rumbling stomach, light headedness, and sensory appeal of food that may draw our attention to the need to eat but do not reflect the real reason we need to eat. Likewise, it is possible that the sleepiness and associated symptoms we feel exist in order to get us to satisfy the underlying need for sleep, but are not themselves the real reason we need to sleep (Meddis 1979).

My own view of the functions of sleep, which is similar to that of Feinberg and Floyd (1982), but also includes dreaming, incorporates most of the ideas presented in Chaps. 10 and 11. Yet, I am struck by evidence that sleep does not seem to be absolutely necessary for anything. People and animals can do without sleep for long periods of time and some animals seem to lack one or more aspects of what is commonly thought of as sleep. Only work from Rechtschaffen's lab (see Box 10.2) has shown that sleep deprivation can have lethal consequences in rats, but this occurred only after a few weeks of continuous sleeplessness. People and animals can survive a few days or even a week of sleep deprivation, then recover after only a couple of rounds of normal sleep. As going without sleep progresses, some components that usually occur during sleep begin to occur when awake. This is not unusual because aspects of sleep such as specific kinds of brain waves, muscle inhibition, and PGO waves have been found to occur outside of sleep in, for example, narcoleptics, people who sleep-walk, and people who are severely sleep deprived. Likewise, the following have been demonstrated regarding REMS and its components (Sakai 1985):

- REMS without PGO waves in animals with lesions in a specific part of the brainstem;
- REMS without muscle paralysis in humans with REM behavior disorder;
- REMS without its characteristic brain waves following administration of the drug atropine.

Each of the aspects thus appears to be an independent process for which sleep is not necessary and therefore not the cause (Fiss 1979).

Yet, without an adequate amount of quality sleep, there is a deviation from the optimal, normal level of functioning. In short, we do not do as well without sleep. Perhaps, then, sleep has no function other than to orchestrate various components and provide a convenient time when they can occur most easily and most efficiently (Adam and Oswald 1983; McGaugh et al. 1979). This statement is not to belittle this function; efficiency is important and in the long run may even be essential, as the Rechtschaffen rat research shows. But, in the short run, it can be sacrificed for other, more pressing needs.

Sleep has a rhythmic character (see Sect. 3.2). In this respect, it is no different from many other rhythms seen in life on our planet and may have evolved out of them. It may have evolved in higher animals out of a simple rest/activity cycle seen in other lower animals, primarily as a behavioral strategy to keep the sleeper out of harm's way and to conserve a little energy at the same time. As warm-blooded animals evolved, sleep may have become more important in the regulation of body temperature. Still later, with the evolution of bigger and more complex brains, sleep also assumed importance in the development and maintenance of this very delicate, yet complex structure. Likewise, sleep, thus evolved, could be a convenient time to perform some cognitive and emotional housekeeping. Thus, dreams were added.

Remnants of this evolutionary history are evident in present day species that have different places on the evolutionary tree (Horne 1988). Remnants are also evident within individual higher species since, during evolution, existing functions of sleep were not simply replaced, but new functions were also added. Later, these add-ons may have gained primary importance, with some of the original functions becoming secondary or even discarded.

Sleep may be likened to an American university. There are many aspects and functions of universities—education, research, extension services, and athletics, to name a few. Each helps define the university and make it what it is; yet, each aspect can exist apart from the university. The assemblage of these various, potentially autonomous, entities not only defines the university but also lends a certain efficiency to each of its parts. Yet, the university can be recognized even if some of its parts are absent. So, too, with sleep. Sleep may, in the end, just be the "recruitment and coupling" of potentially independent elements, including dreams (McGinty 1985).

Just as at the university, educating may be considered a primary function and athletics a secondary function, some of the functions of sleep may be more primary and others secondary (Meddis 1979). Also, the function of the university may differ at different times in history—at one time the primary function of many universities was to produce teachers and preachers—just as the function of sleep has differed throughout evolution (Horne 1983).

Also, the function of the university may differ for different students depending on their attributes and needs just as different animals may get different benefits from sleep. The extent to which sleep is for safety, energy conservation, restoration, or other proposed functions may depend on interrelated characteristics such as the size of the body, degree of cerebral development, and constituents of the diet (Horne 1988). The same is certainly true of other characteristics of animals. Some animals have claws, others hooves, and still others fingers. Some have fins and others have no appendages at all. Likewise, various types of animals may benefit from different functions for sleep according to their own unique needs.

Finally, the function of the university may change for an individual student during the course of study. It is not unusual for US students to change majors for example. In a similar way, the function of sleep may change during the course of its nightly duration (Horne 1988). The greater amounts of N3 early in the human sleep period followed by more REMS toward the end of the sleep period certainly support such a notion.

In the end, then, the function of sleep may be to provide optimal circumstances for many diverse functions. In this sense its function may be summed up in one word—EFFICIENCY.

This statement does not imply that sleep is unimportant. As Webb (1979, p. 31) said very well:

> My position views sleep as a process which evolved to aid us to adapt our behavior to an environment of eons ago. The sleep of Babylon is the sleep of today. For those times

and places it functioned effectively as a biological system. But, modern times have brought the Edison Age of electric lights and is abolishing the natural rhythm of night and day, the jet aircraft tosses sleep across multiple time zones, and drugs have given promises of bending sleep to our momentary demands. Pervasively, we raise our strident cries and push our self-centered demands that sleep be subservient to our whimsy, bend to our needs, pressures and terrors. We ominously move toward viewing our failures of sleep to be "illnesses" to be "cured."

My view point is to the contrary. In a reasonably natural and stable environment sleep will serve its function as a silent and well-trained servant. It is rather our "misbehaviors" in relation to sleep, goaded by a changed environment and a thoroughly anthropomorphic arrogance about "nature", which "fails" sleep as it is pushed beyond its natural limits. From my perspective, anchored in my adaptive theory of sleep, we must rather than learn the proximal causes of sleep, learn the laws of sleep. In turn we must teach ourselves to act in accord with these laws. I agree with Francis Bacon of 500 years ago: "Nature cannot be commanded except by being obeyed."

About the Author

I am often asked about how I got interested in sleep and dreams. I reply with a little story.

> Everyone in the lab is going to the international sleep meeting in Europe. Why don't you come along? The round trip charter flight cost is only $180.00. The meeting lasts for 5 days but the flight does not return for another 25 days after that.

I heard this when I was doing postdoctoral research on the maturation of brain waves in baby rats at the University of Nebraska Medical School shortly after receiving a Ph.D. in psychology, actually psychobiology, from Princeton University. I went. I admit that the main reason was to spend a month in Europe. However, what I learned at the meeting, held in the summer of 1971, fascinated me. It was the beginning of my continuing interest in sleep and all of its ramifications.

Shortly after my return from Europe, I began to teach at Luther College and found myself reading and lecturing frequently about sleep. Within a few years, my research interests shifted away from baby rat brains to sleep. Soon I started a sleep research laboratory at Luther College in which I have studied various aspects of sleep and dreaming. I also kept on attending the meetings (some Europe, others in places like Cape Cod and San Antonio) of what was to become the Sleep Research Society. Later I attended the inaugural meeting of the Association for the Study of Dreams (in San Francisco). In 1980, I learned about sleep disorders and did some research in that area while on sabbatical at the Sleep Disorders Center headed by Rozalind Cartwright of Rush Medical School in Chicago. My interest in dreaming was piqued during this time since Dr. Cartwright had already done landmark research in this area. Later, I was on another sabbatical at the Mayo Medical Center's Sleep Disorders Center in Rochester Minnesota. While at Mayo, I again did some sleep disorders research.

Since my retirement from teaching and research I shifted into a clinical practice of helping people with insomnia, bad dreams and nightmares, and young children with sleep problems by changing thoughts and behaviors rather than by using drugs. To date I have helped close to 500 people to sleep better.

W. H. Moorcroft, *Understanding Sleep and Dreaming*,
DOI: 10.1007/978-1-4614-6467-9,
© Springer Science+Business Media New York 2013

I love sleep and dreams, pun intended. I continue to study, lecture about, write about, and treat sleep, dreaming, and sleep disorders. And of course, I have continued to attend those wonderful meetings. My intention is to keep on keeping on with these things as long as I am able to do so.

References

Adam, K., & Oswald, I. (1983). Protein synthesis, bodily renewal and the sleep-wake cycle. *Clinical Science, 65*, 561–567.

Arden, J. B. (1996). *Consciousness, dreams, and self: a transdisciplinary approach.* Maidson, Connecticut: Psychosocial Press.

Feinberg, I., & Floyd, T. C. (1982). The regulation of human sleep. *Human Neurobiology, 1*, 185–194.

Fiss, H. (1979). Current dream research: A psychobiological perspective. In B. Wolman (Ed.), *Handbook of dreams* (pp. 20–75). New York: Van Nostrand Reinhold.

Horne, J. A. (1983). Mammalian sleep function with particular reference to man. In A. Mayes (Ed.), *Sleep mechanisms and functions in humans and animals—an evolutionary perspective* (pp. 262–312). Birkshire, England: Van Nostrand Reinhold.

Horne, J. A. (1988). *Why we sleep.* New York: Oxford University Press.

McGaugh, J. L., Jensen, R. A., & Martinez, J. L. (1979). Sleep, brain state, and memory. In R. Drucker-Collin, M. Shkurovich, & M. B. Sterman (Eds.), *The functions of sleep* (pp. 295–301). New York: Academic Press.

McGinty, D. J. (1985). Physiological equilibrium and the control of sleep states. In D. J. McGinty, R. Drucker-Colin, A. Morrison, & P. L. Parmeggiani (Eds.), *Brain mechanisms of sleep* (pp. 361–384). New York: Raven Press.

Meddis, R. (1979). The evolution and function of sleep. In D. A. Oakley & H. C. Plotkin (Eds.), *Brain, behavior, and evolution* (pp. 99–125). London: Methuen.

Nicolau, M. C., Akaarir, M., Gamundi, A., Gonzalez, J., & Rial, R. V. (2000). Why we sleep: The evolutionary pathway to the mammalian sleep. *Progress in Neurobiology, 62*, 379–406.

Rechtschaffen, A. (1998). Current perspectives on the function of sleep. *Perspectives in Biology and Medicine, 41*, 359–390.

Sakai, K. (1985). Anatomical and physiological basis of paradoxical sleep. In D. J. McGinty, A. Drucker-Colin, A. Morrison, & P. L. Parmeggiani (Eds.), *Brain mechanisms of sleep* (pp. 111–137). New York: Raven Press.

Sleep Research Society. (1997). *Basics of sleep behavior.* Retrieved from http://www.sleephomepages.org/sleepsyllabus/.

Webb, W. B. (1979). Theories of sleep functions and some clinical implications. In R. Drucker-Colin, M. Shkurovich, & M. B. Sterman (Eds.), *The functions of sleep* (pp. 19–35). New York: Academic Press.

Index

W. H. Moorcroft, *Understanding Sleep and Dreaming*,
DOI: 10.1007/978-1-4614-6467-9,
© Springer Science+Business Media New York 2013

9 781461 464662